A HISTORY OF PLANT MEDICINE

Author of

Herbwise Naturally

Herbcraft Naturally

Herb Sufficient

The Receipt Book of Lady Anne Blencowe

*The Tree Dispensary—The Uses, History and Herbalism
of Native and European Trees*

The Tree Dispensary—The Uses, History and Herbalism of Exotic Trees

A HISTORY OF PLANT MEDICINE
Western Herbal Medicine from the
Ancient Greeks to the Modern Day

Christina Stapley

AEON

First published in 2024 by
Aeon Books

British Library Cataloguing in Publication Data

A C.I.P. for this book is available from the British Library

ISBN-13: 978-1-80-152-041-6

Typeset by Medlar Publishing Solutions Pvt Ltd, India

www.aeonbooks.co.uk

DEDICATION AND ACKNOWLEDGEMENTS

This book is dedicated to the memory of my father who introduced history to me as an exciting and relevant exploration of life and lives. Also, to the memory of Dr Peter Reynolds, who set me searching for herbal history through practical experiment.

I am incredibly indebted to the many scholars who have worked tirelessly in specific areas of history, enabling me to offer detail from translations over such a wide canvas. Huge thanks go to staff at museum sites where I have been privileged to make historical recipes in period conditions. To Barbara Lewis for reading the manuscript and advising, Vicki Pitman for advice on the interpretation of Greek sources, Alison Denham for advice on the period of botanic medicine, Ruth Mannion-Daniels for her thoughts on Arabic medicine and the role of the sea surgeon in the nineteenth century. I am grateful to the following colleagues for discussing their experiences in practising and teaching modern herbal medicine, which are referenced as personal communications; Alison Denham, Alex Laird, Dedj Leibbrandt, Anne McIntyre, Michael McIntyre, Anita Ralph, and Graeme Tobyn. To all at Aeon Books who have encouraged the growth of this book along the writing journey.

CONTENTS

SECTION X: THE FIGHT FOR SURVIVAL OF HERBAL MEDICINE | 1901–2021

FOREWORD

For the many omissions in this history, I apologise; the notes for this work are far, far longer than this book much of which simply had to be laid aside. Fifty years of study and research in the history of Western Herbal Medicine, often through practical methods in testing recipes, preceded the concept of this book. When first asked by Dr Peter Reynolds to think about the Celtic use of herbs at Butser Ancient Farm Experimental Archaeology Centre thirty years ago, I was faced with a lack of written evidence. A multi-disciplinary approach was devised and is explained in Chapter 2. Those first workshops were followed by many more academically-backed explorations of herbal history from the Roman period until the present day.

Celebrating the Millennium at the Weald and Downland Open Air Museum with five workshops exploring herbs in daily life and traditional medical practice over the past thousand years was an important milestone. This research supported the analysis of the most used herbs at different periods, which can be found within this book.

As a history tutor and writer my aim throughout has been to engage students and readers with evidence current to the historical timeline in order to stimulate discussion and thought. It is more a guide to history than a list of facts, including, as it does, a certain amount of experience and practical exploration. Looking at how the herbs are perceived in the light of knowledge and beliefs at particular times will hopefully aid greater understanding of the Western herbal tradition.

While researching history it is possible to see knowledge being lost as well as gained and I have made it my mission to search out effective recipes and practices abandoned in favour of new ideas and foreign herbs. Some of these I have presented to modern herbalists and used myself to treat patients in my own practice. My research coupled with a later scientific training has enabled me to offer patients the best from both sources.

Relating to history fosters identifying with concepts that can be usefully adopted into herbal practice today. British history is a patchwork of invasion and settlement, importation of foreign herbs and ideas. Understanding our roots is especially important at the present uncertain time. In Chapter 13, I have analysed samples of late medieval pharmacy, searching for correspondences and changes since Anglo-Saxon medicine. There are many influences over the centuries, including Norman, Christian, Arabic, and later, American. Each of these has demanded adaptation from what may be described as British herbal medicine with Western herbal tradition as a backdrop.

While Arabic influence resulted in reinforcement of the Ancient Greek philosophy, it had the greatest effects in pharmacy. Our tradition has been a living organic experience shown through the lives of men and women tending the sick and writing of cures and recipes. New patterns of thought emerge throughout history. The role of herbal use has been to respond to changes in living conditions, diet, expectations, and needs. Like a river it has tributaries feeding in different concepts about the origins of disease and streams of responses in terms of herbal preparations distributed by various healers, so that the guardianship of herbal knowledge was spread wide in society. Succeeding chapters explore both increasing sources and who holds the central body of surviving information.

As time passed with the establishment of the Royal College of Physicians, they saw themselves as having a mission to protect Galenic philosophy. This they felt set them apart from the empiric practices of apothecaries, midwives, cunning herb women, and many less educated practitioners. It is ironic that herbalists should be the group who now claim the Hippocratic patient-oriented treatment as theirs, while allopathic medicine has largely discarded it.

While herbalists treat the patient, mainstream medicine treats the disease. That much is easy to see, but who modern herbalists actually descend from is less obvious. In these pages it can be seen that at various times women have been physicians, midwives, surgeons, herb-gatherers, ladies with still rooms dispensing charity, religious ministers' wives or nuns in a similar role, apothecaries, nurses and cunning women, some of whom may have been witches. They all had knowledge of herbs in medicine.

Meanwhile, men have been physicians from Celtic history onwards, as at Myddfai, and the physicians to the households of kings and chiefs in Ireland. As have they been surgeons, barber surgeons, leeches, root gatherers, apothecaries, chemists, druggists, and herbalists. Later in history they became man-midwives and nurses. When botanic medicine came from America with Dr Coffin, the botanic herbal scene appears male dominated, just as the authorship of herbals is male dominated. These practitioners often had shops where they sold herbs and gave advice over the counter, reminding us of the apothecary role.

History is full of answers, but for understanding to take us forward in the knowledge of what herbalism is and needs to be, what makes a true herbalist and whether the nature of a plant is as important as its chemistry, we must find the right questions.

SECTION I

APPROACHES TO UNDERSTANDING HISTORY—THROUGH WRITTEN EVIDENCE AND ALTERNATIVE METHODS

CHAPTER 1

What is History?

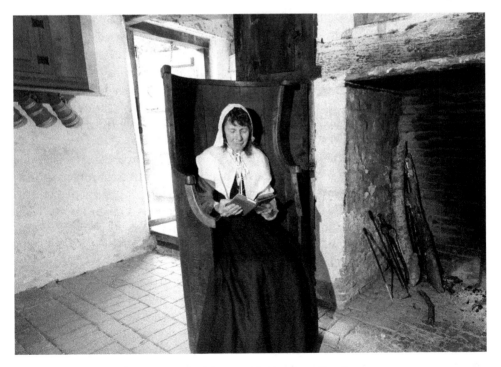

Christina in Walderton. Photo. Sam Stephenson.
Courtesy Weald and Downland Living Museum.

In writing about history, I am struck by how much the interpretation of that word has changed during my lifetime. At school as a child, the aspect of history given most emphasis seemed to be a long line of important dates, reigns of kings and queens and battles. If I had not had a historian and archivist as a father who brought history to life for me, it would have felt a very dry subject indeed. He filled it with real people and a fascination for in-depth research into their lives. His talks and writing were always popular with the public as he loved nothing better than to find an amusing story.

Since then, progress has been made in various scientific disciplines. Fascinating information has come from DNA analysis of bio-archaeological tissue. Examination of human remains, for instance bones and teeth, has been used to give information on where that person originated from which in some cases, even in prehistory is far from where they subsequently lived and died. Reconstructions of physical appearance have been made using skulls and DNA information on skin tones, hair, and eye colour. These have caught the imagination of the general public.

Molecular archaeology has also identified specific diseases, such as plague with *Yersinia pestis* bacterium found in the un-erupted dental pulp within the jawbones of victims, confirming historical references.[1] Erupted teeth can also yield information on the diet of the person.

Recognition of excavated plants has involved the scientific development of archaeo-botany, with the study of pollen and forms of seed preservation in water-logged areas, or through partial burning in a fire, referred to as carbonization. Seeds are also found partly mineralized as calcium salt replaces their decaying tissue. With seeds in each of these conditions DNA of the plants has been identified. Other forms of identification relating to plant residues are possible. The fragments of earthenware containers can be analysed for traces of their contents from hundreds, even more than a thousand years before.

Little did I think as I turned up such pottery fragments on archaeological digs during my childhood that in my lifetime a whole range of spectrographic methods would be developed to reveal traces of what such unglazed pots had actually held. This research can be applied to foods, with even tubers and green leaves being identified by their lipid content[2] and potentially, it may reveal medicines. Such progress has encouraged realisation of the possibility for a deeper understanding and emphasis on social history in daily life in the past.

There is growing evidence of the importance of plants in daily life and their utilisation as foods, medicines, dyes, cosmetics, craft materials, and fragrances throughout history. It has become apparent in my research that the role of herbs has always been about enhancing the quality of life. We may also add an appreciation of the beauty of plants seen reproduced in arts and crafts. The role of plants in medicine, however, has been their greatest contribution. The narrative of this book follows the history of this use through various records, noting influences of other cultures and introductions of foreign herbs as they have affected medicine in Britain. Study of the subject on a small island makes it easier to identify distinct moments of change. The chapters have been arranged in sections to aid in recognition of specific influences.

The plants themselves remain an important focus of attention throughout this book, their energetic classification and roles, familiarity with their identification, so important for quality control, and the effects of introductions on use of native herbs is explored. Following the use of several native herbs by examining their place in recipes from various centuries will give a clear picture of how they have been interpreted and this is finally measured against modern phytochemical evidence.

The island of Britain has been settled or conquered by people from a series of other nations. This, with broadening of experience from British travel and exploration overseas, means that the history of medicine is amazingly inclusive of knowledge and plants from other cultures and parts of the world. It is to be deeply regretted that the search for useful plants led to the evils of war, colonisation, and plunder of herbs in other countries, accompanied by destruction of the cultures and lives of indigenous peoples who had always lived in harmony with their environment.

In the vastness of China an insular medicinal culture has been maintained across millennia. In India there was more interchange of ideas, with awareness of Greek culture through the campaigns of Alexander the Great (c331BC) and trade. Later Greco-Arabic influence saw Unani t'ibb medicine established alongside Ayurveda. By comparison, the medicine of the small island of Britain, meanwhile, has been at the mercy of repeated overwhelming social changes through invasion and settlement and yet the first great influence of humoral medicine from the European continent survived here over many centuries as our dominant system. Taking inspiration from other sources has only gathered pace since the Industrial Revolution and, it might be said, remains a developing situation. Understanding our main tradition then is important. Much of the early Greek concept says more about health than disease. Consequently, the history of the search for health and longevity is an important part of this narrative.

The reader will find plentiful evidence of our ancestors' intimate knowledge of plants. Researching this path requires us to remember we can only work by hypothesis, that is to say when we come up with a likely origin or practice, we may be wrong. Our suppositions need to be tested by comparison with facts, where possible. It is important to recall that we are unable to put ourselves into the minds of our ancestors. Being limited by knowledge that we have and they did not can hamper correct interpretation. Where the opinion of a person writing within that period is available, who often will have had access to information since lost, means attention to their view may prove valuable.

However, within the great weight of written works on plants and medicine from the thinking of Greek philosophers, through our only written evidence on life in early Britain, expressed in Roman propaganda, politics may dictate the image created by using only facts suited to the current cause of the author. This is also true of many later statements where medicinal efficacy of herbs is unjustifiably dismissed. Where there is reason to see a hidden agenda, it is wise to be wary of the conclusions reached. Where indigenous knowledge is either ignored, as with the unrecorded native names of plants, or frankly stolen and used for gain, acknowledgement of these considerations grounds our understanding and informs us of how best to interpret historical information.

THE POOR MAN'S FRIEND.

ASTHMA COUGH.

Take Coltsfoot leaves, Lung wort and Sage of each a small handful, to two quarts of water; boil to three pints; after clearing it, you may add half a pound of brown sugar, and boil it five minutes. Dose—three teacupfuls a day. No. 13.

BILIOUS COMPLAINT.

Take Barberry bark, Dandelion, and Centuary, of each one ounce; water,—three pints, boil to one quart. Dose two or three wineglassfuls a day.   No. 70, 15, and 10

BOWEL COMPLAINT.

Take Tormentil, and Eringo roots, (bruised,) of each one ounce.   Water, one pint, boil to half a pint, adding towards the end, half a pound of lump sugar.   Dose— wineglassful to be taken occasionally.   Nos. 36 and 58.

BLOODY FLUX.

Take one ounce of Tormentil root, (bruised,) a small handful of Shepherd's purse, and Eringo root, half an ounce.   Water two quarts, boil to three pints.   Dose three or four wineglassfuls a day. Nos. 36, 32, and 58.

BLEEDING INWARD AND OUTWARD.

Take Nettles and Cranesbill of each one handful. Boiling water three pints, to be poured upon the herbs. When cold,—take a wineglass every three hours.   No. 29 and 46.

Note.—See Key and Companion, page 21, 8, 19, 17, 9, and 7, for Numbers 70, 15, 10, 36, 32, 58, 29, and 46.

BRUISES AND SPRAINS.

Take of Camphor four scruples, spirits of wine two ounces ; mix these together ; and when the camphor is dissolved, add white wine vinegar half a pint : apply this to the part with linen cloths dipped in it, and keep the cloths wet with

Recipes in *Poor Man's Friend*. Thompson.

With recipes, there is a constant copying of earlier works and many can be followed through various collections for several centuries. There is always the question of whether these are the ones proven by experience, or whether it was simply considered expedient to include them—either because they were originally associated with a well-known physician, or for the sake of completeness. For example, later in history, ladies set down recipes in stillroom books. These could be a record of exchanges of information that may never have been found of sufficient use to actually be made by that person. I find myself thinking of how many recipes I have added to my handwritten book for possible use, and then not found the occasion to make them. Those marked as verified by personal experience are then to be chosen for practical exploration.

When I first decided to write a history of herb use while researching Celtic herbs at Butser Ancient Farm, a unique experimental archaeology site in Hampshire, I realised the challenge ahead. I soon decided that although the role of linguist is paramount when deciphering historical texts, my personal contribution would require the knowledge of the current philosophy behind the medicine and experience of the effects of herbs on patients, to make reasonable deductions and hypotheses about the herbs themselves and their role in a recipe.

It would still be several years before I studied for a degree in herbal medicine and found the career that I should have followed all along. Yet, in that time I also experienced the experimental side of medicine-making, and to a degree, testing historical recipes. This taught me the value of not allowing modern knowledge to over-rule possible outcomes.

For twenty-five years it has been my mission to search for discarded recipes and in them for the gems that work well and can be returned to modern practice. Also, I have aimed to follow the histories of individual herbs noting periods when they were used differently to today so that we may save precious fragments of such knowledge at a point where they could easily be lost. When looking at recipes aimed at treating specific conditions, we must remember that names of conditions and diseases are also interpreted differently in the light of modern medicine. From impetigo and scabies to cancer, certain terms formerly had much broader interpretations. In some cases, the meaning of the term was entirely different.

Other aspects of interpreting history include the pitfalls of translations from one language into another, compilations and abridgements, and the confusion on common names in plants, which is still a problem we can encounter today. Altogether, these bring us to regard written history as truly "his story". In this book I will endeavour to tell "her story" of the past through the women's role too. In fact, the history of herbal medicine is not just about the plants themselves. It is also about the relationship between nations through trade and war, people and plants, and how this has proved beneficial for us, yet not always so for the herbs we depend upon. Attempts at quality control from various angles—of correct identification, harvesting, preparing, and storing—will be seen throughout. Issues in this field remain today.

The history of herbal medicine is a story involving concepts of botany and anatomy, biology and physiology, tales of plant and person, reflections of the universe and our place in it, and explorations of psychology and beliefs—this is a story of the mindful gathering and respect, or lack of it, of discovery and suffering, and of the dedication of so many caring medics of every description who appear in the following pages. Above all, the history of medicine is best appreciated and more intimately understood when viewed through the lens of what was practical and possible at the time, with the knowledge and resources that were available then and there.

By the end of the book, the extent to which herbal knowledge was dispersed within society in Britain, certainly until the social upheavals begun by the Industrial Revolution, may be appreciated. Far from being confined to the wise woman living at the edge of the woods, until recent times it was practised by men and women in mainstream medicine. This was natural, since orthodox physicians also trace their practice back to classical Greece and Rome. The reader will become aware that medicinal herbal knowledge is equally to be found in the stillroom books of charitable ladies in the seventeenth and eighteenth centuries, in the libraries of religious ministers, and books of housekeepers all of whom used herbal remedies for the benefit of others as required. Self-help guides to health and family doctoring written by physicians and others are strong themes during the nineteenth century, offering continued guidance. Although ranging in depth and accuracy, knowledge of herbal medicine has been as widespread in society as the plants growing in the British countryside.

References

1. Martin Jones, *The Molecule Hunt* (London: Allen Lane, The Penguin Press, 2001), 222.
2. Jones, *The Molecule Hunt*, 184.

CHAPTER 2

Celtic Medicine | Largely Iron Age, 300 BC to 43 AD

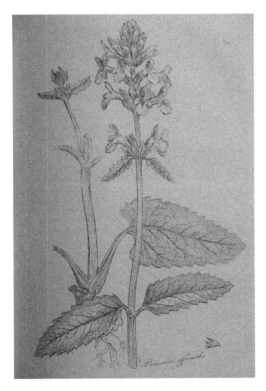

Betony, *Medical Botany*, Woodville.

When it comes to thinking about the origins of our indigenous Celtic medicine, we are faced with an overwhelming lack of early written evidence. We must, therefore, take different approaches.

Key Figures

Information on Britain before the Christian era can be found in the works of the Roman geographer Strabo, (c62–24 BC), writer on Greek philosophers, Diogenes Laertius (whose dates while unknown are placed before 500 AD), and the account of the Greek voyager, Pytheas, who described Britain in 300 BC. Queen Macha, in Ireland, appears in legendary evidence attributed to the early Iron Age.

Key Texts

The Geography of Strabo: Strabo.
Diogenes Laertius Lives of Eminent Philosophers, Diogenes Laertius.
The Red Book of Hergest
The Book of Leinster
Seanchus More, Irish Annal

Roles of Women in Medicine

These are unknown, we may presume the presence of cunning women treating the local sick. Possibly some had roles as a Druid priestess or spiritual healer at holy wells. Women could be powerful in Celtic society, as the lives of Queen Boudicca and others attest.

Quality Control

A good knowledge of herb identification seems likely since daily contact with herbs at this period would be common. There is no evidence on ritual gathering beyond reference to Druids gathering mistletoe, which we find in Pliny.

Archaeology

Archaeological evidence from the Ness of Brodgar, Skara Brae, Glastonbury Lake Villages, Pimperne Dorset, Star Carr, Alpine Wangen, Zug, Marin, and Moringen, Switzerland, The Similaun Glacier on the Austrian–Italian border.

Travel and Trade

There was definitely trade with Europe and some introduction of herbs has been suggested as a consequence of Belgic immigration.

Introduction

Some thirty years ago, Dr Peter Reynolds, a very experienced experimental archaeologist who founded the Butser Experimental Archaeology Project, requested my exploration into herbal use in Britain in pre-history. In recounting this experience, I will refer to archaeobotany, considering surviving evidence of plant distribution, bio-archaeology with evidence of disease conditions, and discuss the pitfalls in interpretation, which can arise from considering archaeological finds. Importantly, I will include knowledge gained from discussion with my mentor, Dr Reynolds, and my own practical exploration of living conditions in a Celtic roundhouse, making recipes using the fire and investigating drying and storage methods for herbs and preparations. This will bring us to hypotheses on which herbs may have been in common use for medicine in the years leading up to the Roman invasion in the first century AD.

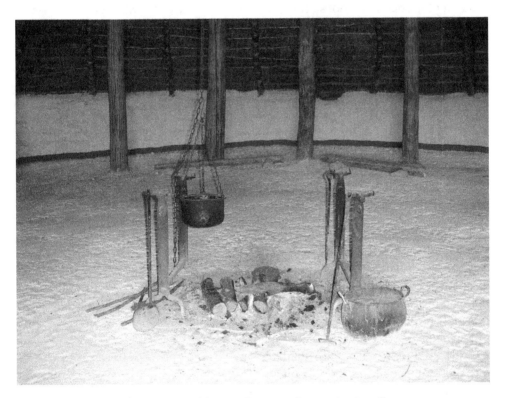

Hearth, Pimperne House. Courtesy Butser Ancient Farm.

Firstly, let us consider what we know. There had been several Celtic migrations from various areas of Continental Gaul to Britain and Ireland at different dates in pre-history. In the later, Iron Age Belgic Celts brought increased trade links, but certainly tin had been exported from Cornwall for a very long time. Some ideas on medicine may have travelled here earlier than has been previously thought. Thanks to scientific development in the field of examining the DNA of human remains, as already mentioned, we are becoming increasingly aware of how much travel there was between the European continent and Britain, certainly in the Bronze and Iron Ages and even before.

Some Hellenistic ideas might even have been part of Druidic lore since the Druids were seen by some Roman writers as "scientists" or philosophers who studied nature. Diogenes Laertius mentions this in the introduction to his *Lives of Eminent Philosophers*. The life of Diogenes himself is unknown. Clearly well educated, he is impartial in his accounts of the different schools of thought and quotes freely from hundreds of sources, mainly from the third and second centuries BC and first century AD.[1] The very survival of his work, containing some valuable references to other books now lost, has made it valued. He debates the point that some people thought philosophy had not started only with the Greeks, but also with barbarians, a view he does not share. He gives references to the Magi in Persia, Gymnosophists in India, Chaldeans in Assyria and Babylon and among the Celts and Gauls with the Druids, or Holy Ones. One source for this was quoted as the *Magicus* of Aristotle.[2]

Diogenes Laertius enlightens us further by writing he is told that the Druids "uttered their philosophy in riddles, bidding men to reverence the gods, to abstain from wrong-doing, and to practise courage".[3]

Writing in 1919 on the history of the Druidic period of medicine in Ireland, Moloney relates passages from legend and states of the three orders of Druidesses, the first lived as a sisterhood of virgins and had supposed powers of divination, healing, and sorcery.[4] It is unfortunate that it is not clear whether this comes from *The Book of Leinster* from 33 AD, which appears on the previous page as reference for information on Druids. He also quotes the Irish Annal *Seanchus Mor*, written centuries later, where it is recorded that Princess Macha founded the first hospital, the Broin Bhearg in 300 BC.[5]

Dioscorides and Galen, both of whose lives and work we will explore in Chapters 5 and 7, had yet to write their influential works setting authoritative standards in medicine, when Julius Caesar made his early forays across the channel to our shores. Therefore, it is at this point that we consider what we can discover of the Celtic medicine which was already established here.

The lack of written evidence on herbs leaves us with physical traces from archaeology on the actual presence of plants. This then is a good source to begin our investigation. Some ground conditions are particularly helpful to survival of plant remains. Excavation at Starr Carr in Yorkshire where the ground at the edge of a lake was waterlogged, revealed the presence of hunters with a domesticated dog from a time earlier than the Neolithic.[6] A collection of rolls of birch bark were found; clearly stored with a purpose in mind. Possible interpretations could include use as containers, or for extraction of their resin.

In the Alps, the discovery of a body revealed by a melting glacier in 1991, which came to be known as the "Ice Man", gives us another use for birch along with a treasure trove of other information. The body was wonderfully preserved with fur and leather clothing, and a grass cloak covering these and his belongings. The finds told us much of his life around 3350–3105 BC. Among his several possessions was an ember carrier for starting a fire quickly, made of birch bark and containing charcoal, including that from the elm. He had been injured and had fractured ribs. Dried fungus found threaded onto fur strips, was also found with him and he is presumed to have worn this around his wrist. The fungus, *Fomes fomentarius*, grows also on birch in Britain and contains an antibiotic substance, polyporic acid.[7] It was assumed that he was carrying this for medicinal use.

In the Neolithic era in Britain, there is evidence of a highly developed society 5000 years ago. Exciting archaeological finds in the Scottish islands over the past decade are likely to re-write our idea of pre-history in Britain. On an archipelago is the central Ness of Brodgar where among fourteen buildings, the largest may have been a temple. It is linked at either end to areas with stone circles, which pre-date Stonehenge and may even have inspired the southern building. Tombs containing skeletons, many of whom had suffered violence, have shown evidence of a healed depressed skull fracture. Links between Neolithic Orkney and Ireland, are now being evaluated. These are concentrated between 3300–2600 BC.[8]

The finds at the once buried village of Skara Brae not far away on Orkney give us exceptionally detailed information. The wonderfully preserved houses with their stone furniture make it easy to imagine life there at a time when the climate supported growing a little wheat and barley and the sea offered meat and fish. After visiting the site some years ago, I was sent a basic list of plant and fungus finds that had been prepared by Camilla Black for the Skara Brae report. One that was highlighted was the finding of at least thirteen mature puffball mushrooms. The number of *Bovista nigrescens* proved that they had been gathered for a specific use.

Puffballs are styptic. Gabrielle Hatfield in her investigation of orally transmitted folk remedies in East Anglia records the common practice of keeping a puffball hanging up in the kitchen or shed for first aid use in case of serious cuts.[9] Such examples of fungal uses were both relatively easy to interpret as, at the very least, they showed evidence of deliberate gathering. However, in both cases the presumptions of the fungi being carried or gathered as medicine were based simply on what we know now. Our knowledge and understanding is not the same as that of previous centuries. Interpretation will always be affected by the understanding of the period.

When I am tempted to make educated suppositions about the past without written support from the period, I am always reminded that in 1694 John Pechey wrote about sugar, "'Tis certain that it increases the Scurvy, for by the frequent use of it the Teeth grow black and rotten, which are certain Signs of the Scurvy".[10] His was a conclusion that fitted the known facts but was still wrong.

When it comes to herbs, it can be a confusing picture. Seeds and pollen micro-fossil debris found on the floor of a living space could have blown in or been trodden in underfoot. Likewise, herbs found in a grave could have been picked as an offering for the dead person as we might do today, rather than for their medicinal properties. With carbonised seeds, which Dr. Peter Reynolds regarded as more often than not occurring as the result of an accidental burning, some are much more easily recognised than others. Godwin discusses pollen analysis[11] and records particular examples of distinctive morphology of pollen as with salad burnet, lime flower, and ribwort plantain. The carpels of meadowsweet, are listed as quite recognisable with an asymmetric, twisted form and Iron Age flax seeds are recorded as being large and generally identified as *Linum usitatissimum*.[12] Waterlogged deposits such as those from the Glastonbury Lake Village, are interesting sources of information, but still require careful interpretation.

The initial discovery of the site later known as the "Glastonbury Lake Village was made by Arthur Bulleid in 1892."[13] He had been inspired to search for evidence of early habitation in the area by the wealth of finds at excavations of the Swiss Lake villages of Wangen, Zug, Marin, and Moringen.[14] His ambition of rivalling the fame of the Swiss finds was realised after four years of searching the peat moors near Glastonbury, followed by years of excavation. Unlike the Swiss villages and the still to be discovered Scottish crannog in Loch Tay, the houses were not on stilts. As with the other habitations at Meare the environment was more of a swamp than an actual lake, with soggy ground built up with layers of brushwood and layers of clay spread on the top.

The Glastonbury site was in use for about 200 years, from 250 BC until wetter conditions saw it abandoned and floodwaters subsequently preserved bone and plant food remains from middens. About forty plants were identified and listed, some foods including chickweed, parsnip, goosefoot, nettle, bindweed, bulrush, bogbean, bur-reed, mustard, water-lily and various berries. There were also many hazelnut shells. Bones retrieved showed a variety of diet far greater than present day with a wide range of fish, meat, and water fowl as well as wheat, barley, Celtic beans and peas, plus wild gathered plants.

Knowledge of diet is always important in thinking about health, and it will be a factor to consider throughout the history of herbal medicine. The prevalence of certain diseases and the corresponding need for particular herbs used in treating those conditions will be marked as we pass through the centuries. The sheer numbers of recipes for treating toothache, worms, rickets, gout, skin eruptions, and fevers in different eras reveal links with both diet and environmental factors. Sometimes the stark differences in diet from rich to poor show not only malnutrition for the poor, but sometimes how their inability to access or afford rich foods actually could work in their favour.

A huge number of sloe stones sufficient to fill a wheelbarrow at the excavation of the Glastonbury Lake Village of the Iron Age are again proof of deliberate gathering. Nettle also was clearly considered useful, having fibres for bindings and textiles and pigment for dyeing. Numerous spindle whorls, bobbins, weaving combs, and loom weights found on the site indicated involvement in weaving cloth.[15] The subject of use of herbs for medicines does not seem to have entered the discussion.

Even the few extracts from the plant foods listed above offer distinct possibilities with chickweed, used in treating skin conditions, bogbean for treating arthritis, nettle as a diuretic and tonic, and mustard for colds to mention a few. It is likely that certain of the medicinal properties of nettle and other herbs were discovered firstly through eating them. On the skin, the heating aspect of the sting is also suggestive of the early use of the seeds externally to warm the limbs. The heat of mustard and cooling effect of chickweed are also apparent to anyone tasting them.

My research into prehistory began before my visit to Skara Brae and my first visit to the Alps and subsequent interest in the Swiss Lake Villages and Glastonbury sites. Shortly after the publication of my first book on growing and using herbs in 1993, I met Dr Peter Reynolds who lived not far from our home. He was director of the Butser Experimental Project, originally set up in 1972 to study agricultural and domestic economy from c400 BC to 400 AD.[16] By then the project was well established and had received such international interest that he had relocated the buildings and fields from the original Iron Age site on the spur of Butser hill to another area.

His scientific experimental archaeology involved careful research using factual knowledge of the archaeology as a basis for reconstructing buildings and tools, and growing crops to estimate Iron Age wheat yields. Results subsequently allowed a more accurate approximation of surplus available for export given the understanding of population at the time and went some way to explain the large number of storage pits found for this period. On an earlier site, a herb garden had been planted for visitors to see, and, more importantly, so that seeds of native herbs could be gathered to establish a viable seed bank for research on identification.

It was planned to use some seeds from this bank for experimental burning, producing known samples which would increase familiarity with the possible appearance of individual species of carbonised seed on excavation. The herb garden had a further aim in learning more about potential uses of the plants.

I had written an article about this garden when we first moved to the area and was already familiar with the guide to native and Roman introductions published by the Butser Ancient Farm Project Trust. This gave only simple descriptions of the herbs, habitat and known uses in later times. The list had no period information to offer for the Iron Age. I therefore found myself in a very different situation to an archaeologist when Dr Reynolds asked me to think about the ways in which the Celts may have used herbs. Despite the scarcity of known facts, he felt my herbal knowledge and deep interest and research into later history might lead, as he put it emphatically, not to re-enactment, but to useful practical experiment.

My work would be based on knowledge of native herbs together with those few indications available to us from archaeology and early traditional use. Some prehistoric introductions could be included as he believed that madder and borage had probably been brought by Belgic tribes in the third century BC. Dr Reynolds also included comparative ethnology in his interpretations of how some implements might have been used, searching for parallels in peasant farming methods in Spain to aid his hypotheses. This would be another similar avenue for me to explore.

Initially, I learnt as much about Iron Age farming and daily life as I could from him. He talked a good deal about the already long history of trade between Britain and Celtic Europe and beyond, emphasising the links. His years of experimental growing and noting yields, confirmed that even on relatively poor ground, such as Butser hill, it was possible to produce a yield much higher than had previously been thought possible. To an extent this explained the numerous storage pits found (although they were not all for grain) and supported the Roman comments on high exports.

We spent time discussing crops, foodstuffs, and weeds that grew among the crops, such as cleavers and black bindweed. Particular attention had been paid to the possibility that some "weed seeds" were gathered and deliberately grown for food value, as with the most likely, fat hen.[17] Dr Reynolds reasoned that black bindweed, vetches, orache, and other inevitable weeds amongst the crops could have been harvested as they came ready before the wheat. It seemed clear in our discussions that all the backbreaking hoeing of weeds from the cereal fields should not be wasted and could readily have resulted in all edible weeds going into the pot as foods.

We considered that where people trade and can understand each other, there will be inevitable talk of medical conditions and remedies. I came to realise that there might be considerable influence from Europe, not least through the Druids. The practice of the Druids of using oral transmission of knowledge, even though Celts in Europe were known to use the Greek alphabet for other writing in daily life, felt as if it was at the centre of my problem. Druids were well known on the European continent for their wisdom in matters of law, settling disputes, and arbitrating in time of war. While Bards were honoured as singers and poets, Vates, who were particularly concerned with herbal healing and Druids, seen more as teachers, were recorded by Strabo as investigators of nature.[18] He further writes of their belief in the eternal nature of the soul and universe, although at some point they predicted fire or water would bring an end. They would seem then to have been philosophers. It would be strange if their investigation of nature did not include medicine as it had with the Greek philosophers.

As in ancient Greece, both in Irish and Welsh tradition early medicine begins with legendary characters and myth. When we reach the early documentary evidence of the medieval period, again the history relates to ancient practice in Greece and other early civilisations with reference to families of hereditary physicians.

In Wales, the legends of physicians of Myddfai appear to refer to a historic family with links to the court of Rhys Gryg.[19] In Ireland, we have abundant evidence of families of physicians in several areas, some attached to the courts of chieftains.[20] At a lower social status, it is likely that the herb woman with cunning or knowledge of herbs treated those in her locality.

Supposition from ancient texts aside, in reality, I would be presenting the possible medicine in everyday life in a rural community with no Druid in sight. I could hardly avoid the subject, however, as I soon had modern Druid Ovates attending my classes. When thinking about comparative ethnology, the work of Juliette de Bairacli Levy, which I was reading at the time was perhaps the best guide.[21] She had travelled extensively in Europe, and learned from nomadic groups of their uses of wayside herbs. So it was that I began thinking towards likely medicinal applications and drinks with what might almost be described as a clean slate, for the certainties were nowhere to be found.

I had first to experience the atmosphere in the reconstruction of the large Pimperne house at Butser, named for the use of planning data from the excavation of a house in Dorset. One possibly to be interpreted as a manor, or feasting house. The roundhouse was sturdily built, giving ingenious support to the massive weight of thatch. With Dr Reynolds I pictured a well-furnished, colourfully-decorated interior of this feasting house. The owner might well have afforded imported Italian wines, glassware and Spanish olive oil traded for excess grain, leather, and hunting dogs.

Roomy inside, despite having no windows it was quite airy and gained light from the open doors. Furnished as in the past, or unfurnished as in the present, I quickly learnt the importance of the fire, and how to make one produce the steadily glowing, fiercely hot, but stable, embers suitable for cooking and making recipes. One of the herbs included in the Project Trust guide to the herb garden, coltsfoot, is a cough herb we find in later times administered by the patient taking in the smoke through a reed as it burns in the fire. This is to treat coughs and breathing difficulties. I have often wondered whether the benefit of this was discovered while using the soft hairy down from the backs of the leaves to light a fire in early times. Anyone blowing on the smouldering fire to encourage flames would also breathe in the smoke and may have decided this was helpful.

Smoke from any fire would also have helped to preserve some food items. Drying racks outside were used for leafy branches for animal fodder and when thinking about drying roots, I settled on cleaning and slicing them to thread on lines and hang to dry in shade. There was much to be explored and I could not apply Dr Reynold's rule when determining identity and use of tool parts, that if you make it and it works, it is likely to be correct.

Pottery was produced on site and other containers, such as baskets for gathering, I could make. When tutoring classes with no ready source of willow, I often used long weavers of ivy growing along the ground and lengths of de-thorned bramble.

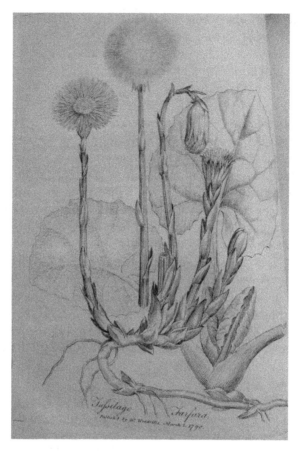

Coltsfoot, *Medical Botany*, Woodville.

Hazel rods had been used in the interwoven roof supports between rafters, and hazel osiers had continued to be grown for ongoing wattle and hurdle require-ments. These are also useful for basketry stakes. Both ivy and bramble weave well in their green state but will shrink as they dry making the basket slightly more open-weave in time, although still durable for regular use.

In later years taking workshops at Flag Fen Bronze Age centre, in a wet environ-ment beside a smaller roundhouse, thatched with sods of earth, we used willow for strong baskets and rushes for other soft baskets and mats. I enjoyed many "golden autumn basketry days" at both of these sites. Perhaps coming closest to the feel of the period when a group of folk singers came on a day course and we sang as we worked in the sunshine.

Other possible containers for herbal preparations were leather bags, perhaps for seeds or dried roots, herbs might also have been involved in preparing the leather. Also horn and wooden boxes could have served. I knew that later in history ointments were kept both in pottery and in wooden boxes. Experiments with wooden boxes for ointments proved them to offer good insulation for the ointment inside against changes in temperature, even in a roundhouse in summer with the fire lit. Wood is additionally antibacterial from the lignin content. I wished I could experiment as to how long preparations would keep in the different containers in the roundhouse—a year, or longer? Unfortunately since there would not be a fire lit in the house through the winter months, it was not possible to carry out a proper trial.

Having come to understand the fire, I still had much more to learn from experience. I recall early in my experiments making an ointment and learning not to set the pot in the embers on the side of the fire towards the open door. By this time, I had discovered the pleasure of using large mullein leaves as pot holders giving good grip and insulation, and begun straining the herbs from the hot oil using wads of cleavers which remove the herb beautifully and protect your hands from the heat at the same time. This method can add some extraction from the cleavers with really hot oil into the bargain.

There are many unexpected lessons from practical experiment, not least those learned from having un-tethered animals and free-range poultry able to access your 'home'. I have experienced sheep eating recipe ingredients when my back was turned and an over confident cockerel running in and knocking a container into the fire. This last made a strong point about having to be able to treat burns and scalds, considering the inevitable small children and dogs of the past were even more likely to cause accidents. Tending animals on a farm also adds exposure to such skin conditions as mange, to say nothing of transference of worms. Watching over the fire on windy days brought me to appreciate how common eye inflammation, sinus and chest problems might have been, even allowing for some acclimatisation. A proportion also filters out through the thatch, but as with all fires you are dependent on atmospheric conditions.

The archaeology of disease reveals that rheumatism and arthritis were definite problems. Gathering thatching materials was done in winter which apart from clear, sunny days must have been a miserable task. Even in a relatively dry environment with age arthritis would have developed simply from working outside in British weather. We have an idea of the weather in the Iron Age and know it was not greatly different to now. The first recorded Greek traveller to explore the land of tin and amber under the Great Bear, later known as Britain, was Pytheas who sailed from Marseilles and landed in Kantion (Kent) on the south coast in about 320 BC. At this point in time Britain was referred to by Pytheas as Prettanike, later, Brettanike. It was considered to be close to the edge of the inhabitable world.[22] The journal written by Pytheas has since been lost but fragments of detail have been quoted by later writers.

This intrepid traveller wrote of the natives living in round houses of logs, evidently with reed thatch, points which had been noted and followed in the building of the house at Butser.[23] His further comment on the people threshing wheat indoors because of the poor weather rings true even today. He did not seem to be impressed by their food, describing a pottage of millet, roots and herbs, along with their drink of honey and grain, mead. It is difficult to believe, since he is thought to have spent at least a year here surveying, that no-one gave him a better meal. We have to remember that only a fragment of his journal has been passed down to us. If he originally wrote about medicinal herbs, this information also has been lost. Pytheas recorded his latitude and distances establishing the truth of his journey north to present day Scotland and on to the Outer Isles, to where there was neither land nor sea, presumably ice.[24]

When thinking of plants, we can start with what we know from archaeology to have been growing in that particular habitat at the time. Later, I tutored herb workshops at Peat Moors Centre, close to the Glastonbury Village sites and the Sweet Track. This is the oldest known timber trackway in the world, dated to c3806 BC.[25] As a result of this connection I also studied the Somerset Levels Papers which gave details of plant finds. Over years my appreciation of probable herb use in different environments grew. On days at Peat Moors we walked along part of the Sweet Track where we could easily gather willow, meadowsweet, and other wetland herbs to use in recipes and I was reminded of the common folklore belief that when a habitat produces specific disease—such as fevers in the fenland and arthritis in wetland—then the herbs to give ease will also be found there.

I also experimented with small scale surveys asking workshop participants, who mainly had no knowledge of medicinal plants to walk around the sites and bring back any plants they felt might be useful. This was quite enlightening as the majority were still in use in herbal medicine today. Having thought about these randomly selected herbs and those mentioned from excavations, I then looked at those native herbs given special notice in the only recipes said to be associated with the Celts in Wales I had access to in the 1990s, the *Herbal Remedies of the Physicians of Myddfai*.[26] There is evidence for such a family of physicians where the knowledge of medicine is handed down the generations and the family owns land which was granted on that basis by princes or chieftains. The practice is also seen in Ireland in early times, as well as in ancient Greece.[27] With my list of probable common conditions to be treated with simple remedies and Juliette de Bairacli Levy to refer to, I came to concentrate on a small group of native herbs in workshops, while at the same time listing some of the many options available.

In particular, the elder offers flowers, berries, and leaves with harvests in spring through to late summer or early autumn. It is thought that farmsteads had a protective bank and ditch that would have been planted with such useful trees, along with hawthorn, hazel, and blackthorn. Sloes have already been mentioned and there has long been use of blackthorn flowers as well as twigs for treating the skin. Elderberries were an obvious food, which did not leave such clear evidence as the sloes.

Elderberries have yeasts on their skins in the same way as grapes, and I have used them to raise bread and start fermentation in wines. Elderberry wine is a favourite of mine and I was interested by the suggestion of Stephen Harrod Buhner[28] that a branch of juniper laid in the base of the vessel of fermenting wine will accumulate grains of yeast and this can be dried for future use. The berries are of course also medicinal.

The flowers can be used to flavour and thicken foods and both the flowers and berries can be used as dyes. Elder could have been used to treat sore eyes, sinus problems, coughs and the skin. Ointment to take home was made at almost every workshop and elderflower ointment was always a great favourite, with reports of efficacy from returning participants who had used it on animals as well as people.

The ditch at Butser also afforded us herbs suited to a wetter environment, along with the brambles for baskets, food, dyes, and medicinal use. Meadowsweet and nettle thrived, both hugely and widely useful. Not surprisingly nettle finds are common in excavations and on the surface above, archaeologists even look for nettle to mark sites of previous habitation, as they like enriched ground. Sometimes in the past, the seeds were boiled in honey and applied to heat cold limbs.[29] Heating the seeds in oil made a less sticky application for rheumatic pain on workshop days. Although olive oil was traded from Spain in return perhaps for grain before the Roman invasion, at that point it was for the wealthy. There is however, abundant

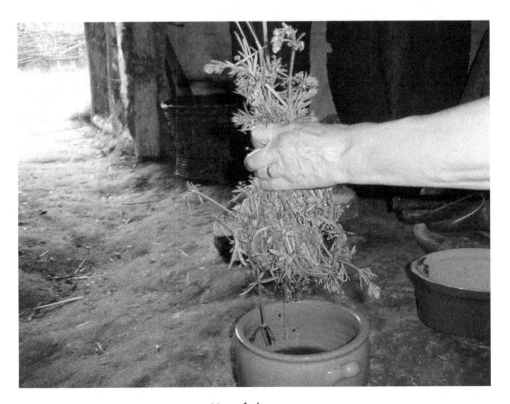

Use of cleavers.

evidence of flax being grown, providing textile fibres, linseed, and oil. How much of the crop was allotted to each use is unknown.

Another herb already mentioned as a common weed of the fields is cleavers. In addition to adding a certain amount of extraction to ointments as I used it to filter hot oil, the herb has long been taken as juice or a tea firstly of the leaves in spring and then the flowering herb in early summer, followed by the seeds to provide a lymphatic tonic.

Chickweed, mints, juniper, and other berries, wild marjoram, dandelion, burdock, wild carrot, wild celery, watercress, certain mushrooms, and wild thyme are all foods or seasonings with potential to become medicine. Yarrow will have been used as a wound herb throughout Europe. There is a beautiful mosaic of Achilles receiving knowledge, in this case playing music, from the centaur, Chiron, in the Museum of Archaeology in Naples. The mosaic came from the basilica in Herculaneum, which was buried along with Pompeii by the eruption of Vesuvius.[30] It adds a context to the legend of Achilles also receiving tuition in medicine from Chiron, and subsequently using yarrow to heal his soldiers. The legend is remembered in the Latin name of the herb, Achillea.

The readily available plantains, both ribwort, and greater plantain, are also given huge praise in later medicine and I felt were likely to have been commonly used herbs for everything from wounds and bites and stings to many internal conditions. Other probable wound herbs are self-heal, shepherd's purse, betony, woad, and, in dire circumstances to staunch bleeding, stinging nettle. The list is by no means exhaustive. Betony I found of particular interest as it was later given the name *bettonica* from the Gaulish tribe the Vettones. The herb was introduced into Roman medicine by Antonius Musa, physician to the Emperor Augustus. This is one of the herbs we will follow through the centuries, including in recipes from the Welsh sources, as it has been much regarded and continues to have Celtic links in destroying dragons in recent folklore.

Home medicine may well have been largely externally applied as poultices, salves, or as a cold compress. We can only suggest that a poultice might be entirely of the crushed or chewed herb, or mixed with animal fats or linseed. Barley flour or oats might keep it in place. Honey would almost certainly have been used to preserve and sometimes apply herbs, or they could have been heated in oil, or butter and milk. Herbs were very possibly used as poultices to draw out thorns, for this hawthorn, agrimony, betony, yarrow, and spear thistle root are possibilities also for removing wood and metal splinters.

Cough medicines might be chosen from coltsfoot, mullein, cowslip, elderberry, marshmallow, sloe, and comfrey. These vary in their chosen habitats and so at least one would always be available.

For treating the eyes, elderflower, eyebright, and greater celandine come to mind. Headaches, whether from sinus problems, or a myriad of other causes and fevers might require herbal drinks, involving beer (Celtic beer was popular during the Roman occupation) or milk of various kinds. Dr. Reynolds' experiments with storage of grain in pits in the ground replicating those found from this period, revealed that grain can be successfully stored without drying it first. This creates conditions where the grain immediately beneath the seal over the storage pit uses up the oxygen and gives off carbon dioxide that then sinks, preserving grain below. In certain conditions, where the seal on the pit is not secure, the grain above ferments, from which stems his hypothesis that brewing beer might have originated from this discovery.

Many published recipes, such as those formerly associated with the Welsh physicians of Myddfai, can be identified as originating either in other medieval manuscripts or sourced as mentioned in the text from works of Dioscorides, Galen, or Avicenna. A few may have had a more local origin and more recent in depth research by Diana Luft has shed considerably more light on the copying, translations and additions that took place over centuries with the recipe collection.[31] We will look again at this subject when we come to the medieval period.

One recipe, which interested me in particular, used coltsfoot and burdock prepared in a very distinctive way. The original source of this recipe does not appear to have been identified as I have not found it among the early Welsh texts translated by Diana Luft.

"For Pain in the Limbs. 463. Take a handful of the herb called colt's foot, and as much of the leaves of burdock, pound and mix with the milk of a one coloured cow, oaten groats and butter being added, the whole being boiled well, and applied as a plaster to the painful parts as hot as you can bear it; it will ease it."[32]

I made this recipe repeatedly after one workshop when we had been out walking and a participant suffering from arthritis was in serious pain. With her agreement on our return to the roundhouse I made the coltsfoot and burdock plaster, using goats' milk. Both of her ankles were quite swollen and inflamed and so I applied the coltsfoot and burdock to one ankle and foot and a control of comfrey and elder leaf to the other. After twenty minutes I removed both applications to find the ankle and foot treated with the coltsfoot and burdock now had no swelling and the inflammation and pain was much relieved, more so than with comfrey and elder, which I had expected to be more effective.

In making the plaster in Iron Age conditions using freshly gathered herbs, pottery containers and the fire for heat, then applying the plaster to the pain in a limb of an actual patient, I felt we had learned something valuable about the recipe which no amount of discussion on reading it could have elicited. Cow's milk would have been more accurate but some from a one coloured cow was just too problematic. The comparison with other suitable herbs was also interesting. Whether it reveals anything about Celtic medicine, I leave the reader to decide. N.B. The comfrey was applied before the later concerns on pyrrolidizine alkaloids were known.

In this chapter, we have followed the available lines of investigation including the meagre written evidence concerning Celtic pre-history with reference to relevant background and conditions for the period. Turning then to practical information from archaeo-botany and bio-archaeology, we have examined the benefits and limitations of what this technology may reveal for us. This has been supplemented with practical information on experiencing the conditions in which herbs would have been dried and stored, and remedies would have been made. A selection of useful native herbs has been completed and details given of preparing a remedy which proved effective. From the selection of herbs we will be following the use of three, betony, nettle, and greater plantain through history with further recipes included in each section.

References

1. R.D Hicks, (trans), *Diogenes Laertius. Lives of Eminent Philosophers* Vol. I. (London: Harvard University Press, 1972), XXI.
2. Hicks, Diogenes Laertius. Lives of Eminent Philosophers, 3.
3. Ibid, 7.
4. Michael Moloney, *Irish Ethno-Botany and the Evolution of Medicine in Ireland* (Litter Press), 54.
5. Moloney, *Irish Ethno-Botany*, 52.
6. Francis Pryor, *Britain BC* (London: Harper Collins, 2003), 84.
7. Konrad Spindler, *The Man in the Ice* (London: Phoenix, 2001), 118.
8. Nick Card, et al. (ed), *The Ness of Brodgar, as it Stands* (Orkney: Kirkwall Press, 2020), 320.
9. Gabrielle Hatfield, *Memory, Wisdom and Healing* (Stroud: Sutton Publishing Ltd, 1999), 96.
10. John Pechey, *The English Herbal of Physical Plants* (London: 1694), 334.
11. Sir Harold Godwin, *History of the British Flora* (London: Cambridge University Press, 2nd edition, 1975), 9.
12. Godwin, *History of the British Flora*, 167.
13. Stephen Minnitt and John Coles, *The Lake Villages of Somerset* (Glastonbury Antiquarian Society, Somerset Levels Project and Somerset County Council Museums Service, 1996), 3.
14. Dr. F. Keller, (trans), E. Lee, *The Lake Dwellings of Switzerland* (London: Longmans Green and Co., 1878), 522.
15. John Coles and Stephen Minitt, *Industrious and Fairly Civilized* (Somerset Levels Project and Somerset County Council Museums Service, 1995 reprint 2000), 149–152.
16. Peter J. Reynolds, *Iron Age Farm. The Butser Experiment* (London: British Museum Publications, 1979), 17.
17. Reynolds, *Iron Age Farm. The Butser Experiment*, 69.
18. D. W. Roller, *The Geography of Strabo: An English Translation, with Introduction and Notes*. Part 4. The Northwestern coast and ethnography. (4).
19. Diana Luft, *Medieval Welsh Medical Texts* (Cardiff: University of Wales Press, 2020), 8.
20. Moloney, *Irish Ethno-botany and the Evolution of Medicine in Ireland*, 58.

21. Juliette De Bairacli-Levy, *The Illustrated Herbal Handbook for Everyone* (London: Faber and Faber, 1991).
22. D. W. Roller, *The Geography of Strabo: An English Translation, with Introduction and Notes.* Part 5. The Nature of the inhabited world. (8).
23. Reynolds, *Iron Age Farm. The Butser Experiment*, 30.
24. Roller, *The Geography of Strabo: An English Translation, with Introduction and Notes.* Part 4. Polybios and the Internal Sea. (1).
25. Pryor, *Britain BC*, 133.
26. John Pughe (trans), *The Herbal Remedies of the Physicians of Myddfai* (Dyfed: Llanerch Press, 1987).
27. Moloney, *Irish Ethno-botany and the Evolution of Medicine in Ireland*, 58.
28. Stephen Harrod Buhner, *Sacred and Herbal Healing Beers* (Boulder U.S.A: Siris Books, 1998), 65.
29. Pughe, *The Herbal Remedies of the Physicians of Myddfai*, 71 (427).
30. Francesco P. Maulucci, *The National Archaeological Museum of Naples* (Naples: Carcavallo), 50–51.
31. Luft, *Medieval Welsh Medical Texts*, Introduction.
32. Pughe, *The Herbal Remedies of the Physicians of Myddfai*, 74 (463).

SECTION II

THE ANCIENT GREEK BACKGROUND
TO MEDICINE

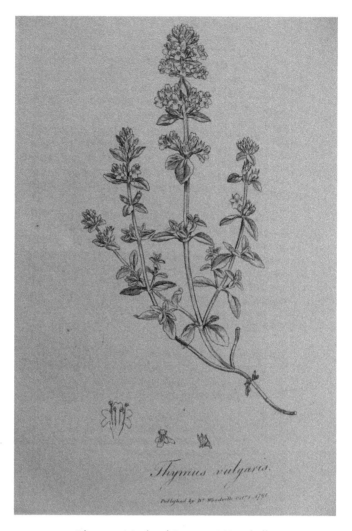

Thyme, *Medical Botany*, Woodville

It is difficult to place too much emphasis on the influence of early Greek thought when writing about the development of herbal medicine in Britain. This influence arrived initially with the Roman troops and once adopted became the standard philosophy behind practical medicine. It was subsequently re-inforced over several centuries through the spread of classical medical works.

Key Figures

Anaximander, (6th century BC), Asclepius, (dates unknown), Pythagoras, (c570–c500 BC), Hippocrates, (460–375 BC), Aristotle, (384–322 BC), Theophrastus, (c372–c287), Apollodorus, (c180–post-143 BC). Aesclepiades, (124–40 BC).

Key Texts

Theophrastus Enquiry into Plants, Theophrastus.
On the Nature of Man, Regimen I–III, Aphorisms, Hippocrates, Hippocratic Corpus.

Roles of Women in Medicine

A stele to Peseshet in the tomb of Akhet-hotep records her (allowing for translation difficulties) as 'female overseer of female physicians'. Dated to the old kingdom of the fifth to sixth dynasty, this statement supports her as the first known lady doctor.[1] I have found no evidence in Greece for female physicians, but experienced women acting as midwives may be presumed. The role of temple priestess in various cults would have been likely to have included healing of some kind.

Quality Control

Emphasis is laid on the quality of what we would now term the consultation. Knowing the patient, their lifestyle, diet, and exercise is seen as key to understanding the problem. The qualities of foods and herbs are considered to be important.

Herb Energetics

The rules for these are being thought through during this period. There is emphasis on the heating, drying, moistening and cooling effects of foods in the Hippocratic corpus. We will see observations leading to the development of the concept of energetic relating to the humoral system.

Archaeology

Stele and papyrus from Egyptian tombs. A copper tablet from Cyprus.

Travel and Trade

It is good to remember that ancient Greece was not isolated from other cultures. Even as early as 610 BC when Anaximander was born in the city of Miletus in Ionia, that area had strong connections with Egypt, shown by influence on the architecture, and with the East, including India due to its coastal position for trade. Later the campaigns of Alexander the Great (356–323 BC) would extend the Greek Empire to cover an area from Greece to the Indian Punjab, south as far as Egypt and north to the Danube. Aged only twenty-five, he became King of Persia and Pharoah of Egypt. Following the long history of trade this would have given the Greeks even closer contact with other well developed civilizations.

Introduction

Cures had been carried out for many thousands of years already as we see in the written evidence in the cultures of Persia, India, China, Egypt, Assyria, and Babylon. The Egyptologist, Wallis Budge was convinced that Greek medicine was rooted in Egyptian practice. He wrote "an examination of the medical literature of Egypt proves that they were the founders of the chief systems of medicine which were, with modifications and improvements in use throughout Greece, Arabia, Syria, and many other parts of Western Asia, down to the Middle Ages".[2] Scholars have since differed on this point. The reader will come to appreciate there are many unresolved questions and opinions about history.

Anaximander who lived in the sixth century BC was the first to write in prose about natural phenomena in *On Nature*. He is looked upon by the modern physicist Carlo Rovelli as the founder of scientific thinking. From his established models of the time, Anaximander concluded that the earth was a stone hanging in space with nothing beneath and it was spherical in shape. He began lines of thought that nature could be explained and that man was part of nature. This was followed by a long line of philosophers who viewed the universe, and the place of man in it in new ways. Aristotle (384–322 BC), discussed his ideas and Theophrastus, (born c372 BC) known to us for his work on classification of plants, also wrote a history, sadly now lost, which included Anaximanders' theories.[3] The ancient Greeks did not invent cures for disease. Their contribution was largely one of philosophy, a new way of thinking about the world, health, and why disease happened. They were not alone in progressing this, for at about the same time, possibly the sixth to fifth century BC, a similar process has been noted in both India and China.

In India this led to the Ayurvedic observations and advice. In her book, *The Nature of the Whole, Holism in Ancient Greek and Indian Medicine*, Vicki Pitman has made interesting comparisons between principal texts of Ayurveda, such as the *Caraka-Samhitā* and the Greek text *Ancient Medicine* from the Hippocratic Corpus. She concludes that there is much common ground relating to doshas and humours as constituents of the human body. In both cases, they can become pathogenic when out of balance with each other. Pitman finds seven such correspondences, including constitutional types and similar therapeutic methods. She concludes finally that although using different terms, according to their cultures, "the experience which generated the concepts, that of the human body-mind-spirit whole, was the same."[4]

As discussion on medicine provoked new thought, inevitably several different theories attracted followers. Serapion in the first century BC and those members of the School of thought called Empirici believed that medicine should be founded on experience and practice. He declared reasoning was no part of medicine. The Empirici did accept that evident causes should be taken into account, but felt that those more obscure imbalances were in their view incomprehensible, so of little use anyway. This view is found in a treatise that is part of the Hippocratic Corpus, *Tradition in Medicine*.[5]

The Methodists looked upon disease as coming from outside the body but turned to diet, exercise, emetics, blood-letting, and bathing as treatments. For the mentally sick, music therapy was recommended and this could be tailored to treat other diseases too. Celsus, author of a first century encyclopedia of medicine, the subject of Chapter 6, writes the Methodici observed that if the patient had overly relaxed tissues due to disease then tightening astringent remedies should be given and with constriction, relaxing remedies. He pours scorn on how general and ineffective this theory is, pointing out that where there is flux or discharge from relaxing disease this may be due to quite different conditions, for instance with vomiting, whether blood or bile is vomited. Likewise diarrhoea and dysentery are not the same. These specific cases he insisted need different treatments.[6] The Empirics pointed out that since the various schools of thought reached different conclusions, and argued amongst themselves, time would be better spent treating the patient with remedies already proven to work in that situation.

Physicians treating patients were often peripatetic and we find in the texts observations on differences of climate and other conditions to be considered in different countries. They might be paid by a city for a set time, or, if found to be exceptional, given land on which herbs grew in addition to payment, to induce them to settle. This was recorded on a copper tablet from Cyprus from the fifth century BC.[7] There are also references to knowledge of medicine being passed down in families, both practices we have already seen in Celtic lands.

The Hippocratic Corpus contains seven books of immensely detailed case notes, taken sometimes on ten or more consecutive days.[8] Often there appear to be daily visits for at least a week. These set a high standard of observation including the appearance and manner of the patient, their urine, stools, etc. The examination did not include the pulse, as the importance of this was not yet recognised. Despite many arguments on the causes of disease, names for particular disease conditions seem to have been standard. With remedies some texts give precise measurements for a dose. Forty-four species of plants account for half of the 380 references to different species in Hippocratic texts and most of these would have been easily obtainable in Greece. Hellebore, (*Helleborus cyclophyllus*) is prescribed sixty-three times in recipes.[9]

With concentration on the development of thought about medicine and detail of the consultation taking a large role in this section as a main influence for a considerable era in British plant medicine, we look first at thinking about the plants themselves with Theophrastus. Again this is a beginning for the scientific presentation of their forms and relationships, which informs botany and quality control in centuries to come.

References

1. John F. Nunn, *Ancient Egyptian Medicine* (London: British Museum Press, 1996), 124.
2. E. A. Wallis Budge, *Syrian Anatomy, Pathology, and Therapeutics* Vol. I (Alpha Editions, 2020), CXXX.
3. Carlo Rovelli, *Anaximander and the Nature of Science* (London: Penguin Books, 2023), 30, 31.
4. Vicki Pitman, *The Nature of the Whole Holism in Ancient Greek and Indian Medicine* (Delhi: Motilal Banarsidass Publishers Private Ltd., 2006), 218.
5. G.E.R. Lloyd, *Hippocratic Writings* (London: Penguin Classics, 1983), 40.
6. W.G. Spencer (trans), *Celsus De Medicina* Books I–IV (London: William Heinnemann, 1971), Prooemium 65–69, 37.
7. Robin L. Fox, *The Invention of Medicine from Homer to Hippocrates* (London: Penguin Books, 2022), 45.
8. Lloyd, *Hippocratic Writings*, 130.
9. Fox, *The Invention of Medicine From Homer to Hippocrates*, 92–94.

CHAPTER 3

The Beginnings of Botany

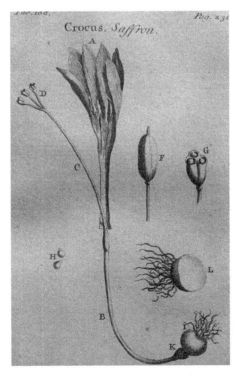

Saffron, *The Compleat Herbal*, Tournefort.

As we have seen in the introduction, Egyptian medicine was already long established at the first stirrings of innovative thought by the Greeks on the subject—for we can trace their drugs and recipes through written texts back to the period of the Ebers Papyrus, dated by a passage within it to the reign of Amenhotep I about 1534 BC. The papyrus was said to have been discovered with a mummy in a tomb presumed to have belonged to a physician and mentions anatomy, diseases, and remedies in 110 pages.[1] This level of Egyptian knowledge must surely have been recognised in ancient Greece.[2] Indeed, traces of Egyptian medicine are to be found in the form of prescription writing, mix of magical ritual, and medicine and numerous individual recipes still to be found in the medieval period.[3]

The contribution of Greek philosophy and science as a cradle from which the system both of Western herbal and mainstream medicine emerged, is almost impossible to over emphasise. The unceasing search for order and reason in the natural world consumed the lives of men who are remembered to this day and stood as authorities in their subject for more than a thousand years. Theophrastus, in the company of Hippocrates, Dioscorides and Galen, is one of these.

Theophrastus was born on the Greek island of Lesbos c370 BC. Originally named Tyrtamos, he was well educated and already a student of philosophy when he left the island for Athens. There he studied at Plato's academy where he met Aristotle, who later became his mentor and gave him the name of Theophrastus, because of his graceful style.[4] Aristotle was working on a classification of animals and it was perhaps knowledge of this task that inspired Theophrastus to begin the unbelievably massive enterprise of constructing a framework of classification of plants. Others had of course already given much thought to important questions about plants. In his *Enquiry into Plants* which runs to fifteen books including minor works on odours and weather, Theophrastus quotes several earlier authorities. These include Anaxagoras who lived c500–428 BC and Diogenes, the Ionian philosopher, in his discussion of the origins of seeds. He also quotes Kleidemos who believed that plants and animals were made of the same elements.[5]

What is a plant? His questions on the basic premise of what constitutes a plant reveal how he began his train of thought by comparison with animals. This is something he must have discussed with Aristotle, perhaps many times as he searched for analogies. Looking for similarities, he notes that all plants have moisture and warmth as being necessary to life. Going further, he identifies veins containing moisture, tissues corresponding to muscle, and writes that some call the middle of the wood of a tree, "heart" or "marrow".[6]

He is uncertain as to whether parts of plants can be identified in the same way as parts of the body of an animal, and asks whether a fruit born of a plant is still part of it. Much later in his work he compares plants that live near water with animals that are aquatic and notes that both seem to have shorter lives than those living on dry land. Again when writing of bedstraw flowers maturing into seeds within the plant, he likens this to weasels and sharks producing eggs, and bearing their young alive. These examples are stark illustrations of the gap between our thinking with all the botanical information we have on plants today and his journey of investigation long ago.

Theophrastus conducted research through minute examination of all parts of the plants he knew, constantly making comparisons of leaf shapes, heights, habits of growth of plants, and so on. He also gathered information from other people, such as those who went on campaign into India with Alexander in 327–326 BC. He writes in detail of the Indian fig tree and several others, adding there are many more which are "different to those found among the Hellenes, but they have no names".[7] That his source in the legions has not obtained the names of the trees is not really surprising. The army was not there to talk to locals, or research plants. When comparing how a plant grew and whether it flourished from one area to another for instance, he quotes the words of the Macedonians as against the opinion of the people of Mount Ida. Theophrastus may have travelled in Macedonia with Aristotle while young. He gives many references to plants in Egypt and Syria and through his contacts was able to include plants he would never have seen, from the Arabian penninsula to Ethiopia and India. His geographical range of plants is considerable.

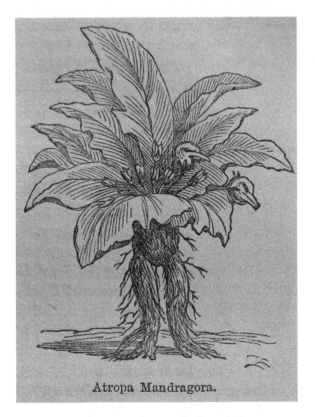

Atropa Mandragora.

Mandrake, *The Complete Herbalist*, Phelps Brown.

Sometimes the lack of agreement among his sources on far off plants gives him problems as in the case of frankincense and myrrh. Some have told him that frankincense has leaves like bay, others that they are reddish and the fruit is like that of mastic. Even more confusing are the completely contradictory reports of the weather and therefore the soil where frankincense and myrrh grow. When he is told that the portion of harvested cinnamon left behind as it is allotted from the harvest as a tribute to the sun catches fire as harvesters leave, Theophrastus is not to be taken in and writes that it is "sheer fable".[8]

He is equally discerning when it comes to writing of medicinal plants and statements on special methods and precautions during harvesting made by herb-diggers and druggists. While acknowledging some as sensible, Theophrastus gives several examples of what he regards as the far-fetched. These include danger from attack by a woodpecker if peony is harvested during the day. Inevitably the ritual of gathering mandrake is related. This is elaborately carried out using a sword to draw three preliminary circles around the plant, being sure to cut it when facing west. A second cut required dancing around the mandrake while reciting everything known about the mysteries of love.[9] He concludes that the stories are made up by those wishing to increase the importance of their craft.

In the first nine of his books he begins by setting down basic divisions of trees, shrubs, under-shrubs, and herbs. A tree, he writes, has a single stem, whilst a shrub has several. An under-shrub is so called because it has many woody stems and small leaves, this includes some pot herbs. Herbs he describes as coming up from the root with leaves and only the flower on a stem.

Herbaceous plants are divided again into wild and cultivated, and every aspect of the propagation and growth of cultivated forms is examined. He puts some plants into groups and it is tempting to suggest that the group of ferula-like plants[10] may be the embryonic *Umbelliferae* family, although he is actually more interested in the fibrous stems than umbels. While hemlock is included in this class, he also describes aconite along with them, which does not have umbels. Most attention for the ferula-like plants is given to Silphium and Papyrus from Egypt, which he has evidently received reports about as he is quoting the people of Cyreneas on when silphium first appeared there. Again when he is writing about plants with spinous leaves, Theophrastus notes that the largest class is thistle-like. Reading his work it is clear he understood the importance of different soils and habitat and questions the effects of climate on the speed of germination.

When describing the saffron crocus, Theophrastus gives it as having narrow "hair-like"[11] leaves and blooming for only a few days after the rising of the Pleiad (autumn). Use of the rising and setting of stars to give the season is a regular reminder in the text of the importance of the heavens as a calendar in antiquity and of his acute observation of the relationship of plants with their environment. Differences in the form of plants are of importance and he often emphasises this. While discussing eccentricities in specific plants he writes, " … as has been repeatedly said, we must only observe the peculiarities and differences which one plant has as compared with others".[12]

In writing of medicinal plants he indicates which part or parts of the plant are used and different methods of preparation—e.g. in plasters, as a pessary, olive oil applications, taken in wine, mixed with honey, or vinegar. In fact, with several we have what may be described as short monographs of the plants with a physical description, preferred habitat, harvesting, preparation with other ingredients as necessary, and both the action and dose. A good example may be found under the various kinds of *tithymallos*, which are spurge plants.[13]

With localities identified in a list of countries and districts that specialised in producing medicinal herbs, including parts of Egypt, Ethiopia, Scythia, India, Thrace, and Crete, the *Enquiry into Plants* demonstrates the impressive extent of his knowledge. Theophrastus further comments on repeated use of drugs reducing their efficacy in the patient. He has been particularly impressed by how taking repeated small doses of poisons could render them harmless. His work revealed his curiosity about the way in which gum Arabic and marshmallow act on water, thickening it. Constantly questioning, Theophrastus carefully researched how plants may affect the mind—suggesting the root of oleander taken in wine made the drinker more cheerful. He warned that the plant *strykhnos*, translated by Hort as thorn-apple, causes madness.[14] He further muses over the lack of understanding as to how certain plants cause similar effects to others. Do they have "some virtue" in common?[15]

After the death of Aristotle he became head of the famous Lyceum school, founded in 335 BC, a role which he filled for another thirty-five years. The school is said to have had 2000 students and we can imagine he will have taught with enthusiasm and passion for his subject. His amazing works written over a lifetime of dedication are a truly valuable record for posterity. Theophrastus died shortly after ceasing teaching in 290 BC and was buried in the gardens where he had lectured.

References

1. John F. Nunn, *Ancient Egyptian Medicine* (British Museum Press, 1996), 31–34.
2. E.A. Wallis Budge, *Syrian Anatomy, Pathology, And Therapeutics* Vol. I (Alpha Editions, 2020), CXXX.
3. Warren Dawson, (ed), *A Leechbook of the XVth Century* (London: Macmillan and Co. Ltd, 1934), 14–15.
4. R.D. Hicks, (trans), *Diogenes Laertius. Lives of Eminent Philosophers* Vol. 1. (London: Harvard University Press, 1972), 485.
5. A.F. Hort, Theophrastus *Enquiry into Plants* Vol. I (London: William Heinnemann, 1999), Book III, Chapter I, Verses 3–5, 163.
6. Hort, *Enquiry into Plants,* Vol. I, Book I, Chapter II, Verse 6, 23.
7. Ibid, Book IV, Chapter IV, Verses 5–8, 317.
8. Hort, *Enquiry into Plants* Vol. II (London: William Heinnemann, 1980), Book IX Chapter V, Verse 2, 243.

9. Hort, *Enquiry into Plants,* Vol. II, Book IX, Chapter VIII, Verses 7–8, 259.
10. Ibid, Vol. II, Book VI, Chapter II, Verses 6–8, 13.
11. Ibid, Vol. II, Book VI, Chapter VI, Verses 8, 43.
12. Ibid, Vol. II, Book VII, Chapter XV, Verses 2–4, 139.
13. Ibid, Vol. II, Book IX, Chapter XI, Verses 7–9, 275.
14. Ibid, Vol. II, Book IX, Chapter XI, Verses 5–6, 273.
15. Ibid, Vol. II, Book IX, Chapter XIX, Verse 4, 315.

CHAPTER 4

Development of Greek Medicine

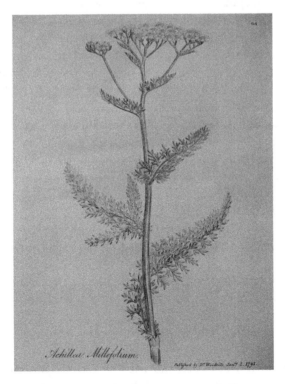

Yarrow, *Medical Botany*, Woodville.

The long-established, thriving drug trade between the Ganges and Karnak, as well as from the Arabian Peninsula by sea and land, continues as we follow myth and legend through to recorded, if still with some scholars, debatable facts, and text. Much had already taken place in the field of thought on medicine by the time of Theophrastus. We are fortunate in that a first century AD writer on the subject, Cornelius Celsus, opens his work with a "potted history" of these developments. With his account we are taken back in time to before the life of Theophrastus. He tells us that the art of medicine has been cultivated among the Greeks more than anywhere else and refers to Homer, writing in *The Iliad,* around 750 BC, as his source that Aesculapius was the first authority on medicine.[1]

Asclepius (spellings of his name vary in Greek and Roman references), appears first in Greek history as a hero who was mortal and healed the sick in a kindly way, with gentle hands, even bringing patients back from the jaws of death. His life is dated by involvement in the Trojan Wars, and is mentioned in the Hesiodic Catalogue written about 600 BC. Apollodorus had served as a librarian at the great library of Alexandria. He is later described as "of Athens" by Diogenes, who refers to his four books of *Chronology* as sources for some of his information.[2] These works covered the period from the fall of Troy 1184 BC to 119 BC. In the *Chronology,* Apollodorus adds that Asclepius was taught by Chiron the centaur.[3] Chiron in turn was believed to have been the inventor of medicine and very first physician.[4]

As time passed, the legend of Asclepius was embroidered and we find conflicting versions about his birth, although his father was consistently said to be Apollo, who variously operated on his mother to take him from her womb, or otherwise saved him. The earliest version has Coronis as his mother, and his birthplace the city of Epidaurus. All legends, including those in Diodorus' *Bibliotheca Historica* IV and Ovid, agree that Zeus killed him with a thunderbolt for bringing back the dead. Different areas claimed to be his birthplace and gave his mother different names to support this. If he had truly come from Thessaly, an idea that can be traced back to the fourth century BC, then this gave him a background shared with Chiron. The truly verdant surroundings near Mount Pelion had their own legend to explain the richness of medicinal herbs growing there.

As to where Asclepius actually came from originally, the honour was sufficiently important for the matter to be settled by the Delphic oracle. Even then, commentators J. and L. Edelstein in a work that collected and interpreted material on Asclepius, believe it was a matter of political expediency that Epidaurus won.[5] Over centuries his reputation, which was surprisingly without a long list of famous patients or detailed achievements, grew, and he was raised in status to a demigod of medicine. An inscription to him in this role was found in Athens, dated to 420 BC. Many temples were built and dedicated to him where patients were cured by him in dreams or trances. Later oracles revealed his prescriptions to patients. As a mortal physician, yet son of a god, his abilities were compared to those of Jesus. For this reason he was hated by early Christians. To the ordinary physician, however, he became an honoured ancestor; in Homer's time physicians described themselves as Paeonii, sons of the Greek god of medicine, Paeon, later they called themselves Asclepiads to identify themselves with Asclepius.

As a god, Asclepius was portrayed with a snake—a symbol of the patient shaking off age and being restored after disease, in the way a snake sloughs off its skin. The snake was also a symbol of wisdom and its representation as twisting around the staff, symbolised the support Asclepius gave to his patients.

Was Asclepius a real person? It is impossible to prove one way or the other. His son Macheon is referred to in the Iliad first as a healer, then as a surgeon.[6] As the story of Asclepius unfolded in the fourth century BC, his daughters joined him in his practice of medicine. Their names include Hygeia, Aceso, Iaso, Aegle, and Panacea. However, Iaso, Hygeia, and Panacea had all been healing deities in their own right when Asclepius the hero achieved divine status, and Edelstein's interpretation was that they seem to have been added to the myth to extend his power.[7] Perhaps the status and inspiration he gave to early Greek medicine is the most important fact.

Celsus continues his history stating that there followed a time when herbal knowledge was simply handed down from one generation to the next until men spent more time studying for the sake of their souls as philosophers. This "restless thinking and night watching"[8] was, Celsus writes, good for the spirit but bad for their bodies, and it was his opinion that those whose health suffered as a result began to study the science of healing. He gives names of famous philosophers, (the etymology is Greek, meaning lover of wisdom), such as Pythagoras (better known today as a mathematician) and Democritus as experts in medicine. The division of medicine into three parts; curing by diet, medicaments, and by hand (surgery), came early. The followers of curing by diet were divided into those who prescribed diet based on reasoning and those who depended simply on the results shown by practice.[9]

Hippocrates was born on the island of Cos about 460 BC and became a strong influence in Greek thought on medicine. Celsus records him as a pupil of Democritus. Possibly this idea came from the influence of Democritus appearing in a Hippocratic treatise. The Hippocratic Corpus as the collection of writings is known, consists of around seventy manuscripts, varying in length and quality. While some, notably the Aphorisms—a selection of observations concerning patients, diseases, and likely outcomes—are accepted by some scholars as most likely to have been the work of Hippocrates, other writings in the Corpus are not. In the introduction to his translation of these works for the Loeb Classics Library, Jones suggests some possibilities, namely that certain parts of the Corpus may have been notes made by students at lectures, as can be seen to apply particularly to Humours i–iv. Alternatively, they may have been added later.[10] For the remainder of this chapter, when the name Hippocrates is used it can also be read as standing for the Hippocratic Corpus, since what follows may, or may not be attributed directly to him.

The reasoning of Hippocrates will, of course have been affected by knowledge and theories contributed by his predecessor. We find ideas from Homer who was familiar with Egyptian drugs, and Jones notes some from Plato's *Timaeus*. Plato in turn was influenced by Pythagoras (580–489 BC) whose legendary teacher was Un-Nefer of Heliopolis.[11] The work of Empedocles and his theory of the four elements, air, fire, earth, and water is also acknowledged by Hippocrates. However, he does not use the two active forces of love and strife that in Empedocles' theory explains how these four elements are mixed and separated to affect health.

There are passages of the Hippocratic Corpus that can be difficult to follow but this may be deliberate, possibly to make sure only the initiated fully understand the text. Translators have noted this as a common ancient Greek technique to emphasise how mysterious the workings of nature are. From this it can be appreciated that philosophy with a basis in poetry and science was still an art. While travel added to the physician's knowledge, physics, philosophy, and medicine were combined in his rhetoric. The Hippocratic texts show a particular emphasis on clinical observations of the course of the disease and understanding the patient as an individual. In this way, the formulation of a prognosis was supported by judging the ability of that person to regain health through the resilience of their own body.

Hippocrates states at the outset that the body contains many constituents and multiple changes amongst these of moisture or heat can produce different diseases and therefore, require different treatments. He writes, "Now all animals, including man, are composed of two things, different in power but working together in their use, namely, fire and water"[12] and that "fire has the hot and the dry, water the cold and the moist".[13] However, each is seen as containing some of the other so that the intermingling and separation of these opposites, is a constant ebb and flow. He includes life and death as an example of opposites, each of which contains the other. In the Hippocratic view, there is no new creation, only a constant re-cycling of all things.

Hippocrates uses the forces of fire and water to explain the content of the soul, how the body is formed and the separation between male and female. "Females, inclining more to water, grow from foods, drinks and pursuits that are cold, moist and gentle. Males, inclining to fire, grow from foods and regimen that are dry and warm".[14]

This statement is followed by advice to both potential parents to act accordingly to influence the sex of their future child. So we see that men and women are viewed very differently as to their basic essence.

Different blends of fire and water giving the various combinations of temperature and moisture are set out as basic constitutions for men and women. These are then interpreted to predict when in the year and at what ages in their lives that person might be likely to fall ill. With each patient their temperament is given with the corresponding balances of rest or exercise and diet to counteract the tendency towards illness from their constitution. Various treatments such as vapour baths, purges, and emetics are suggested along with advice on walking, athletics, and sexual intercourse.

This might seem sufficient to consider about a patient when assessing their needs but it is only the beginning. The Hippocratic author is clearly aware of the differences in the patients' environment that affect how their body responds. Personal experience has, I am sure, brought this to the attention of many herbalists even today. The influence of a predominantly wet, cold climate as opposed to a dry, warm one may decide whether a patient recovers quickly, or the problem becomes chronic. It is unsurprising to see the statement that climate is different in different countries, but the detail of asking or observing the predominant wind direction, and whether this comes off the sea or land, comes as reminder to the modern reader of important points that would not occur to a physician today.

Inevitably, a large section on diet confirms the huge importance of this aspect of lifestyle for health. In the Regimen it is pointed out that dividing foods into those

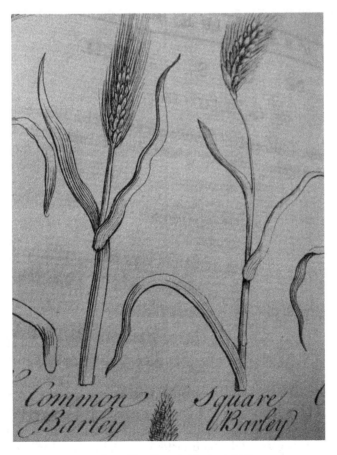

Barley, *The British Herbal*, Hill.

that are sweet or salty does not give accurate information on their action in the body. For instance, it is suggested that some sweet things may be laxative, while others have the opposite effect. Hippocrates, therefore, undertakes to give details on individual items, beginning with grains.

Barley, he relates, can be purgative when eaten with the husks, but cooling and astringent as barley meal. Several instances are related of the use of barley, including in a food called *cyceon* with preparations using various milks with the barley added either to honey or to wine. This is followed by comments on wheat, spelts, beans, and meats. Whether the animal is wild or has been tamed is deemed important to the effect of the meat in the patient's diet. This is a concept just beginning to be appreciated today. The flesh of various animals from lamb to wild boar is compared as to how heavy, dry, or strengthening it is, and whether it passes easily by stool. Almost all birds are considered to be drier in their meat than animals, with fish the driest of all. Where the fish feeds, whether in stony water or in mud is recorded. Of wines the sweet and dark are stated to be moist in their effects on the body and also weaker than acid wines, causing flatulence. Acid wines were appreciated as cooling. Although acid wines moisten from their water content, it was stated that they also empty the body of moisture. Whether they pass better by stool or urine is always recorded.

In another text, *Nature of Man* blood, phlegm, yellow bile, and black bile are named as making up the body.[15] These four humours will become very familiar to readers as we continue through time. The exact number of humours was debated by early philosophers and recorded in other texts as three or five, and the actual nature of the humours as bodily fluids has also been questioned. This text however appears to set a pattern of belief that held sway for over a thousand years and is, therefore, important for our narrative.

Nature of Man explains that if these four humours are not in balance pain results. The imbalance might be caused, it tells us, when a large quantity of one of them is lost out of the body, or flows into a part of the body where it does not belong. Having established what these four substances look like and whether they feel hot or cold, moist or dry to the touch, our source supports the argument that they are all contained in everyone by the evidence observed from giving certain drugs to extract one or other from the body.

Reading this following passage, it is difficult not to feel alarm for any patient given emetics, which was common practice. Hippocrates states that after the initial substance closely related to the drug is vomited, the other substances can follow, as with a drug to withdraw phlegm, "First they vomit phlegm, then yellow bile, then black, and finally pure blood, whereon they die."[16] This statement is made in order to stress that all four substances or humours are present in everyone.

The Hippocratic Corpus contains information on over 350 herbs. Of the drugs, it is written that just as plants take their tastes of acid, bitter, sweet, and salt from the nourishment of the earth, they also take of the element closest to them in nature, equipping each one to draw a particular element in man, whether phlegm, bile etc.

The text goes on to relate the increase of phlegm in winter, as observed particularly in the older person. Certainly, it is the time of colds and chest infections so something we might agree on today, as a generalisation. The association of blood with spring is less obvious but he asserts that nosebleeds and dysenteries are more common—dysentery as we understand the condition is rare in temperate countries nowadays. The interpretation of dysentery in terms of symptoms was not necessarily the same then. Yellow bile increasing in summer he supports by saying that it is vomited in this season even without taking a purge and with purges the discharges are more bilious.

Bilious attacks are a familiar condition from my own childhood—when friends were sick and had diarrhoea it was not termed a "stomach bug" or "virus" but a bilious attack. I recall that some friends were more prone to them than others, usually in summer. Black bile, he notes, increases in autumn but does not offer such a graphic description for illustration.

So, we see the basis of humoral theory being grounded in specific observations.[17] There are many references in the Aphorisms of signs to watch for. These are intensely practical observations, clearly recording extensive experience as a practitioner. Some include influences of the seasons, with lists of conditions most likely to arise at a particular time of year. These are also related to the age of the person and we see the expanded theories on humours and humoral types condensed in these brief statements. Everything from a sign in the heavens, such as the rising of a star, to the patients' appetite at different stages of the illness, is considered.

Many of these pointers from the Aphorisms are brought together in the instruction to compose a full understanding of the patient through their lifestyle, how much food they eat, and whether this is balanced by exercise taken. We have already seen the needs to know the patient's age, and whether where they live is a damp plain or on a windy hill, to include the prevailing air and wind direction as relevant to recovery. Also considered are the season and climate. All of this gives a picture of the patient as a whole and assists identification of imbalance within that person's life that might have caused disease. We can already see the basis for humoral theory of four humours being related to the four elements. Now the text gives advice on balancing the humours within the four seasons. In winter, he prescribes drying and warming foods in one meal a day only or with a light lunch if the person has a very dry constitution. Much exercise of all kinds is recommended, sexual intercourse to be more frequent for old men and taking emetics three times a month. He notes that as spring approaches milder foods and exercise are appropriate, just as a tree prepares itself for summer by providing shade with leaves, he feels man should prepare extra healthy flesh. He goes on into detail with each season, using the rising and settings of stars to indicate timings.

This wide and deep approach is one a modern herbalist can readily identify with. It also enables the identification of aspects of the patients' diet, personal constitution, and lifestyle that make them likely to develop disease. With the appreciation that disease does not spring from nowhere, comes the valuable concept of preventive medicine and the opportunity to advise on balancing measures to be taken in declining health. It is only when this advice does not work that prescribing herbs will be resorted to in addition to regimen. An experienced practitioner today will prescribe strengthening and restorative herbs to prepare a chronic patient in the weeks preceding a season that has proved difficult for them before.

Birds' eggs and cheese are deemed strong foods through being concerned with the nourishing foods of young creatures. Honey is given different effects on the bowels of the bilious type of person to the phlegmatic. Pure honey is described as laxative to the first and having a binding effect to the second degree. Vegetables and their effects have detailed consideration as to whether they are heating or cooling, pass readily by stool or urine, and have specific curative or unwanted effects. It is noted of garlic also that when raw it is more powerful and while it warms the body, it is considered bad for the eyes. Onions on the other hand are classified as good for sight, but their degree of heat is greater and so bad for the body.

While mustard, rocket and coriander are all hot herbs, lettuce, mint and fresh purslane are cooling. Drying herbs are those we regard as astringent such as sage and moistening vegetables include pumpkin and turnip.[18] A general guide to wild vegetables follows and depends on determining their sweet or strong smell and their acidic, sharp, or warming effects on the taste buds. There is again a detailed list of fruits, with special notice taken of apples. The effects of sweet and sour apples, cultivated apples, wild apples, apple juice, and even the beneficial effect of the smell of apples are related.

The extreme importance of an intimate knowledge of dietary matters is emphasised when later in the text instruction is given on effects of foods not only in the abdomen but on the veins.[19] Important points in advising treatment were clearly which foods can give strength without eating a larger amount, and that the country a food had come from affected the strength of that food. It was judged that hotter, drier regions produced more compact and nutritious foods than moist ones.

There is also instruction and observations on bathing, oiling the skin, sexual intercourse, sweats, vomits, sleep, and methods of exercise. Exercises are interestingly divided into natural and violent. "Natural exercises are those of sight, hearing, voice and thought."[20] The effects of natural exercises are described as being warming and drying on the soul.

His closing comment will resonate with the modern practitioners' experience of those around us—"such is my advice to the great mass of mankind, who of necessity live a haphazard life without the chance of neglecting everything to concentrate on taking care of their health".[21]

Our examination of the selected texts, *Nature of Man, Aphorisms*, and *Regimen I–III*, has highlighted the development of Greek thought on matters pertaining to health and, therefore, the patients' natural resilience and ability to recover from disease. We have centred on the detailed Hippocratic methods of examining the patient, assessing their strengths and weaknesses due to individual constitution and lifestyle. These rules are important considerations that will come to inform medicine in Britain for well over a thousand years. They became our traditional system. In particular, we have set a focus on the four humours, first clearly stated by Empedocles and appearing only in *Nature of Man*.[22] Along this journey through the ages, we will follow how these are interpreted, noting the role of ideas about them in medicine and daily life.

References

1. W.G. Spencer (trans), *Celsus De Medicina* Volume I (London: William Heinnemann, 1971), 3.
2. R.D. Hicks, Diogenes Laertius *Lives of Eminent Philosophers* Vol. I. (London: Harvard University Press, 1972), 39.
3. E.J. & L. Edelstein, *Asclepius. A Collection and Interpretation of the Testimonies* Vol. I. (Baltimore: The John Hopkins Press, 1945), 11.
4. Edelstein, *Asclepius. A Collection and Interpretation of the Testimonies* Vol. II. 5.
5. Ibid, 71.
6. Homer, *The Iliad* (Oxford: Oxford University Press, 2008), 202. Iliad II. Verse 38, (714–83), Verse 193, (449–520).
7. Edelstein, *Asclepius. A Collection and Interpretation of the Testimonies* Vol. II, 88–89.
8. Spencer, *Celsus De Medicina* Vol. I, Prooemium, Verses 4–8, 5.
9. Ibid, 8–12, 7.
10. W.H.S. Jones (trans), *Hippocrates Volume IV*. (London: Harvard University Press, 1st published 1931), Introduction, XIX–XXI.
11. E.A. Wallis Budge, *Syrian Anatomy, Pathology, And Therapeutics* Vol. I (Alpha Editions, 2020), CLI.
12. Jones, *Hippocrates Volume IV*. Regimen I. Chapter III. 231.
13. Ibid, Regimen I, Chapter IV. 233.
14. Ibid, Regimen I, Chapter XXVII. 265.
15. Ibid, Nature of Man, Chapter IV. 11.
16. Ibid, Nature of Man, Chapter VI. 17.
17. Ibid, Nature of Man, Chapter VII. 19.
18. Ibid, Regimen II, Chapters LIV–LV. 331.
19. Ibid, Regimen II, Chapter LVI. 341.
20. Ibid, Regimen II, Chapter LXI. 349.
21. Ibid, Regimen III, Chapter LXIX. 381.
22. Jones, *Hippocrates Volume IV*. Nature of Man. IV–V.13.

SECTION III

BACKGROUND TO ROMAN MEDICINE AND OCCUPATION OF FIRST CENTURY BRITAIN

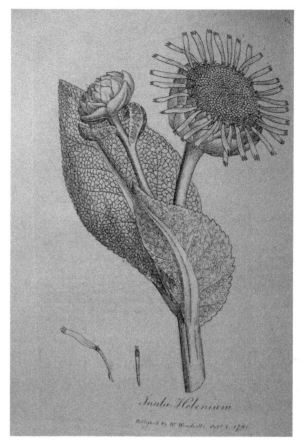

Elecampane, *Medical Botany*, Woodville.

Key Figures

Dioscorides, Celsus, Galen, Cunobelinus, Claudius, Scribonius Largus, Hadrian, Pliny, Tacitus, Vortigern, Cunedda. (All first century).

Key Texts

De Materia Medica, Dioscorides.
Celsi de Medicina, Vols. I–IV. Celsus.
Galen Natural Faculties, Galen.
The Periplus of the Erythræan Sea.
Compositiones Medicamentorum, Scribonius Largus,
Tacitus on Agricola and Germania, Tacitus.

Roles of Women in Medicine

Many women, including some from Greece, became physicians in the early centuries AD; some, we know to have been very successful. In Lycia, Antiochus, daughter of Diodotus, who was possibly also a doctor, was honoured with a statue in recognition of her skill.[1] Although from epitaphs we see that a noble disposition was appreciated, practice was not restricted to a single social class. Freed enslaved people could also be physicians and while one epitaph was to "Julia Pieris obstetrix"[2] and women are known to have specialised in breast disorders, they were not necessarily only treating women. Galen dedicated his work *Anatomy of the Uterus* to a midwife who had helped him. Pliny also noted that women had long occupied a pre-eminent position in folk medicine. Midwives were expected to be able to read medical treatises and were clearly well qualified for the time.[3] A midwife might also be called in for advice on wider health problems simply because they were known to the family.

Quality Control

Dioscorides sets the standards for identification and names of herbs, habitats, drying, storage, and quality of preparations. In Britain we may presume some quality control of herbs being applied where they are used under Roman administration. However, there is no evidence from this period to put forward.

Herb Energetics

Energetics of herbs are repeated and further revealed in Galen with hot, cold, dry, and moist in various combinations.

Archaeology

Funerary epitaphs occasionally supply useful information on professional status. Surgical instruments and stone collyrium identification stamps extend our knowledge on surgical techniques and ingredients in eye medicines. The remains of the Roman towns are evidence of the temples, forums, and baths typical of Roman life. Villas also give evidence of the Roman lifestyle with floor mosaics showing Greek myths and Christian symbols. Timber-framed shops in the grid pattern streets have revealed finds of spices and herbs on sale and possible bakers' shops in southern towns, such as Canterbury.[4] Wooden tablets from Vindolanda on Hadrian's wall offer us a detailed look at some aspects of army life during the early occupation.[5] Indications of changes in diet come from excavated latrines and other finds all over Britain.

Travel and Trade

An immensely useful modern book on the spice trade during the rule of ancient Rome offers not only maps of the extensive trade routes, but detail of various herbs, where they were sourced, and how they reached the centres of drug trade, such as Alexandria.[6] Sources of the spices, such as Arabia were made rich by trade of goods rare in the Mediterranean. The southern Arabian confederacy controlled the Incense road across the desert and sea routes at the end of the Red Sea corridor.[7]

From Britain, extensive travel was possible with the Roman presence encouraging imports and exports of Celtic produce, such as grain. With the Roman infrastructure travel was easier around the country and there is evidence of manufacture of goods and transporting them between forts in the written records on the Vindolanda tablets. The Celts already had roads, but the Romans made them straighter and stronger. Trade became very important in the later period. Roman control did not extend to Ireland and the Irish raided western Britain taking captives as enslaved people. Exactly when particular herbs, vegetables, and trees were first imported is difficult to assess as the remains, often in latrines or under collapsed buildings, may be associated in the archaeology with datable items from a later period.[8]

Introduction

In the Greek world we have seen that physicians were respected and could earn well, although they also had to be prepared sometimes to treat a patient with no monetary reward. The Roman view was different, if we believe some authors, we find them often looking down on physicians and there was a clear element of suspicion when physicians were of Greek origin, as many were. This influx of Greek physicians had been encouraged by Julius Caesar when he granted citizenship to foreign doctors willing to work in Rome.[9]

Dentistry was adopted from the Etruscan civilization and flourished. Numerous surgical instruments of bronze or copper alloy were found in the house of the surgeon in Pompeii, including a vascular clamp, a catheter, pincers, forceps, scalpels, and needles. In another house of a physician on the Via dell'Abbondanza, instruments for obstetrics and gynaecological examination, such as the specula uteris with screws and levers for dilation, were found.[10] The work of Celsus describes surgery in great detail.

Medicine before the Roman conquest of Greece in the first century BC, however, seems to have been largely dependent on prayer to the gods and magical ritual. We still find much superstitious ritual and belief in the works of Pliny. In following the development of medicine, I have, therefore, chosen to rely on the more discerning work of Celsus, who certainly spent a great deal of time and study on his research. With him, we are able to find out about diseases and how the herbs were used to treat them.

Before we look at the effects of the Roman invasion and settlement of Britain, it is helpful to understand the stage of knowledge and interpretation of Greek medicine being adopted in Rome in the first century. We will then consider how elements of this medicine might have been experienced in Britain with the Roman administration and those herb introductions which were made and whether they were included in foods or medicinal preparations.

References

1. Ralph Jackson, *Doctors and Diseases in the Roman Empire* (London: British Museum Press, 1998), 86.
2. Jackson, *Doctors and Diseases*, 97.
3. Ibid, 87.
4. Joan P. Alcock, *Food in Roman Britain* (Stroud: Tempus, 2001), 30.
5. Alan K. Bowman, *Life and Letters on the Roman Frontier* (London: The British Museum Press, 1998), 6.
6. J. Innes Miller, *The Spice Trade of the Roman Empire* (Oxford: Oxford University Press, 1998).
7. Miller, *The Spice Trade of the Roman Empire*, 13.
8. Alcock, *Food in Roman Britain*, 15.
9. Jackson, *Doctors and Diseases*, 56.
10. Annamaria Ciarallo and Ernesto De Carolis, (ed), *Pompeii Life in a Roman Town*, (Milan: Electa, 1999), (Antonio Cascino et al, Medicine and Surgery), 227.

CHAPTER 5

Dioscorides and Drugs | c70 AD

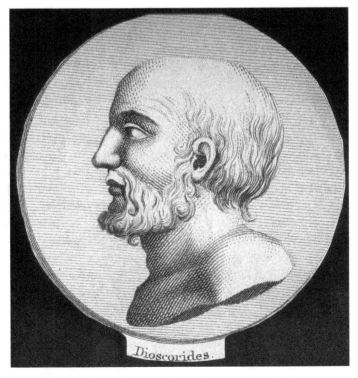

Portrait of Pedanius Dioscorides. Line Engraving.

The popularity and relevance of Dioscorides *De Re Medica* in a way outlasted the works of Galen, whose mistaken ideas on certain points of anatomy and, in particular, physiology, finally saw his downfall. Dioscorides' breadth of plant knowledge, recording their names, instruction on identification of plants and his standards of quality in drugs and preparations are still appreciated. We will see him constantly referred to as an authority over centuries, as it appears few texts were considered to be complete without reference to his work, all the way to Mrs Grieve in the twentieth century. His herbal has been part of the training of physicians, apothecaries, and botanists alike.

We know very little of the life of Dioscorides, in reality, only what can be deduced from his own words. Biographies were written for him after his death but are not considered dependable. They do, however, agree that he came from Anazarbus, a town then in the Roman province of Cilicia, which is now in Turkey. That he wrote in the same period as Pliny, around 70 AD, is taken partly from the authorities he quotes, and partly from Pliny not quoting him. Had Dioscorides' *De Re Medica* been available to him, Pliny would undoubtedly have used it. It is presumed from this that he wrote immediately before Pliny finished his works in 77 AD. It was a time when the Roman Empire was still expanding and trade and travel was extensive within it. The Mediterranean was an exciting place for anyone interested in plants.

He writes of his enquiries about herbs in the regions where they grew as he travelled from one area to another. In this chapter we will look at why he has been so revered by exploring his background so far as it is known, his text and its relevance to modern herbal medicine. The puzzle of why he put the herbs in the order he did, which is neither alphabetical nor according to any other obvious rule may just have been solved. This makes his work even more interesting and topical, in fact, ripe for fresh study.

Of all the accepted historical "authorities" on medicine, I relate most to Dioscorides and I have treasured my copy of his *De Materia Medica* for twenty-five years. This facsimile of the 1934 edition of one of the numerous translations, is perhaps the one I turn to most, as it was "Englished" by the botanist John Goodyer in 1655.[1] John Goodyer counted John Parkinson among his friends and sent material and corrections to another friend, Thomas Johnson for inclusion in his enlarged edition of Gerard's herbal. In his younger life, he had travelled the countryside identifying plants and was respected as "unquestionably the best botanist in England"[2] after the death of Parkinson in 1650.

Aged over sixty years, Goodyer became more sedentary and spent his time with his considerable library of books and manuscripts, all carefully dated with the day he bought them. These included the works of Dioscorides with many others and having already translated those of Theophrastus, he began diligently writing out the Greek text of the Materia Medica from his 1499 edition, making an interlinear translation. His attention to detail can be judged from the six volumes of his work in which he notes the dates he began and finished writing and the time he spent on revision of the 4540 pages.[3] In the 1630s John Goodyer moved to Petersfield and was a familiar historical figure to me, as I often walked past his home with its neat blue plaque on my way to work at the nearby hospital.

On his death, his books and papers were left to Magdalen College Oxford. This included his translation of *De Materia Medica*, which lay neglected among them for centuries. I have imagined him sitting in his study in that house writing out the whole of the text with an interlinear translation over the three years between the twenty seventh of April 1652 and the twenty ninth of August 1655. Reading his translation of Dioscorides, it is easy to see how a man with his deep interest in plants would have been fascinated by the detail there. Perhaps sometimes excited by what he read and sometimes puzzled. It must have been a work of love. The accuracy of the translation has been harshly judged in this century, but for me, it remains of value as a piece of history in itself.

There have been a number of other translations and over the many centuries no doubt some parts of Dioscorides treatise have been lost, and many slight and sometimes much larger changes have been made to his original work. This has increased the controversy about certain aspects of the book. Unlike many writers since, Dioscorides did not use the alphabetical order of the plant names for his classification. His ordering makes it difficult to find specific plants or other ingredients and so it is understandable that we are given the following information in the preface to my copy.

The illustrations in this edition are those drawn by a Byzantine artist in 512 AD at which time an alphabetical version was presented to Princess Juliana Alicia, daughter of Emperor Anicius Olybrius, Emperor of the Western Roman Empire. With no earlier manuscript available for comparison we do not know whether the illustrations were originally better or even different in some cases. It is quite possible some early ones had been lost by then. In the appendix to Goodyer's translation, there is the statement taken from a lecture by Professor Charles Daubney in 1857 that with the help of Mr Masters, lecturer on botany at St Georges Hospital, a survey had been conducted of the illustrations. Of those with the text now, ninety three are regarded as good depictions of the plant and thirty six fictitious, with the others placed somewhere in between.[4]

The Byzantine illustrator appears to have based his drawings on those in turn resembling the illustrations in the herbal by Crateuas, whose plant descriptions are sometimes quoted by Dioscorides himself. Certainly eleven illustrations have been credited by Singer with being identical with his. Crateuas was experienced as a rhizotomist—one who gathered roots and herbs and expressed the juices of plants for medicine. He wrote and illustrated his herbal for Mithridates VI Eupator (120–63 BC) King of Pontus in northern Anatolia, as his physician.

Pliny informs us that the king also wrote about plants and had the reputation of being expert in poisons and their antidotes. Agrimony takes its second name to honour him—*Agrimonia eupatoria*. This was a time when poison served in food or drink was a real threat to rulers and Eupator had taken tiny doses of poisons, gradually increasing them every day over years, for protection. The famed Mithridatium antidote to poisons and pestilence containing at least thirty-six ingredients was prepared for him by Crateuas. When defeat of his armies finally came and he administered poison to others and then himself to avoid capture, he did not die and was forced to use his sword. This story ensured he was remembered through many centuries to the end of the Middle Ages and the fame of Mithridatium meant it continued to be made. The recipe containing spices, gums, agaric, and castorei from the glands of the beaver was recorded by physicians and apothecaries from Scribonius Largus in Britain with the Roman legions in the first century AD to Culpeper.

After struggling to find what I was looking for in the *De Re Medica* on many occasions, I confess to sometimes wishing I had an alphabetical version of Dioscorides. Instead, the book keeps to the five main groupings of his classifications, aromatics, with oils, ointments, trees and shrubs in the first; living creatures, fats, dairy, cereals, pot and sharp herbs in the second; roots, thistles, and herbs for juice in the third; more herbs and roots in the fourth; and vines and wines, metallic ores, and earths in the fifth. Within these categories I have made a list of individual items and their page numbers. This I keep inside the front cover for convenience. Many scholars, and no doubt practising medics, have tried to work out why the materials are ordered as they are in this all-encompassing treatise.

In the preface, Dioscorides dedicates his work to his teacher Areius of Tarsus. He makes it plain by his remark, if John Goodyer has translated it correctly, that he is grateful for the affection shown to him by Areius as he does to all led by learning and especially those of the same profession. Since Areius was known to lecture on the use of drugs this appears to suggest Dioscorides as a physician. Some scholars have also wondered whether he might have traded in drugs or been a rhizomatomi or root cutter. However, his mastery of his subject covers acute observation not only of drug quality but of the effects on patients, and he emphasises personal observation as the source of his considerable knowledge. He is also keen to point out tests for detecting adulteration of various kinds.

In addition to teaching history to students of herbal medicine, I teach pharmacognosy and I present Dioscorides to my classes as the father of quality control. He gives us the perfect guide when he writes that the most important task is care in the gathering and storage of herbs. His first instruction covers observing the correct maturity of the plant. Dry weather is noted as most important on the day of gathering, but he also mentions the weather on the preceding days. It can be observed particularly with mucilage rich herbs, such as marshmallow, that they dry best if there has been dry weather for two days, but we now know also that weather prior to gathering has a wider effect on certain constituents. For instance, the anthocyanin content of bilberries (*Vaccinium myrtillus*), which are important to the antioxidant properties, show not just seasonal and geographical variations from different areas of growth, but are affected by light intensity and temperature.[5]

Dioscorides takes into account the locality, giving different strengths to those herbs growing where they are not open to the wind and pointing out that in some countries the same plant may ripen earlier or keep its leaves longer. Leaf shape may also differ. This knowledge as he tells us has come from his careful observations and questioning of local inhabitants as he has travelled about.

One short phrase, as he describes his travelling life, is open to more than one translation and could refer to a career as a physician in the Roman legions. Several writers have taken it to confirm that his experience was gained in this way. Others believe that whereas he may have been in the army his main journeys were as a civilian, since it was usual at the time for physicians to be peripatetic, going from one city to another. Riddle points out that many of the places he mentions in relation to the herbs alongside what appear to be personally observed comments were centres of trade in drugs, rather than where a legion would have been stationed.[6] The area covered by those countries mentioned alongside herbs is almost as wide as the Roman Empire with Syria, Libya, Egypt, and Macedonia.

Recognition of the correct herb when gathering is paramount, and for those aspiring to be skilful as herbalists, he advises that they need to observe the plant at all stages of growth, from emerging seedling to maturity. Dioscorides writes of mistakes made by those who have confused one plant for another because they have never seen the plant at that season. This remark could well be more pertinent to root gatherers than a physician, but as was the case with Crateaus, it was possible to be both. He also makes it clear in his preface and by including subjects such as the great variety of wines listed, that this work is written for a wider readership.

On the right stage of maturity of the part of the plant to be gathered, he again gives detail. With seeds he advises, "when they begin to be dry, and before they fall out".[7] Timing on seeds is critical as some, especially certain *Umbelliferae* members are likely to be infested with insect eggs if left too long. Dioscorides directs that if roots have earth stuck to them this needs to be washed away before drying, juicing, or peeling away the bark. Drying is carried out in the shade with a linen thread passed through them to hang root pieces. Reference is made to roots bought ready-dried, and sensory markers, of touch, taste and smell are described to identify the best quality roots in individual cases.

Storage is equally important. For moist medicines, wood is given at the end of a list of other materials, with silver, glass, horn, and earthenware coming first. One wonders exactly what is meant by 'moist medicines'. Certainly, juices are included as at the end of the entry on wild lettuce in Dioscorides given as *Lactuca scariola*, he notes that the isolated milky juice is stored in new earthen vessels.[8] I have wondered whether it could include ointments. Perhaps not, since he stores fats in tin.

It is not surprising, given his intimate knowledge of trees, that when Dioscorides mentions wooden boxes, he names two specific woods for storing very different items. These are flowers and moist medicines. Lime is chosen for storing delicate flowers. Lime wood is soft to carve and light in weight, it does not have a strong

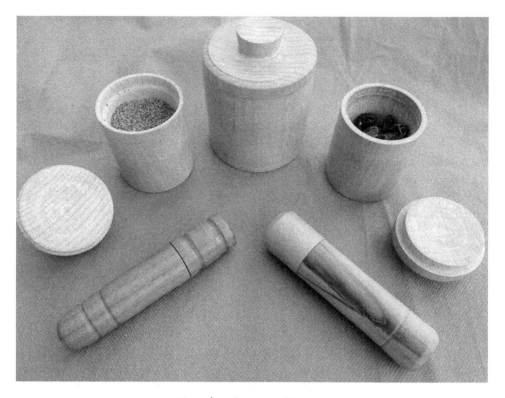

Wooden Ointment Boxes.

scent or character to impart to easily spoilt flowers. Then box wood is specified. This is a wood of very different character to the lime. Boxwood is heavy and solid, it has been used for pestles, however the name is presumed to have come from the frequent use in the Roman period and beyond for boxes to contain jewels, toiletries, or drugs. They were turned on a bow lathe and some similarly made have been found at Vindolanda used as needle cases with tight fitting lids.[9]

After my own positive experience using wooden boxes for storing all parts of dried herbs over long periods, as well as ointments and the solid jelly of quince membrillo, which even today is properly stored and exported in wooden boxes; I would like to see more experimental research before discounting wood as a proper storage medium.

With preparations, Dioscorides sets out his method and then with some, such as castor oil he gives the alternative method followed by the Egyptians, commenting they can do this because they have a plentiful supply. The books are so rich in information I would just like to pick out a few entries which contain ideas, herbs, or recipes we will see given importance and repeated across the centuries to show the huge influence Dioscorides' work has.

Reading the headings within the books, it is almost as if Dioscorides is working his way along shelves in his dispensary beginning with aromatics. Under resins in Book I, he writes of the mastic tree as "a knowne tree".[10] This is a term that appears often. He is able to remark that all parts of the tree are of equal force and describes soaking the leaves in water until it has the consistency of honey.

If I had not seen the tree and split a leaf to be rewarded by the intense citrus and pine fragrance of the oil, quite as powerful as the resin I tasted from harvesting from the trunk, I might not believe in the honey consistency. Chios would surely have been a place he visited for even then, as now it was the centre of excellence for mastic production. The uses of the resin for treating coughs and the stomach, in cosmetics and especially for dental use, sweetening the breath and strengthening gums is exactly the same. His description of the clear white resin shows his recognition of the best quality. I found it interesting that he records mastic, which has always been prized as it all comes from a very small area, as being adulterated with the more plentiful frankincense.

In the section on trees, he is less complimentary about the fruit of the walnut, accusing them of hurting the stomach and bringing on headaches, but good as an emetic on an empty stomach. Here the role of walnuts is recommended in antidotes to various poisons when they are eaten with figs and rue. This same prescription turns up as long as over a thousand years later. He does not give a botanical description of the walnut, presuming that of course everyone knows what it looks like. He also uses it to liken the forms of lesser-known plants to.

The use of raw egg white as a cooling agent for burns[11] and inflammations continues through history and is particularly useful, as it would be sterile if applied directly from the shell. Burns are also eased using powdered old leather, which clearly has the benefit of the tannins it would contain. Leather is used in later times also to apply plasters and hold them in place.

Among the pot herbs are several together that would be regarded as cooling, with three types of sow thistle and endive, described as a good refrigerant.[12] Cucumber, melon, pompion, lettuce, and wild lettuce fall into the same category. Shortly afterwards violently heating rocket, the seed of which is suggested as an alternative to mustard, is followed by basil, another hot herb.[13] Of interest, in that in my experience today it is viewed simply as a salad vegetable, we have the radish.

In interpreting recipes in later periods, I have preferred the Spanish black radish as this is still used in Eastern Europe for treating chesty coughs. Here, Dioscorides warns that radishes should be eaten after food in order not to interfere with concoction (digestion). He used it medicinally to treat a long-standing cough and adds more preparations, such as with oxymel (honey and water), smeared on or taken with vinegar or simply with honey. Each of these forms was for different conditions from black eyes and gangrene when applied, to encouraging menstruation and urination, or treating the spleen with internal medicine.

Ribwort and greater plantains have a long entry and as we pass on through history this emphasis on their usefulness will be ever present for over a thousand years.[14] Here botanical detail is given to separate the lesser from the greater form clearly for the reader. The greater being the broad leaved and more recommended for use. The leaves are described as having a binding quality for stopping blood and healing ulcers, dog bites, and inflammations. Taken internally the list of actions of the herb covers everything from epilepsy to asthma and dropsy to dysentery. The seeds are taken in wine for spitting blood and a drink made for those with consumption—tuberculosis of the lungs. The root can be chewed for toothache, or a mouthwash made by soaking the root. Dioscorides quotes the Magi (followers of Zoroaster, generally regarded as originally from Persia), Egyptians, Spaniards, French, Africans, and Syrians on plantain, and you might be tempted to think the range of treatments exaggerated, until you read a modern evaluation of constituents and actions.

Greater plantain reaches a zenith of appreciation in the Anglo-Saxon period and we will appreciate more of the properties in later chapters. It is interesting that in Goodyer's translation Dioscorides repeats a recipe for the herb with calaminth and honey for curing paralysis. He opens his comment with the words "The Syrians say",[15] which going by his sparse entries on preparations means that he sees what follows as magical and far-fetched, and implies he does not believe it will work. However at the end he writes "… but take this as a secret, for it is most true and according to experience".[16]

Betony, a herb we have noted as adopted from the Celts by the Romans, we find under wines. The whole, seeding plant is soaked in water for seven months, before being decanted into another vessel as the wine he calls "Psychotrophon". [17] Dioscorides specifies it is not given where there is fever, but is good for many ills, which he does not stipulate, but we learn from observing the entries that he gives only that information he thinks important. The wines section is not directed at physicians, but perhaps those caring for family members, therefore it is enough to say the wine will be helpful. We will meet the herb again in Celsus.

Dioscorides refers not to the stinging nettle *Urtica dioica*, common in Britain, but the nettles of his experience, the small *Urtica urens* and *Urtica pilulifera* and he describes one as wilder and having darker leaves than the other. There is no mention of the sting. Both are wound herbs applied not only to stop bleeding, as with a nosebleed, in the same way we find stinging nettle used in Britain, but to treat gangrene and malignant ulcers. He gives nettle expectorant and digestive qualities, as well as encouraging menstrual flow.[18] *Urtica urens* is the annual nettle with male and female on the same plant, brought to Britain by the Romans.

Four more herbs of interest throughout our history are elecampane ginger liquorice, and henbane Elecampane, supposedly named for Helen of Troy, Dioscorides tells us in a concise paragraph, has a shallow root that is sharp to taste. Elecampane root certainly has a powerfully hot taste with sharpness to it.

He recommends a drink of elecampane against serpents' poison, a common recommendation at this time, which we find repeated in England later, where it is barely of relevance. He also mentions the hairs for the same use.[19] The underside of elecampane leaves is soft and hairy, as is the case with several anti-cough herbs. In the past, elecampane was eaten and it is a valuable herb for the digestion, as a bitter tonic and to encourage the blood supply for the stomach wall.

The use of elecampane for digestion, although not mentioned by Dioscorides, was certainly known already. Columella's important book on husbandry *De Re Rustica*, written in the first century near Rome, gives three recipes for pickling elecampane root. My preference is to harvest the root in October as he instructs, but I use a later recipe to make extremely effective cough sweets. In two pickles, the dried, sliced root is put with wild marjoram firstly into vinegar, and then honeywine. One variation of Columella's third recipe would be interesting to try as a treatment for the stomach. He writes, "Some after they have pickled the elecampane" (in brine), "dry it, and mix it with bruised quinces, which they have boiled before in honey, or in must, (freshly crushed grape juice for wine-making, still containing the skins), sodden into one third; and so pour raisin wine, or must, sodden in to one third, upon them; and, when they have put the lid upon the vessel, cover it with leather".[20]

Returning to Dioscorides another root we will be following is ginger. Dioscorides writes that the plant grows in Troglodyticall Arabia, which is on the west coast of the Red Sea. He notes the roots have a hot taste and smell sweet, but go rotten quickly and so are imported in earthen jars, already as a preserve. He compares the strength of ginger to that of pepper, informing us that the root is included in antidotes and is a warming digestive for the stomach.[21]

Our third chosen root is liquorice, next to the entry for "Glukoriza,"[22] Goodyer has noted that the illustration does not resemble liquorice. The description, however, compares the leaves to the Lentisk, which is of the same pea family as liquorice, and says the plant has little cods with seeds like lentils. Likening the flowers to the hyacinth, however, would not have occurred to me. The properties of liquorice for quenching thirst, and being chewed to comfort the stomach, kidneys, and liver will become familiar from later history. I am not sure how to interpret liquorice being good for the sharpness of the arteries, but it certainly can have an effect on blood pressure. The root and the juice of the root are already established as the parts to be used.

The fourth herb of considerable interest is henbane. Dioscorides devotes over a page of detail to the three different forms of henbane recognised, (*Hyoscyamus niger*, *H. albus*, and *H. aureus*). He gives us one with a purple flower and one with yellowish flowers. These two he classes as too strong in causing "frenzies, & of sleep".[23]

The last form with white flowers and seeds he recommends as the most gentle and suitable. From the fresh seed and other parts of the plant, juice is extracted and he gives us the detail that it is dried in the hot sun, but will only keep for a year.

This is made into Collyries (salves) and trochisci, a Greek term referring to emollient plasters with a liquid ingredient, or pastils—dry applications for pain relief. The pains specified are varied, from ear-ache to inflammations in any part of the body, from the eyes to the feet.

The seed is listed as helpful for coughs, catarrhs, gouts, stopping bleeding, including reducing menorrhagia, inflamed genitals, and soothing swollen breasts after childbirth. In short, whether in salves, troches, or mixed into cataplasms (plasters), henbane was looked to for dependable pain relief. Sometimes it was simply the fresh leaves that were smeared on and at others henbane might be mixed with polenta to apply. There is a final warning that eating the leaves will disturb the sense, indicating for the first time that henbane is a hypnotic drug, affecting the mind. The last use is the root sodden in vinegar for toothache.

Use of henbane will continue through time, either alone, or, as is often the case together with other narcotic herbs such as white poppy and mandrake, either for powerful pain relief or, taking their properties further, as anaesthetics for operations. It will still be sufficiently important for supplies to be of concern in the first World War.

Dioscorides does not confine himself to including herbs and the list of animal parts used in medicine is particularly varied. Honey, milk from different animals and eggs are the more innocent but not many patients today would be happy to drink dried locusts in wine, much less swallow bed bugs with their food. Animal parts include the lungs of a fox and liver of a goat. Having given a highly knowledgeable account of the minerals used in medicine, which has been judged to rank him as an expert on the subject, Dioscorides lists the medicinal earths. This is an interesting subject that, together with preparation of sea sponges for inserting into wounds and ulcers to dry them, we will return to when we look at the period of the apothecary shop in later times. He recommends whitening them under the moon, moistened with sea water, or burning them for more astringency in stopping bleeding.[24] Burnt sponge was a treatment in the eighteenth century for scrofula.

We have examined some of the range and variety of materials in this important herbal. There are of course many more items of interest to be found, including the medicinal properties of fats, a subject that will be raised later in history. We have considered a number of selected herbs and points of interest to show the depth of useful knowledge which may be called on, even today. Before we leave Dioscorides it is needful to return to his preface and the question of the ordering of the herbs and other items. He states that his reason for writing is to record his personal practical experience, offering the evidence of his own eyes to support his statements, while others largely copied the work of earlier writers. He describes his diligent searching for the truth about plants and states he will make a new arrangement "… and also to describe the kinds and forces of every one of them".[25]

Just as it has been with Hippocrates and Galen, Dioscorides' work has produced considerable controversy. Bearing in mind the hazards of translation, politics, and not being able to put our thinking into the minds of people in the past, there is a new interpretation and hypothesis from John Riddle.

His painstaking work in identifying a possible solution has revealed that Dioscorides placed plants and other items next to each other, sometimes just two together, sometimes in larger groups according to their precise physiological effects on the patient. Certainly, detailed observation Dioscorides excelled in, and Riddle supports his discovery with extensive evidence from all five books. The identification of these effects with metallic ores containing sodium, calcium, sulphur, and so on in book five is especially impressive. This is an exceptional study.[26]

References

1. Robert T. Gunther, (ed), *Dioscorides Greek Herbal*, (London: Hafner, 1968), title page.
2. Robert T. Gunther, *Early British Botanists* (Oxford: University Press, 1922), 82.
3. Gunther, *Early British Botanists*, 84–85.
4. Gunther, *Dioscorides Greek Herbal*, Appendix.
5. Yan Zhang, (ed), *Pharmacognosy* (Virginia: Cognella Academic Publishing, 2021), 177.
6. John M. Riddle, *Dioscorides on Pharmacy and Medicine* (Texas: University of Texas Press, 2011).
7. Gunther, *Dioscorides Greek Herbal*, 4.
8. Ibid, 177.
9. Robin Wood, *The Wooden Bowl*, (Ammanford: Stobart Davies Ltd., 2005), 58.
10. Gunther, *Dioscorides Greek Herbal*, 48.
11. Gunther, *Dioscorides Greek Herbal*, 104.
12. Ibid, 148.
13. Ibid, 171–182.
14. Ibid, 165.
15. Ibid, 166.
16. Ibid, 166.
17. Ibid, 618.
18. Ibid, 491.
19. Ibid, 293.
20. Julius Moderatus Columella, *Of Husbandry in Twelve Books* (London: A. Millar, 1745), 552.
21. Gunther, *Dioscorides Greek Herbal*, 200.
22. Ibid, 238.
23. Ibid, 464–5.
24. Ibid, 649.
25. Ibid, 2.
26. Riddle, *Dioscorides on Pharmacy and Medicine*.

CHAPTER 6

Roman Medicine in Celsus

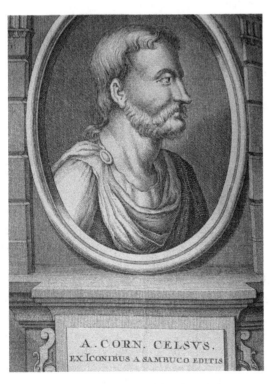

Portrait of Cornelius Celsus, *Celsi de Medicina*, 1746.

It was a considerable loss to the appreciation of Roman medicine that while the work of Pliny became well known and his folk cures, often involving superstition and magic, were widely available, the scholarly books on medicine by Celsus were almost lost in obscurity for centuries. It is commonly known that Pliny wrote on many subjects in an encyclopaedic way. We have no factual evidence of his personal life except that Celsus also wrote on a range of subjects, but his work on medicine alone survives. It is presumed to have been written in the second or third decades of the first century. His *De Medicina* does not appear to have been available to the Arabic writers on medicine.

As he began writing his first book on medicine Celsus compared the role of agriculture in producing nourishment to the art of medicine in promising health to sick patients.[1] This reference to agriculture links to his previous work, for Quintilian, seen as an expert on education and rhetoric after writing his *Institutio oratoria*, writes that Celsus wrote on many other subjects—agriculture, philosophy, rhetoric, military art, and jurisprudence.[2] Quintillian refers to the work of Celsus disparagingly as mediocre. He did not always follow popular opinion in his judgments. In contrast James Grieve, who made the first translation of Celsus into English in the eighteenth century, writes that in his own time Celsus was admired for the quality of his writing, and describes it as elegant.

If we think back to his history of the development of Greek medicine and the three divisions of regimen and dietetics—foods to build strength, herbal medicaments, and surgery—we find all three are well represented in the books of *De Medicina*. The study necessary to bring together this body of concentrated information is remarkable and it is accepted as one of the most important medical works of the period. Hence, I have included the work of Celsus to represent Roman medicine and omitted Pliny who is a lighter read for more general interest.

At the end of his history Celsus states, "I am of opinion that the Art of Medicine ought to be rational, but to draw instruction from evident causes, all obscure ones being rejected from the practice of the Art, although not from the practitioner's study".[3]

There has been discussion as to whether Celsus was a physician or not. The range and depth of instruction in his books on medicine and surgery has convinced some readers that he has been a practitioner. He makes an interesting comment that before taking the pulse of a patient it may be helpful to talk quietly with them for a few minutes, as the presence of the physician can increase the rate—this suggests experience. He later notes that the pulse can be deceptive as it is altered by sex, age, constitution, fever, bathing, and exercise.[4]

His detail on diet, prescriptions and even on surgery is precise. On the other hand the number of subjects he is recorded as writing about suggests he has simply compiled this encyclopaedia, if it can be called that, from the works of others, acting as an editor. In either case his frequent use of the aphorisms of Hippocrates marks the Corpus as a major source of his information. Given that the aphorisms would surely have been a widely known source of inspiration for practitioners, perhaps this is hardly surprising. At the start he writes that he will have no hesitation in repeating the advice of former authorities, such as Hippocrates, as they were better at prognosis. Prognosis here means being able to predict likely causes of illness before it happens, and so be able to give advice on avoiding disease.

Roman medicine in the view of Celsus entirely adopted the Greek ideals of health and preventive medicine. The most important initial advice is therefore not on treating a disease, but is directed to a healthy man. The regimen for health concerns the same essential factors which we will note in passing being recommended century after century. How to remain healthy has been, and remains, the most consistent message to the general population. It is also the most persistently ignored by the majority.

There is guidance for the strong person and the comment that many of those who are weak reside in towns—weakness is especially noticed in those who study. The weak require far more instruction. This includes their diet, exercises, movement of bowels, bathing, sleep, and every aspect of lifestyle and possible regimen such as rubbing, (massage), vomits, or purging. Celsus also, as one might expect, relates warnings and changes in lifestyle to the seasons of the year. A life with a variety of exercise and wholesome food, lived at least partly in the countryside with healthy air, and planning daily routine in tune with the seasons is recommended in a comprehensive guide.

If we compare the opinions of Celsus with those expressed in the Hippocratic Corpus we find the approach is different. The importance of fasting for instance is passed over with brief attention. Celsus puts all foods into one of three classes according to the strength of nourishment offered. Centuries earlier, the Hippocratic text had begun by warning not to make generalisations based on tastes or power and then immediately considered individual foods. In some respects, for instance on the strength of nourishment of beef and wheat being strongest,[5] they agree, but they differ on other matters.[6] After listing physiological effects of foods, Celsus lists those of good juice and then those of bad juice. There is no comparable list in Hippocrates and they seem to have different opinions on garlic and barley. Celsus puts garlic in the bad juice list while in the Corpus garlic is regarded as warming, although there is the remark that it is bad for the eyes.[6] Hippocrates pays a good deal of attention to barley, in Regimen II XL and XLI.[7] Celsus includes bread made from barley as alien to the stomach.[8] Upholding the belief in treating every patient individually, he states that the quality of the food should be administered according to the patient's strength, with weak patients receiving light foods. The quantity of food given in this case should also be in accordance, meaning a small amount.[9]

The detail is impressive and reflects what we are only just coming to appreciate today in that the life an animal leads can affect the quality of the meat when it is killed. Whether an animal was wild or tamed, and whether fish came from the sea or river water mattered. Eggs, milk, and cheese (as a milk product), were all seen as giving the strongest nourishment along with grain and meat because they were providing foods for young close to birth. This is followed by medicinal effects from foods, such as inducing sleep, action on the bowels, acting as diuretics and even being applied as poultices.

Regarding Regimen observances for protection when pestilence strikes is another theme that we will find repeated through history, and one we have just formulated for ourselves in recent times with the pandemic. Historically, certain cleansing practices have been very pertinent and the first recommendation of leaving the area to take a voyage might certainly avoid catching the infection. Beyond that the bath is to be avoided as well as walking barefoot, becoming overtired, sweating, and indigestion. Eating only once a day and drinking one day water, then the next wine, is given precedence.[10]

In talking about pestilence, autumn is identified as the most likely time of year for this to appear and naturally the wind direction that has brought disease is viewed as important. Each individual season is seen in terms of the illness it may encourage in those who are not careful of their health. Knowing what to look out for may be helpful and he also lists such warnings as the north wind irritating the throat, causing coughs.

Celsus cautions that not only the weather on the day the disease begins is relevant, but that of the preceding days. Many symptom patterns and what they portend as far as the prognosis is concerned show real depth of observations. For instance, there is also guidance on early symptoms that should cause concern, and he adds that if the patient has had these symptoms before, enquiry should be made as to what followed. This is a useful practice today.

Diseases of the mind affecting behaviour in various ways are described and thoughtful treatments prescribed. Celsus writes about relieving empty fears with steady reassurances, removing melancholy thoughts with music, and awakening the patient's interest in books. On insanity he disagrees with Asclepiades that patients should always be kept in the light as he thinks that with some who are fettered so as not to harm themselves, they might be calmed by darkness.[11] In all, he recommends tailoring approaches to the individual patient.

Asclepiades, who died in the previous century to Celsus opposed humoral doctrine, following instead theory derived from Democritus and the atomists. Taking a more naturopathic view on treatments, including massage and diet, he treated tissue states seen as relaxed or constricted in disease. He believed that nearly all drugs "harm the stomach and contain bad juices".[12] However, Celsus notes that there are times for use of diet and times when medicaments are necessary. When chronic diseases affect the body as a whole, he points out that chronic disease gives time to adjust remedies if necessary, as the same remedies do not suit all patients.

Roman historians suggest a familiar belief that still survives to this day that the more exotic and difficult a herb is to come by the more effective it will be. Herbs growing by the garden gate have never had the same attraction to the masses as those from another country. As such, venerated herbs were imported, the seplasarii, dealers in unguents and drugs who sold them to physicians, kept them in their shops in the same way as apothecaries in later centuries and so their role of dispensing for physicians was born. In Pliny's opinion, the seplasiarii were often adulterating their medicines and selling drugs to physicians when they were past their useful date.[13] Dioscorides too gives many tests for possible adulteration, clearly with just cause. This is a problem that accompanies the herb trade throughout history and we will return to quality control many times.

Through this book we will be looking at and comparing herbal treatments for specific conditions. This will allow us to assess which herbs are unchanging and popular in their main use. While we are following selected herbs in their wider historical applications, we may also consider the proven worth in traditional use of a greater number. I have chosen certain simple conditions that occur in daily life even to otherwise healthy people. With the range of prescriptions in *De Medicina*, Celsus has provided us with plentiful material on Roman use. Some of these can be checked against those in the Compendium written by Scribonius Largus, a surgeon with the Roman legions in Britain in the first century.

The chosen conditions are: eye inflammation, coughs, toothache, headache, burns, joint pain, boils, and fevers. Of course, coughs, fevers, eye inflammation and headache can also be symptoms relating to more serious conditions. The eyes seem to have been very problematic in this period, particularly inflammation in ophthalmia and many treatments are suggested. Evidence comes also from stone collyrium stamps bearing names and ingredients of these applications.

Treatments

Eye Conditions—Use saffron, myrrh, and poppy tears most often. Some ointments include long pepper, or white pepper, and acacia gum along with zinc oxide and other minerals. An example quoted is of Indian nard, poppy tears, gum, saffron, and fresh rose leaves (petals) in mild wine.[14]

Ophthalmia in all its forms and range of symptoms might initially be addressed through diet, blood-letting, complete rest, and clysters. A clyster consists of a pouch possibly made from the bladder of an animal, filled with a fluid that was then directed into an orifice through a metal tube when the pouch was squeezed. They were used for injecting enemas and irrigating parts of the body. Various diseases of the eyes are listed. Cataract was treated surgically when it had been established for some time. A regimen to make the phlegm thin and anointing the eyes with acrid medicaments are suggested before the cataract has reached the stage necessary for surgery.[15]

Coughs—Horehound, plantain juice garlic, hyssop, myrrh, squill, poppy tears or pepper. Eating moist, cooked figs is also recommended. Often a bland diet of mallows, and nettle-tops, followed by garlic in milk may be suggested.

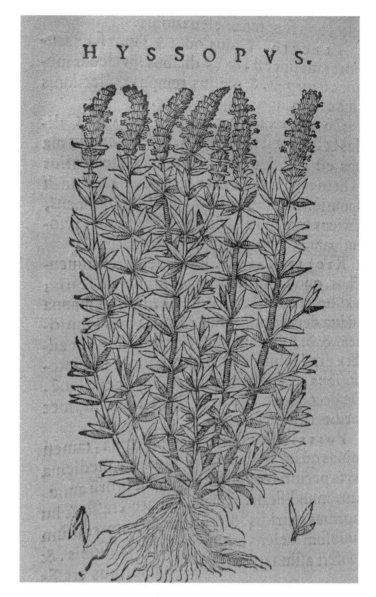

Hyssop, *Opera de Medicamentorum*, Mesue.

Both minor, dry coughs and more serious conditions are treated. For a dry cough, hyssop is to be taken every other day.[16] The accompanying exercise of running while holding your breath has thankfully been abandoned. Juice of horehound is also given if the cough is very troublesome. This would be incredibly bitter. Alternatives are squill in vinegar and bruised garlic in wine.[17] In his instructions for treating phthisis (chronic pulmonary TB), he writes of this as a dangerous malady that he believes starts in the head and drips down into the lungs which become ulcerated.

Celsus describes the cough and instructs to put the patient's sputum on the fire when the resulting smell will confirm the diagnosis (according to Hippocrates, indicating destruction of bronchioles, as they contain sulphur). If the patient"s strength allows he recommends a long sea voyage, if not, then rocking on board ship without going far. The patient should rest and sleep more, be given ewe's or goat's milk, take moderate exercise, avoid bathing, and keep warmly wrapped. Following dietary recommendations, the unfortunate patient endures application of hot cautery irons in four areas of the throat and chest to set up ulceration, which is kept open all the while the patient is coughing. Plantain juice is given alone, or with horehound juice cooked with honey.[18]

Toothache—Described as "the greatest of torments"[19], herbs used include cinquefoil, henbane root, poppy, and mandrake root, which are powerful pain killers. Among many herbs suggested, we find astringent pomegranate rind, oak-galls, and pine bark. Also used are the anodyne herbs of saffron, myrrh, and chamomile. To extract a tooth, either a peppercorn or ivy berry with the outer coat removed is inserted into the cavity, causing the tooth to split and fall out in pieces.[20]

Headaches—There are many causes that attract different approaches accordingly. Sneezing, bleeding and cupping the temples, or shaving and bathing the head are some. For headache with fever, rose oil mixed with vinegar is applied, or bread soaked in a poppy head decoction. Snuff of thyme, or dill, is also suggested.[21]

Burns—Treated with lily, hound's tongue, or beet leaves. These are first boiled in wine or oil. Serious burns were treated in different stages, firstly checking blisters and roughening the skin before soothing and healing. Lentil meal with honey or myrrh with wine might begin the process with greasy yolk of egg sometimes following.[22]

Joint Pain—May be treated with dried fig and catmint black bryony berry, without the seeds, pennyroyal or pounded henbane and nettle seeds in fat rubbed on and fomented with sulphur. Joint pain, especially that of the hip, would be first fomented with bags of hot water and salt, or perhaps a leather bottle filled with hot oil then a plaster, sometimes of caper bark and fig applied. The most effective application according to Celsus, however, was one of pounded elecampane root boiled in dry wine.[23] For severe joint pain, the rind of poppy heads was boiled in wine and then made into a salve with rose oil and wax.[24] The most drastic treatment mentioned was hot cautery irons covered in salt that dripped onto the affected sinews.

Boils—Often considered to treat themselves by bursting. The specific treatment was galbanum,[25] a gum which was tapped from *Ferula galbaniflua*, also known as all-heal.[26] For boils slow to burst, we find sulphur, soda, myrrh, frankincense soot (from burning the resin), ammoniac salt, and wax.

Fevers—Given a great deal of attention through regimen—diet, bathing, vomits, etc. Individual treatments to suit the patient and individual symptoms are paramount. A good deal of attention is paid to all aspects of fevers, with special notice of those produced by pestilence.[27] When writing of the necessity sometimes to give food to a feverish patient, he gives the practices of other physicians, then writes, "For these reasons I delay until midnight".[28] This comment underlines the need for the physician of a seriously ill patient to be with him, sometimes through the night in order to judge the right moment for treatment of some kind. This and other examples, confirm that a physician could not have been caring for many patients at once.

Commenting on hemi-tertian fevers he writes, "Many die suddenly from error one way or the other on the part of the practitioner".[29] A reminder that treatments such as vomits, purges, and clysters were to be used with discretion according to the condition of the patient. Applications using clysters ranged from the more gentle enemas with fenugreek and mallow to the more drastic with soda. Black hellebore root was commonly used over many centuries for purging the body and in this era white hellebore root was given for chronic and violent disease when there was no fever. Both require warnings on how they are used.

The main body of prescriptions are in Books V and VI, beginning with an alphabetical list of ingredients that runs from southernwood, which grew in the Mediterranean, through to ginger which was recorded by Dioscorides as growing plentifully in Trogodyticall Arabia on the west coast of the Red Sea.[30] He recommends it for digestion and comments it is mixed with antidotes. The list ends with the name of a salve, Zmilion.

There is also a useful list of surgical instruments and appliances used in treatment, including items such as woollen bandages, ear syringes, and splints. Celsus classifies the full list of medicaments we have seen in Dioscorides, as to their action on the body from stopping bleeding to caustics. Those to suppress bleeding include acacia, frankincense, and iron and copper scales. To agglutinate the wound he gives gums, linseed, white of egg, and if the wound is slight, cobwebs. Alum or quince oil are listed amongst anti-inflammatories, while the list of cleansers is very long, beginning with verdigris- and ending with bitter vetch.[31]

Having set out these lists he explains the mixtures of these he gives is to be restricted to the best known. He writes of emollients that these are made chiefly from flower essences or their shoots, while plasters and pastils contain certain metallic materials. A plaster always contains a liquid ingredient, is soft and applied over intact skin. Pastils are entirely made of dry ingredients laboriously made fine in order not to irritate the wound. In a dried plaster vinegar or some other fat-free liquid was used to bring the powders together. As an example of an emollient unusually being used for cooling rather than heating to disperse or extract diseased matter, he gives a cupful of oak-galls, with carefully specified amounts of coriander seed, hemlock, dried poppy-tears, gum, and washed cerate.[32]

His details of mixtures and compositions include multiple recipes, each specifying quantities of their ingredients. Many are sourced from Greek medicine with names given of those who first invented them, such as the black plaster of Diogenes, and the compound of Heras. We also find the compound of Judaeus, a recipe said to have been prepared by Zopyrus for King Ptolemy.[33] Additionally, the famous Antidote of Mithridates, which almost defies belief in its complexity of thirty-six to fifty-seven ingredients according to different sources but was still being made, as we will see, over 1600 years later. The king of that name had already become a legend at this period for taking a small dose of the mixture every day as protection from possible attempts to poison him.

Having discussed dietetics and medicaments, we come lastly to the third category of medicine, *surgery*. It is clear that the source of knowledge on surgery was most certainly the Hippocratic corpus, as so many passages are similar. All of the detail is there, preparation of the patient beforehand, exact positioning of the patient with restraint, possible complications and aftercare in minute detail. Parts of them so graphically described as to be painful to read. He describes operations for removing stones from the bladder in male and female patients, removing a dead foetus, varicose veins, and small tumours. On amputation in the cases of gangrene, Celsus writes that patients often die under the operation, but makes the pragmatic comment that safety does not matter since it is the only remedy.[34]

We have now reviewed the whole of Roman medicine through the writings of Celsus, taking in along the way matters of ongoing concern, such as a detailed consultation with the patient, a healthy regimen or lifestyle, longevity, avoiding catching pestilence, quality control of herbs and drugs, and our survey of herbs treating specific conditions. Throughout his writing Celsus shows the typical Roman sense of order and flair for recording, with attention to detail, which we see exhibited in the army records available to us from the Vindolanda tablets recovered in Britain. Perhaps the disparaging comments by Quintillian, which we noted at the beginning of this chapter refer to him acting more as an editor, which he definitely and understandably was on the medicaments, rather than adding any new philosophy of his own. Certainly the number of parallels with Hippocratic texts supports this. Nevertheless, his writing was an important source on the subject of medicine to those who had access to it in the following centuries. With use and advice from several sources, we have to acknowledge that this was a re-working of the texts with more re-workings to come.

References

1. W.G. Spencer, (trans), *Celsus de Medicina*, Vol. I. Books I–IV. (Loeb Classical Library. 1971), 3.
2. Spencer, *Celsus de Medicina*, Books I–IV. Introduction VII.
3. Ibid, Books I–IV. Prooemium 41, 72–75.
4. Ibid, Book III. Chapter 6. Verses 5–7, 253–255.
5. Ibid, Book II. Chapters 17–19, 191–201.
6. Ibid. Book II. Chapter 21, 203.

7. W.H.S. Jones, (trans), Hippocrates, Vol. IV (London: Harvard University Press, 1st published 1931) Regimen II Chapters XL and XLI. 307–311.
8. Spencer, *Celsus de Medicina*, Vol. I. Books I–IV. 25, 205.
9. Spencer, *Celsus de Medicina*, Vol. II. Chapter 18, 199.
10. Ibid, Book 1. Chapter 9, Verses 5–10, 79.
11. Ibid, Book III. Chapter 18, 291.
12. Spencer, *Celsus de Medicina*, Vol. II. Books V–VI. Book V, 3.
13. C.J.S. Thompson, *The Mystery and Art of the Apothecary*, (Philadelphia: J.B. Lippincott Co., 1929), 25.
14. Spencer, *Celsus de Medicina*, Vol. II. Books V–VI. Book VI. Chapter 6, Verse 9, 201.
15. Ibid, Book VI. Chapter 6, Verses 34–36, 223.
16. Spencer, *Celsus de Medicina*, Vol. I. Books I–IV. Book IV. Chapter 9, Verse 10, 389.
17. Ibid, Book IV. Chapter 10, Verse 10, 391.
18. Spencer, *Celsus de Medicina*, Vol. II. Books I–IV. Book III. Chapter 22, 331–333.
19. Spencer *Celsus de Medicina*, Vol. II. Books V–VI. Book VI. Chapter 8, Verse 9, 247.
20. Ibid, Book VI. Chapter 9, Verse 10, 251.
21. Spencer, *Celsus de Medicina*, Vol. II. Books I–IV. Book III. Chapter 9, Verse 10, 271.
22. Spencer, *Celsus de Medicina*, Vol. II. Books V–VI. Book V. Chapter 27, Verse 27, 125.
23. Spencer, *Celsus de Medicina*, Vol. I. Books I–IV. Book IV. Chapter 28, Verse 9, 453.
24. Ibid, Book IV. Chapter 31, Verse 5, 459.
25. Spencer, *Celsus de Medicina*, Vol. II. Books V–VI. Book V. Chapter 28, Verse 9, 143.
26. J. Innes Miller, *The Spice Trade of the Roman Empire* (Oxford: Oxford University Press, 1998), 99.
27. Spencer, *Celsus de Medicina*, Vol. I. Book III. Chapter 6, Verse 7, 263.
28. Ibid, Book III. Chapter 5, Verses 4–7, 247.
29. Ibid, Book III. Chapter 7, Verse 8, 267.
30. Robert T. Gunther, *Dioscorides Greek Herbal*, (London: Hafner, 1968), 200.
31. Spencer, *Celsus de Medicina*, Vol. II. Books V–VI. Book V. Chapter 3, Verse 5, 7.
32. Ibid, Book V. Chapter 17, Verse 18, 17.
33. Ibid, Book V. Chapter 22, Verses 3–9, 53.
34. Spencer, *Celsus de Medicina*, Books VII–VIII. Book VII. Chapter 31, Verse 33, 469.

The Essence of Galen's Medicine |
2nd Century AD

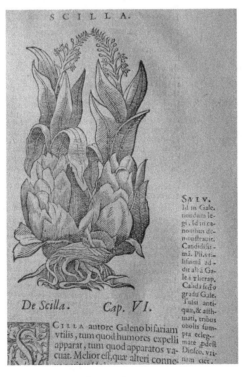

Squill, *Opera de Medicamentorum*, Mesue.

T he influence of Galen has been so broad and deep over the centuries, one could easily write a whole book about it, and so we will, necessarily, be comparatively brief. He was born c131 AD in the city of Pergamum to wealthy parents. His father, an architect, expected him to become a philosopher or politician. Galen was interested in healing from an early age. He had a strong belief that in order to be a good physician it was necessary to be a good philosopher. He began learning from the lectures of local philosophers from various schools of thought, Stoic, Platonist, and Epicurean from the end of his fourteenth year, guided by his father.[1]

At the local temple of Aesculapius, natural methods of healing would have included massage, psychotherapy, and a regime similar to those followed in later sanatoriums with fresh air and bathing. After his father"s death, he travelled to Smyrna, where he studied with Doctor Pelops and Albinus the Platonist, and to Alexandria to further increase his knowledge. On his return to Pergamum, he was appointed surgeon to the gladiators giving him valuable experience in trauma medicine. Four years later, he moved to Rome where he first made a favourable impression through his public lectures and by demonstrating his now detailed knowledge of anatomy and physiology. This brought him to the attention of the Emperor, Marcus Aurelius.[2] However, his fiery criticism of the opinions of other physicians, showing contempt freely expressed, encouraged so much bad feeling against him he was finally forced to return to Pergamum. Now aged thirty-six, he continued writing and his extensive works were to cover almost the whole of the philosophy and practice of medicine in his time. The Emperor Antoninus summoned a reluctant Galen to join him as he went to fight the Germans, but on arriving in Aquileia plague broke out and Antoninus fled to Rome leaving Galen there with the sick. He afterwards relented on taking Galen on campaign, having been given the idea that the god Asclepius did not want this. He then appointed Galen to stay as physician to his small son, Commodus until his return, giving him time to research and write *The Usefulness of the Parts of the Body* and other works.[3]

In his writing, he was just as forceful in his opinions and denigration of others, incorporating long arguments as to why named individuals were wrong. This can make his books quite difficult to read and perhaps comes from the practice of the time when physicians were also orators, establishing their reputations and attracting important patients through public argument. The main predecessor he gave real credit to appears to be Hippocrates. Of him Galen acknowledged, "he was the first to recognise what nature does".[4]

His book, *On the Natural Faculties*, shows him as following the Hippocratic humoral theory on which he expounds. Perhaps it was his early experience treating seriously wounded gladiators and the anatomy demonstrations that he undertook that made him constantly curious about human physiology. In that period, Galen was unable to carry out dissection of human bodies and so used animals.

His favourite, as appearing to be closest to man, was the Barbary ape. Partly due to this he came to certain strange conclusions in some cases, as with the digestive system, which was much discussed and little understood at the time. Later physicians appear to have assumed that he had dissected human bodies, and it was not until over a thousand years later that the famous anatomist Vesalius was to successfully dispel some of his anatomical and largely physiological errors.

Galen was by no means always wrong and he was not averse to using vivisection without anaesthetic simply to prove his point. This was so when he correctly argued that urine flowed through the ureters into the bladder, but could not flow back up towards the kidney. This procedure, which must have been terrible for the animal, involved cutting the peritoneum to expose the organs and first applying, then removing ligatures around the penis, or one then the other ureter, in a series of restrictions while squeezing the bladder or ureters where the urine was being held as necessary for the demonstration. It would have taken an agonizing time and is fully described, ending with him encouraging others to repeat the same process for further proof.[5]

His eager patients provided a constant source of case studies with which to illustrate his theories and treatment experiments. When it came to obstetrics he was evidently not above respecting and working with an experienced female midwife as he dedicated his *Anatomy of the Uterus* to one.[6] Galen also travelled when necessary in order to source good quality medicinal earths as well as herbs.

Anaximander who readers may recall as an important Greek philosopher-scientist from the sixth century BC, wrote the first prose text about natural phenomena and drew the first map of the known world. He began a new way of thinking in looking upon nature as something that can be explained. This encouraged those philosophers who came after him to see man as part of nature. Gradually a series of links were made which led to the humoral doctrine. At the centre of all considerations in this doctrine is the constitution or balance of elements or humours within each individual person—we were introduced to these in the Hippocratic corpus. Empedocles begins with four elements air, fire, earth, and water. In Hippocrates fire and water are described as elements within each of us, with fire being hot and dry and water being cold and moist.

Galen had studied the Hippocratic teachings—that the four humours in the body of blood, yellow bile, black bile and phlegm are present in each one of us in differing amounts from birth. In many people one humour may predominate throughout life, thus dictating their basic constitution and the type of person they are. The influence of each of the humours within the body systems however can be increased or decreased according to factors of age, season, diet, locality, and lifestyle. Their individual strengths and balance, one with another, determines the health of the patient. He sought to prove, explain, and further these ideas. In order to understand his views, it may be helpful to have a simple table to illustrate the connections being made.

Element	Humour	Energetics	Period in life when strongest	Season when increased
Air	Blood	Hot and moist	Infancy	Spring
Fire	Yellow bile	Hot and dry	Youth	Summer
Earth	Black bile	Cold and dry	Middle age	Autumn
Water	Phlegm	Cold and moist	Old age	Winter

The four humours, blood, yellow bile, black bile, and phlegm are identifiable as body fluids and each have their corresponding links to the qualities of the elements. We can readily, I think, agree on some of the connections made.

Blood can be felt to be actually hot and moist, and imagining a baby as hot and moist is not difficult. However, the moistness refers to the softness of the solid parts of the body, including the bones at this early stage of life.[7] As growth takes place, this moistness is used up so that by youth the bones are established as dry. Spring is a time of new life and naturally is linked in our thoughts to infancy. That hot and moist is partnered with the season of spring has long caused discussion. Galen himself points out that philosophers were mistaken to try to make the four categories of the elements fit the four seasons. He looks upon spring as a well-balanced season in terms of moisture and dryness. He repeats the Aphorism of Hippocrates, that spring and early summer is most healthy for the young.[8] The name of the constitution in which blood is the dominant humour is sanguine from the Latin *sanguis* meaning blood. A sanguine person came to mean a hopeful, positive one, as well as someone having red cheeks.

The example given in Chapter 4 is of hot and dry conditions, which come from the element Fire and may encourage stomach upsets in summer. I suggested that this links summer to bilious attacks and yellow bile. The classification of hot and dry applied to summer is an easy one, when applied to bile it may be more difficult to understand.

Galen addresses this by referring to the experience of having an unquenchable thirst from a large quantity of yellow bile collecting in the stomach. He points out that vomiting it up removes that thirst as no amount of drinking water can.[9] His case sets a clear illustration of his perception of the hot and dry qualities of yellow bile. The phrase hot-headed youth may occur to minds today in order to establish the age when yellow bile is dominant, but there is a deeper reasoning too. The innate heat of life remains strong, while moisture has been used up in growth producing a new dryness. The constitution of the person with a dominance of yellow bile is choleric, from the Latin cholera, meaning bile.

Black bile, classed as from the Earth element is even harder to relate to. Galen writes that intelligent physicians find more evidence for it being dominant in autumn and mainly in those who have passed their prime. He identifies the organ which clears away the excess of this humour as the spleen which cleanses the blood, quoting Hippocrates on the danger in dysentery, if it proceeds from black bile. This, he writes, proves it to be more acrid than yellow bile.[10] The cold and dry classification seems to be one of elimination, in that he writes phlegm is cold and moist, yellow bile hot and dry, blood can be felt as hot and moist, therefore he is left with cold and dry. The name of the constitution that corresponds to dominance of black bile is melancholic.

In Chapter 4, the links between winter with coughs and colds increasing production of phlegm were set out from the work of Hippocrates. Galen writes of phlegm, or mucus collecting in old people and that "not even a lunatic could say that this was anything else than cold and moist".[11] He also links it with those who are chilled. That winter accords with old age, follows from spring being a time of new birth. It can be observed that some people are more affected by colds and chest infections than others in winter and this fits with a predominantly phlegmatic constitution.

Although people are seen as predominantly one of the four types, the constant interplay of the humours due to age and season is seen to alter the balance and these changes in turn affect the patients' health. Galen regards changes of season, or changes within a season as causing illness, for the human body is always subject to change and as he writes change will always be towards the opposite of the present state.

Autumn, being subject to larger drops in temperature after the heat of summer, brought a greater danger than from a cooler day in spring when the body has already adapted to the cold. The heat and moisture that we see allocated to spring are not a healthy combination as can be appreciated when they occur in summer and are associated with epidemics of plague, in his book of that name.

Always the four interacting qualities of heat, cold, dryness, and moisture arising from fire and water were behind Galen's convictions and his questioning. He applied these qualities in various proportions to the parts of the body when a foetus is formed. With the anatomical difference between veins and arteries he writes, "it appears to me, then, that the vein, as well as each of the other parts, functions in such and such a way according to the manner in which *the four qualities* are mixed".[12] Therefore he believed that any change in these balances in one part of the body could cause disease.

Accepting the four humours as fluids or conditions within the body, he then wanted to be able to explain how they are increased. He discussed at some length whether they were present in food when it is eaten, or the body makes them from food substances. Galen wrote that Hippocrates, Aristotle, and others had already demonstrated that when food was altered in the veins, a secondary digestion after concoction in the stomach and a further stage in the liver, by the innate heat of the person, if it is in moderation then blood is produced. If it is not in proper proportion then other humours are produced. He considered that warmer foods are more productive of bile and colder foods more productive of phlegm.[13]

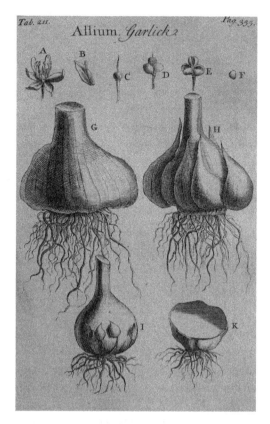

Garlic, *The Compleat Herbal*, Tournefort.

Galen constantly reviewed the opinions of others, writing some contended that yellow bile was made in the liver, others that it came from honey. He considers the nature of bile as being very bitter, which honey is not, suggesting that could not be right. His detailed observation of the effect of honey on patients served him here as he noted that with the young patient, already rich in yellow bile, their natural heat assists the conversion of honey into more bile, and is unhelpful. He has further seen that the opposite is the case for the older person who is cold and phlegmatic in whom it produces more blood.[14] This relation of cause to effect referring to humours we find also originates with the Hippocratic Corpus. He further states that an excess of phlegm produces cold diseases, while an excess of yellow bile results in warmer diseases.[15]

We see Galen extending his questioning on foods into the action of drugs on the body. For this he had a theory of attraction in which each drug attracted the humour that was proper to it. He maintained that in summer yellow bile, which is hot and dry, is evacuated in greater quantity by some drugs. In winter the emphasis would be on cold and wet phlegm. To carry this argument further, he claimed that the same drug would evacuate more bile in a younger man and more phlegm in an older one who has more a moist and cold constitution due to his age.[16]

Galen further notes that warmth can also be affected by the patient's occupation, their locality, and age. He refers back to Aristotle who had previously interpreted Hippocrates correctly on this in his view. His aim with medicine was to learn from the ancients and then by testing, evaluate their philosophy and methods, practising those he found best.

As for the individual, naturally he believed that everyone was at all ages and in all seasons made up of a blend of all four humours. Whether this is a balanced blend within the person or not depends on many factors. Clearly their base constitution and age may predominate while factors of season, locality, diet, and much more can influence whether the four humours are balanced, giving health referred to as *eucrasia,* or unbalanced, causing disease, known as *dyskrasia.* Galen related particular dyskrasias to particular conditions. He gives the example of a young man spending time out in the hot sun of summer, taking in heating and drying foods and similar medicating drinks, indulging in frequent sexual activity, becoming prone to developing a fever as a result.[17]

Treatments are always aimed at restoring *eukrasia* and to that end herbs are also classified as heating, cooling, drying, or moistening. These terms refer to potential actions on the human body and are later translated in part into the terminology of diuretic, carminative, narcotic, and so on. When standing in the sun the person is actually heated by it, with drugs they mostly need to be partially digested and travel within the body before they take effect, therefore, they have potential actions which may vary with the condition of the patient. This has to be remembered.

Many Mediterranean herbs are seen as hot and dry, for instance thyme. An example of hot and moist would be elecampane, which opens and warms the chest, producing expectoration. For a cold and dry herb, we have chicory, and cold and moist can be illustrated by purslane. It is also evident that while one part of a plant can have one classification, it is not always the same for all parts of the plant. Just as some plants can actually be therapeutic in one part and poisonous in another. Galen favoured complex prescriptions using the polypharmacy of his day.

In writing of treatments in *Methods of Medicine,* he goes into considerable detail and additionally refers his readers to his other works—for instance, his classification of eight diseases in *On the Differentiae of Diseases.* He also refers readers to his earlier works such as *On Krasias, On the Affected Parts* and *The Medical Art.* These references encourage the idea that diverse as his books are, together they form a complete system of medicine. The text continues with his advice on the specific condition. He stresses that while being grateful to the teachers of the past such as Hippocrates, he has discovered many particulars for himself. Galen states that he is the first person to set out method in treatment with every consideration in the right order.[18] He also gives the order in which to read many of his books in a long list in *The Art of Medicine.*[19]

He sees the therapeutic indicators as coming from the disease, the krasis or balance of humours in the body, and the surrounding air or environment the patient is in, which includes location, season, and climate. If the ambient air is hot when the patient is suffering from a fever then it is contributing to it. If it is cool in this situation it can be regarded as helpful. Understanding at what level cooling treatments should be applied to an overheated patient, or heating remedies to a cold dyskrasia for health to be restored, is clearly vital for success. This requires a deep understanding of the nature of the individual patient and their surroundings. He therefore encourages others to be methodical in their reasoning and above all to relate their approach in this way.

When writing about a particular case where rubbing and bathing the patient are being described detail of the temperature of the room and the timing are given. These instructions are followed by a re-iteration that there is no one form of regimen to suit everyone. A restorative regimen is recommended and the general guidance from his work, *On The Preservation of Health* is suggested.

Plato wrote of the body as containing three vital capacities, or souls. The term soul does not relate to what is later understood by the word. These capacities govern the organism in different ways and are in fact essential organs when it comes to supporting life. Galen agrees with Plato that the first, which is essential for nourishing the organism and he believes is in common with that of a plant, is the liver. He writes that the veins run as conduits from this organ, distributing nourishment all over the body—I am at a loss to identify the liver in a plant, but there are certainly veins. The second soul, in plants animals and humans, is the heart. This is the source of innate heat and actually adds heat to the blood. The arteries are the conduits of this fount, which has many names and among them, passionate soul. The third, the rational soul is in the brain. This governs movement and sensation through the conduits of nerves.[20]

Plato also considered the rational soul in the brain to be immortal, but Galen is unable to commit himself on this. Following his earlier thinking on the importance of the balance of heat, cold, wetness, and dryness in how body parts work, Galen writes that the substance of each soul must also be a mixture of the four qualities. Differing balances of these qualities due to changes in the humours would then affect them. He thinks about dark moods experienced by the mentally ill and assumes that when a patient sinks into melancholy and sadness, this must have a physical cause.

The cause obvious to him is an accumulation of black bile or black humour, and so this in turn proves that changes in the humours have the power to affect the rational soul, or brain.[21] Affections of the soul may thus have an emotional as well as physical context. He further refers to the Hippocratic discussion of waters and of mixtures of the seasons to show that all three souls depend on the mixtures of the body.[22]

The heart, liver, and brain must all be supported in order to maintain life. Galen notes that when considering treatments involving strong bleeding or purging this should be remembered. The health of these three souls and their likely responses to powerful treatments should dictate whether or not the treatment should happen. The liver, heart, or brain might need to be strengthened using herbs, before strong treatments to evacuate humours from the body, such as bleeding or purging, were carried out. To illustrate this, he relates having seen two patients bled excessively. This exhausted one of their three souls (main organs) and caused their deaths.[23]

We will be returning to Galenic theory through the work of others over the centuries, particularly with Avicenna. This brief introduction has been designed to give a basis for understanding the more detailed interpretations of others and to give an idea of this highly experienced practical man who at the same time sets down a whole philosophy of medicine in his lifetime. He writes, "For producing health is, in fact, nothing other than to bring the condition contrary to nature, which is now present in the body, to an accord with nature".[24]

References

1. P.N. Singer, (trans), *Galen. Selected Works*, (Oxford: Oxford University Press, 1997), 119.
2. A.J. Brock, *Galen on the Natural Faculties*, (London: Harvard University Press, 1971), Introduction, XVII.
3. Singer, *Galen. Selected Works*, 8.
4. Brock, *Galen on the Natural Faculties*, XXV.
5. Ibid, Book I. Chapter XIII. 59.
6. Ralph Jackson, *Doctors and Diseases in the Roman Empire*, (London: British Museum Publications, 1988), 87.
7. Singer, *Galen. Selected Works*, 233.
8. W.H.S. Jones, *Hippocrates*, Vol. IV. (London: Harvard University Press, Ist published, 1931), Aphorisms Section III. Verse XVIII. 129.
9. Brock, *Galen on the Natural Faculties*, Book II. Chapter IX. 201.
10. Brock, *Natural Faculties*, Book II. Chapter IX. 205.
11. Brock, *Natural Faculties*, Book II. Chapter IX. 203.
12. Brock, *Natural Faculties*, Book I. Chapter III. 13–15.
13. Brock, *Natural Faculties*, Book II. Chapter VIII. 183.
14. Brock, *Natural Faculties*, Book II. Chapter VIII. 181.
15. Brock, *Natural Faculties*, Book II. Chapter VIII. 185.
16. Brock, *Natural Faculties*, Book I. Chapter XIII. 69.
17. Ian Johnston and G.H.R. Horsley, *Method of Medicine*, Books 5–9, (London: Harvard University Press, 2011), VIII. 7, 429–31.
18. Johnston & Horsley, *Method of Medicine* Books 5–9, Book IX. Chapter 8, 499.
19. P.N., Singer, *Galen. Selected Works*, 394–6.
20. Johnston & Horsley, *Method of Medicine*, Books 5–9, Book IX. Chapter 10, 505.
21. Singer, *Galen. Selected Works*, 154.
22. Ibid, 167.
23. Johnston & Horsley, *Method of Medicine*, Books 5–9, Book IX. Chapter 10, 507.
24. Johnston & Horsley, *Method of Medicine*, Books 5–9, Book IX. Chapter 15, 525.

Roman Invasion and Settlement | 1st–5th Centuries

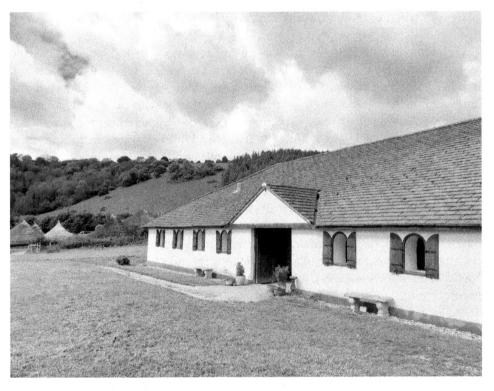

Roman Villa, Butser, Courtesy Butser Ancient Farm.

A little background information may help understanding of how Roman medicine may have been encountered and perceived by the indigenous population and those troops stationed in Britain. It is easy to think that the Roman legionaries stationed here were mainly Italian, and in the first century eighty percent of the troops did come from Rome. By the second century, however, things had changed considerably. Evidence from written material and inscriptions confirms men from across the continent, from Belgium to Austria, including Spaniards and Gauls, as well as from North Africa with Syrians were stationed here.[1] Britain as a multi-cultural country begins at this point.

As the Empire spread, two methods were part of the strategy to maintain control of such large regions. The first was to negotiate with and accept friendly native rulers of small kingdoms, giving them subservient roles as client kings with their own autonomy. Contacts had already been made with some tribal rulers in Britain. According to Strabo, the geographer and historian, some British Rulers were allowed to send embassies to Rome, possibly Cunobelinus was one, who introduced Roman ways and imported luxuries to his court of Colchester while expanding the territory of the Catuvellauni. Pre-Roman Colchester has been confirmed as a well-developed town by recent archaeology. Any acceptance of friendly relations did not last long after his death in 40 AD, as revealed by events just three years later when Claudius launched his invasion and attacked Colchester, making it his new Roman capital.[2]

Cogidubnus, king of the Regni was given Roman citizenship, retained his role as local client king and became a deputy for the Emperor in his capital, Chichester. In other areas the story was very different; for instance, with the Brigantes in the north and the Iceni who, having initially been friendly, with the dire treatment of Boudicca, changed their minds. Without becoming distracted by the patchwork history of the invasion we should note that with Wales offering sanctuary for the resistance, the island of Anglesey became a refuge for freedom fighters in addition to being a stronghold of the Druids, who were seen by the Romans as holding power through their network of priests and belief.

The second strategy was to recruit natives into the Roman army early in the period of an occupying force. In the second century the legions had not only reached but built forts in northern Britain. We already find Germanic Gauls, who might be considered by some to be brothers to the local population (since they were only lately conquered themselves), were stationed there. Along Hadrian's Wall, reminders of the multi-cultural worship of various gods and goddesses have been found. These include the surviving relief of the torchbearer for Mithras, for his worshippers from Housesteads Fort and the shrine of a Celtic water nymph, Coventina.[3] Of particular relevance is the sculptured relief of the three Celtic Genii Cucullan, hooded godlets of healing, fertility, and after-life from a domestic shrine nearby.[4] By the end of the century there were already British units being posted abroad.[5]

Early Roman centres such as Colchester were quickly developed on Roman lines with a temple to Claudius and baths at Colchester funded by heavy taxation on the local people. A settlement of Roman citizens was established nearby and two other coloniae, were built at Lincoln and Gloucester. Retiring legionaries could choose to settle in one of these coloniae in Britain or return home with payment, rather than being given land to live on. Timber framed houses and shops selling a variety of imported goods supplied their lifestyle in retirement.[6] There is no reason not to think that medicus, a term applied to physicians or their assistants, were not also able to do this. Roman citizens (citizenship came automatically on retirement with twenty-five years of army service), would have welcomed their services.

Of course, health care would have been available from both Roman and native sources. Archaeology has revealed a temple complex at Lydney in the Cotswolds built at the end of the third century. It was dedicated to a Celtic god, Nodens, and the finds of a miniature bronze hand left in thanks for healing and an oculist's stamp for an eye salve, confirm medicine was practised on that site.[7] There are other similar Romano British pagan sites around the country possibly built as this one was, close to villas of the wealthier class. No doubt British and Welsh healers, whether connected to temples or healing wells, midwives, and cunning women also cared for the sick.

The army took care of the health of the military with hospitals at some forts and veterinary care would be available for the horses where cavalry units were stationed. In the senior ranks of the equestrian troops, families accompanied soldiers and so women and children were also housed at forts and visited each other. A wealth of personal information has been recovered from the documents and letters written in ink on thin leaves of wood found at the fort of Vindolanda on Hadrian's Wall, confirming the lifestyle enjoyed by those of higher rank.

There we find proof of daily documentation of those who were sick and unavailable for duty. Eye problems seem to have been frequent with ophthalmia accounting for ten of the men on sick leave in a strength report for a unit at the wall, with fifteen sick of all other causes.[8] An eye test was part of the medical for acceptance into the army but ophthalmia, a serious problem centuries later in the Navy, was contagious and hard to treat.[9] Eye salves are one of the treatments better represented in archaeology by small stone stamps used for stamping the identification into the salve itself. These bear the names either of the maker or main ingredient and what it was for.

So, from Bedfordshire, we have salves to treat running eyes, cloudy vision, or inflammation. From Kenchester, Herefordshire there is a stamp reading "frankincense ointment," with the name of the oculist, Titus Vindacius Arnovistus and three other eye preparations.[10] From Cirencester another four-sided stamp reads both Atticus' quince ointment as one of two for soreness of the eyes, and gives us two ointments for pain.[11] Stamps found in Chester detail ointments, drops and a saffron salve.[12]

In addition to the mix of local suppliers of foodstuffs, specialist foods were imported, and the wealthier class, whether officers in the army, Roman citizens, or local elite, would no doubt have had access to imported medicines. Army supply systems seem to have been well run and involve items from other garrisons in Britain as well as goods imported from abroad. The alcoholic drinks range from Celtic beer, which would have been brewed locally and appears in one of the longest accounts of foodstuffs, to imported wine.[13] Leatherworkers are recorded in the Vindolanda workshops and there is reference to hides from Catterick where the site has produced evidence of tanning.[14]

Some of the medical prescriptions of Hippocrates and Dioscorides may have been known through the work of Scribonius Largus, a physician who arrived with Claudius in AD 43.[15] So far, the archaeology shows hospitals to have been few and far between, sometimes serving several forts. Medics such as travelling oculists who specialised just in treating eye conditions would have been available for a wider, if wealthier public. It is possible some members of the general population who were part of the families of soldiers were treated medically. The written work of Scribonius Largus on medicine meanwhile, containing a variety of Greek and Roman prescriptions survived in Latin to return later. It has never been translated and tends to gain mentions but no more than that, in British history.

From later comments on herbs growing where the Roman way of life was followed, particularly along parts of Hadrian's Wall, they clearly grew some of the medicinal plants of the Mediterranean here. We have evidence in Britain also for probable Roman introduction of "culinary" herbs. This comes from archaeobotany—finds from London, various forts around the country as well as written lists. Waterlogged conditions give the best chance of gaining information on fruits, herbs, and vegetables and so these and evidence of mineralised samples from cesspits and latrines offer the best evidence for understanding the area of most interest for herbalism.

A report on the archaeo-botany of Roman Britain published in 2007 pointed out, however, that data from late Iron Age waterlogged sites was limited from the south east of Britain and more information was needed to be sure that foods such as cherries, plums, and turnips had not been introduced before the Roman invasion.[16] Dill, fennel, marjoram, a variety of mint, sage, rosemary, rue, and a variety of thyme are listed as being introduced by the Romans.[17] There is mention of lovage on one of the Vindolanda tablets but that could have been imported seed.[18] Even this short list of culinary herbs is also a list of potential medicines.

Additionally, the Romans brought Alexanders. This herb still grows as a naturalised plant by the sea and is much in evidence on the south and west coasts and on the Isle of Wight. The leaves not only provided tasty greens in January and February, which can be eaten in pottage when they were understood to heat the stomach as a digestive, the seeds were also used to treat the urinary system. Anise seeds are listed on Vindolanda Tablet III 591 with other prescription ingredients.[19] Wild celery found at Calleva (Silchester), could have been used as a flavouring, a diuretic, or to reduce swelling.

Bay leaves were used by the Romans for cookery and medicine. They appear as *folium lauri* in the only surviving book on Roman cookery that bears the name of one, or possibly more men, called Apicius.[20] In medicine the crushed berries gave an oil used for treating the liver and included in an extractive plaster, *diadaphnidon*.[21] In Ancient Greece, bay was dedicated to Apollo, god of medicine and the leaves used in making prophesies and charms in temples. In Rome, wreaths of bay were awarded to victors and worn by Emperors. The herb was looked upon as protective from evil spirits and lightning.[22] John Harvey regards it as undoubted that bay became naturalised in the south of England by late Roman times.[23] Bay is mentioned later along with fruit trees in the plan of St Gall for monastery gardens. In the Medieval period, it became very popular so that the native word for berry (bay) became the name adopted for the tree rather than calling it laurel. The list of Roman introductions is considerable and bears witness to the changes in kitchen and garden to come.

There are more herbs recorded on Vindolanda tablets, and knowledge of others comes from archaeological finds. Caraway, chervil, cumin, garlic, hyssop, and *Rosa gallica off.* were found at Calleva.[24,25,26] Purslane and parsley are both culinary herbs with medicinal properties, while rosemary and white mustard found at Silchester and London have even more obvious medicinal use alongside being seasonings.

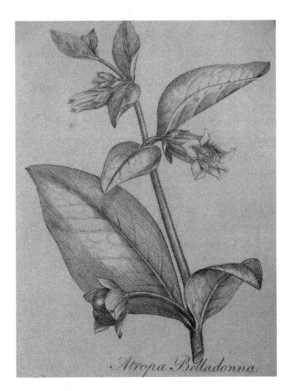

Belladonna, *Medical Botany*, Woodville.

Some herbs maintained hugely important roles in pain relief and primitive anaesthesia into the twentieth century. Evidence of these came when the seeds of *Atropa Belladonna* were found at a Roman site. Hemlock occurs as a fossil associated with a Roman site. Henbane is regarded as Roman from a find at Pevensey, but there is also an Iron Age find from Aldwick Barley.[27] Lastly, remains of opium poppies have been recovered from Hadrian's Wall.

The Romans also brought fruit and nut trees, some of which, the mulberry, medlar, and fig, have medicinal roles. The mulberry was recommended by Celsus for encouraging sleep and as a mild laxative, and the medlar fruits were valued for normalising the bowel action after diarrhoea, without causing constipation. The laxative uses of the fig, a popular Roman food, were extended in later periods to other conditions besides constipation.[28] It can easily be appreciated from this list that the Roman influence in diet and medicine over the following centuries was massive.

As ever, knowledge of the way in which lifestyle and diet influence health is important in understanding the popularity of particular treatments and use of herbs at any point in time. A physical experience of these can offer greater understanding of the past as the history of the plants is entwined with human need as well as cultivation, trade, and beliefs.

The beginning of my own research of this period followed a few years after establishing Celtic herb workshops at Butser. I had been further inspired by the plans Dr Reynolds had for building a reconstruction of a Roman villa, based on the archaeology of a villa at Sparsholt, also in Hampshire. He had already begun work on constructing a hypocaust for underfloor heating, discovering along the way more about how these constructions worked. By 1998, I had begun taking days on Roman herbal medicine at Butser using the works of Celsus, Dioscorides, and Pliny. It felt wonderful to have actual recipes to interpret, even though at this stage they were made in the round house.

Sadly, Peter was not to live to see his dream come to fruition, but four years later in 2002 work began for a team of dedicated people who had to face and overcome the many hurdles of research with construction materials and methods the archaeology left open to interpretation. A full account of these stages over the period from starting the build in 2002 to the opening of the villa, a building twenty-three by thirteen metres in October 2003, can be found in *Rebuilding the Past*.[29] I was eager to follow new developments at each of my visits.

Progress of the mosaic for the hypocaust room was the most fascinating. Once again I needed to research and think about who would have lived in such a villa and which herbs might be involved in their lifestyle and therefore grown in their garden. I loved the wall paintings which included faces of people associated with the project and was delighted to be able to cook and make recipes using a charcoal fire in a brazier or even better over iron supports resembling the rings of a cooker from my childhood with charcoal beneath. This was luxury indeed. I made recipes in the room identified possibly as the kitchen from the Sparsholt excavation floor-plan, which gave us a corridor villa with eight rooms.

The following details from workshops serve merely to show an attempt to gain an experiential glimpse of a backdrop to what is still sparse written evidence for the period. Participants enjoyed making and eating adapted dishes from the cookery of Apicius using imported herbs. Onion and lovage dressing over cold tuna also contained cumin, mint, rosemary, mustard, and dates. The lentils and chestnuts in a coriander wine sauce, again using pepper, cumin, mint, and rosemary, this time with fennel and a little pennyroyal, was always a favourite.[30] I chose these as simpler dishes from the only source we have, even though there is no proof these recipes were used in Britain. We made scented beads. These were Rhodides slightly adapted from Dioscorides' *Rosaceum*[31] using red *Rosa gallica* petals, spikenard, myrrh, orris root, and mixing the dry ingredients with a very little of my home made, rather than Chian wine, and honey. The result was slightly sticky at first but beautifully fragrant.

For medicine, the simple and effective cooling of pounded marshmallow root left in water to produce gel over a low heat from charcoal for several hours was appreciated in treating a case of painful sunburn for one participant at the end of the day. We made the bitter wormwood and myrrh pills from the medicinal recipes from Celsus and a more ambitious tonsillitis recipe containing frankincense, garlic, saffron, and myrrh gently heated in sweet raisin wine.[32] My home made wines were often useful in recipes and the days containing also more serious sessions of discussing treatments and recipes, were filled with fragrance.

Salves were a popular item as these could be poured into jars and taken home. A really impressive one for colour was of orris and alkanet roots, prepared in olive oil and thickened with wax. This red application was to be spread on burns. I suspect it was more likely used as a lip salve by eager participants. White horehound in honey for the chest, an oxymel of thyme in honey and vinegar for melancholy, and a paste of mint and honey to freshen the breath were a few of the recipes we explored over several years.

Since then I have been able to access recipes from the *Compositiones Medicorum* of Scribonius Largus,[33] which are perhaps even more relevant than those from Celsus in that he appears to have been stationed with the Roman army in Britain in the first century AD. His work contains 271 recipes, some accompanied by anecdotes and personal comments. He dedicated the collection to Caio Julio Callisto, a Greek who had been made a freedman by Caligula, who went on to have wealth and influence and died in 54 AD, which confirms completion of the work before that date.

As might be expected Hippocrates is referred to, as well as Asclepiades of Bithynia but this is clearly the work of a practising physician rather than a record of medicines from the past. Scribonius begins, as would many collections of remedies to follow, with treatments for pain in the head varying from clearing the nasal passages with his early snuff, a blend including white pepper to make the patient sneeze, to more soothing and elaborate compositions. As may be expected from the emphasis on eye medicines found elsewhere, these are followed by sections on first soothing collyria and then the more piercing to address scar tissue.

It is worth noting that collyria could be liquid or solid. If solid the paste was formed into sticks for convenience. Lengths could be detached as needed for use with the eyes but a different formulation might also be used for keeping a fistula open, or inserted in the manner of a suppository. We find this other use referred to later in the recipes when treating the intestines.

Aloes, saffron, opium, myrrh and greater plantain juice are part of one eye recipe for swelling and pain.[34] In another, alum, frankincense, aloes, saffron, opium, and dried rose leaves (actually petals but the word had not yet been invented) are used, again with plantain juice.[35] As we journey through history, we will see these same herbs and resins continually associated with eye treatments. Earache receives comparatively little attention, although success with patients is noted and with recipe forty Scribonius notes this has succeeded where others he has tried on his own problem have failed.[36]

When it comes to the teeth there is more advice and Scribonius, not averse to name dropping, involves Octavia, sister of Emperor Augustus as using his recipe. He has already named Augustus using collyria. Augustus appears again with Messalina supporting an excellent strengthening powder for his teeth. Here the presence of mastic from Chios would recommend it to anyone with experience of using this resin in toothpaste or alone, which gives excellent results.

The pattern of remedies treating areas gradually moving down the body continues with the throat and we read of those herbs for coughs—saffron, myrrh, frankincense and opium—prescribed again, this time for dry coughs. Antidotes follow—these are a large group of medicines used both to treat venomous bites from a variety of animals and as a general panacea for infectious diseases. They are very complex and containing so many ingredients, it was thought they could be given in small quantities at regular intervals.

Among these are three possible versions of Theriac, often referred to as treacle. In the first of these, the ingredients listed include cumin specified as from the Thebaic region of Egypt and cumin from Aethiopia, which clearly were expected to have slightly different properties. Including provenance of recipes was evidently important to Scribonius, whether this involved famous authorities or not. Some antidotes bear the name of the physician responsible for them, and he cannot resist bringing the Emperor Tiberius into the Antidote Hiera Pacchii Antiochi. Although not naming the African woman who sold him recipe 122, he nevertheless makes us aware of her as a source and her success with it.

There are also some short notes on substances regarded as toxic. These include the plant sources of hemlock as *Cicutam*, opium as *Opii*, henbane as *Altercum*, and aconite as *Aconitum*.[37,38,39] Regarding stones, gypsum, used as a bright, white granulated styptic powder, which can be burnt to produce plaster of Paris, is a surprise.[40] In 1751, Hill notes he does not understand why the ancients saw it as a poison. It had long been dug out of the ground near Paris at that time.[41] However, toxic results can be ascribed to the use of ceruse or cerussa. This is white lead powder, produced by suspending plates of lead over sharp vinegar in a covered earthen vessel.[41,42] Representing animal ingredients, there are also notes on the salamander,[43] which was burned to ash because this produced a substance rich in lime, and cantharides or Spanish flies.[36,44] These bright green and gold beetles with wings more like flies were collected in large numbers from bushes in France and Spain and dried mostly for external use in blisters.[45] Taken internally they would be incredibly acrid.

Of those chosen conditions that we looked at in Celsus, we find the herbs in eye recipes, as recorded above, correspond well with those in Scribonius. As far as treating coughs and toothache are concerned, there are no identical recipes. Rose is again used for headache with fever in the first recipe in Scribonius.[46] The highest number of recipes in his compendium are for the eyes, antidotes for bites or other poisons, digestive remedies, and emplasters to apply.

Herbs included in the remedies that we value today as Roman introductions include hyssop, elecampane, rue, white horehound, thyme and the powerful narcotics already mentioned. These are often overshadowed in the recipes by resins and gums, myrrh appears in several forms from different sources, *opobalsamum* and *xylobalsamum* are both from *Commiphora* species. Frankincense is listed as thus or thuris. Bdellium resin is from *Commiphora mukul*, storax *Acacia* spp., these and Indian spikenard are all used, and mastic has already been mentioned. Then there is gum tragacanth and gummi, pine resin and the solid element, colophony from species of pine, and the Mediterranean plant galbanum from *Ferula galbanum*.

Roman medicine was rich in a great variety of ingredients and we have already seen how many of these—the spices, such as cinnamon, cardamom, and cumin and some resins in particular—came to the Roman Empire over vast distances. They crossed continents from India, Persia, and Arabia, China, and south-east Asia. How much of this entered the experience of the general public is difficult to say. We have looked also at the herbs definitely introduced for use in Roman cookery. Over the almost four hundred years the army was here, the separate populations of foreign troops and British residents merged to a greater or lesser extent in different areas of the country. The population became one of Romano-British as people moved into towns where they had a greater dependence on shops perhaps, than on plants from their own gardens, whether for cookery or medicine. Difficulties in dating archaeological finds exactly, has been noted, but the considerable contribution to a wider herb use during the occupation and settlement period is undeniable.

References

1. https://ancientworldsmanchester.wordpress.com/2013/03/04/dna-and-the-roman-army-in-britain/
2. H.H. Scullard, *Roman Britain Outpost of the Empire* (London: Thames and Hudson, 1979), 38.

3. Roger Wilson, *A Guide to the Roman Remains in Britain* (London: Constable, 2002), 484–5.
4. Scullard, *Roman Britain*, 158.
5. A.K. Bowman *Life and Letters on the Roman Frontier* (London: The British Museum Press, 2003), 23.
6. Scullard, *Roman Britain*, 52.
7. Wilson, *A Guide to the Roman Remains in Britain*, 202.
8. Bowman, *Life and Letters on the Roman Frontier*, 16.
9. William Turnbull, *The Naval Surgeon* (2020), Diseases of the Mediterranean Station. Ophthalmia.
10. S. Ireland, *Roman Britain A Sourcebook* (London: Routledge, 1996), (554), 247.
11. Ireland, *Roman Britain*, (556), 247.
12. Scullard, Roman Britain, 144–145,
13. Bowman, *Life and Letters on the Roman Frontier*, 111–113.
14. Ibid, 38.
15. Scribonius Largus, *Compositiones Medicorum*, Scholars Select Facsimile, 1786. (Franklin Classics Trade Press), X.
16. M. Van der Veen et al., *The Archaeobotany of Roman Britain: current state and identification of research priorities*, Vol. 38, Britannia, (The Society for the Promotion of Roman Studies, 2007), 206–7.
17. Joan Alcock, *Food in Roman Britain* (Stroud: Tempus, 2001), 69.
18. Bowman, *Life and Letters on the Roman Frontier*, 64.
19. Ibid, 125.
20. Christopher Grocock and Sally Grainger, Apicius (Prospect Books, 2006), 347
21. Spencer, *Celsus De Medicina*, II Books V–VI List of Medicamenta. Laurus; XXXIX.
22. Christina Stapley, *The Tree Dispensary. The Uses, History and Herbalism of Native European Trees* (London: Aeon, 2021), 275.
23. John Harvey, *Mediaeval Gardens* (London: Batsford, 1990), 30.
24. Bowman, Life and Letters on the Roman Frontier, 69.
25. Ibid, Vindolanda tablet 679.
26. Ibid, Vindolanda tablet 233, Appendix II, 129.
27. Harold Godwin, *History of the British Flora* (Cambridge: Cambridge University Press, 1975), 316–317.
28. Christina Stapley, *The Tree Dispensary. The Uses, History and Herbalism of Native European Trees* (London: Aeon, 2021), 141, 230, 166.
29. Dai Morgan Evans, et al, *Rebuilding the Past. A Roman Villa* (London: Methuen, 2003).
30. Christopher Grocock and Sally Grainger, *Apicius* (Devon: Prospect Books, 2007), 295, 209.
31. Robert Gunther (ed), *Dioscorides Greek Herbal* (London: Hafner, 1968), Book I. Item 53, 31–32.
32. W.G. Spencer, (trans), *Celsus De Medicina*, Books V–VI. (London: William Heinnemann, 1971), Book VI. Chapter 10, Verse 4, 255.
33. Largus, *Compositiones Medicorum*, (1786).
34. Largus, *Compositiones Medicorum*, 27, (21).
35. Ibid, 32, (31).

36. Ibid, 36, (40).
37. Ibid, 100, (179, 180).
38. Ibid, 101, (181).
39. Ibid, 104, (188).
40. Ibid, 101, (182).
41. M.D. John Hill, *A History of the Materia Medica* (London: Longman, Hitch & Hawes, 1751), 254–255.
42. Hill, *A History of the Materia Medica*, 22.
43. Largus, *Compositiones Medicorum*, 104, (187).
44. Ibid, 105, (189).
45 Hill, *A History of the Materia Medica*, 822–823.
46. Largus, *Compositiones Medicorum*, b3 (1).

SECTION IV

CULTURAL INFLUENCES IN POST-ROMAN BRITAIN | 407–1066

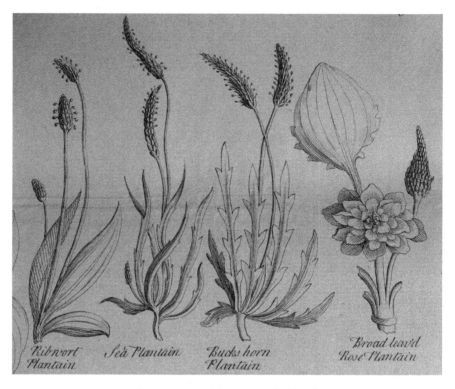

Plantains, *The British Herbal*, Hill.

Key Figures

Saint Augustine, (354–430 AD), Theodore, Archbishop of Canterbury, (c602–690), Abbess Hilda, (c614–680), Alfred the Great. (640–690), Bede, (c673–735), Walahfrid Strabo (c808–849), Bald, Dun, Oxa, (dates unknown).

Key Texts

Dioscorides Greek Herbal, Dioscorides.
Medical Collections, Oribasius.
Medical Works of Alexander of Tralles, Alexander of Tralles.
Seven Books of Paulus Aeginata, Paulus Aeginata.
Macer Floribus de Viribus Herbarium.
Lacnunga.
Books of Bald.
Old English Herbarium.
Bede's History of the English Church and People, Bede.
The Anglo-Saxon Chronicles.

Roles of Women

These might be as a midwife, healer, or leech. This last term can be translated as a healer using charms, herbalist, or someone acting as a physician without classical training.

Quality Control

Information on the best months of the year, sometimes particular days to gather specific herbs can be found in Leechbooks and other records. It is clearly understood that this relates to their efficacy.

Herb Energetics

These are set beside most of the herbs in the *Macer Floribus de Viribus Herbarum*, A number of copies of this main text for the period have survived. We will be noting herbal energetics in this and other Latin sources in the following chapters.

Archaeology

The archaeology of settlements is rich and more is being learned about the later period all the time. Cemeteries offer information on disease such as arthritis from the evidence of skeletons. Identification of residues in pots is also becoming more available.

Travel and Trade

After the Roman army left, Saxon incursion in the south east steadily pushed the Celts to the west of Britain, including Cumberland and south-west Scotland.[1] There were centuries of fighting and famine ahead. Angles, Saxons, Jutes, Vikings, Picts, and Irish all raided Britain. The western sea routes between Wales and mainland Europe were revived after the collapse of the Roman Empire.[2] Since trade was seen as of great importance by all, trading continued amid the difficult times of the sixth century with the Franks and Scandinavia.[3] This could not always be the case however and in some periods trading was interrupted. Various agreements were made and in the tenth century Aethelred promised peace for all trading ships, even from areas not covered by the truce. In return, Vikings were not to attack English traders in Continental ports.[4]

Introduction

The mass conversion to Christianity began in earnest with the mission of St Augustine in 597. The following year saw the first monastery established and the monasteries and church schools kept the classical medicine alive, copying manuscripts and conveying knowledge. Raids persistently destroyed books and robbed the wealthy Church, but documents were often replaced from mother houses on the Continent. Bede (673–735), a monk whose reputation as a scholar was known in Europe, wrote his history of the English Church and people. Writing in the monastery at Jarrow in his old age, he was able to quote from classical writers whose works were in the library there such as Pliny, from copies of Papal archives brought from Rome and Church records from Canterbury and various bishoprics.[5] His work, completed in 731 is a main source of information on this period. He begins by describing the length and breadth of the island and writing of the five languages spoken by the English, British, Scots, and Picts, which also included Latin. Then he gives the origins of the Britons as from Armorica (Brittany), the Picts from Scythia (perhaps Scandinavia), the Scots from Hibernia (Ireland) and writes of the intermarriage of Scots with Picts.[6] Later in his account, following that of the Roman occupation, he describes the Angles as Germanic, from Angulus, between the regions of the Jutes and Saxons.[7]

It is not until the century following Bede's death that Alfred the Great succeeded in bringing a large part of Britain from the River Thames to the River Tees under his control and formed Angle-land, the basis for the England to be. North of the River Tees was still under Danelaw and ruled by Vikings who had come originally as raiders. Alfred loved learning and encouraged writing in the Anglo-Saxon language; it is believed that he made the first translation of Bede's history from Latin himself.[8] Our other source of information from this period is the Anglo-Saxon Chronicles. Of these there are two Chronicles quoted in the following pages. The Parker manuscript was written in Anglo-Saxon in the same book over a period of 200 years by more than ten different scribes through all the trials of fighting and famine. This gives us continuity. Also the Laud Chronicle which did not have a single source.[9]

References

1. Baldick et al. (ed), *Bede A History of the English Church and People* (London: Penguin Classics, 1968), 21.
2. John Davies, *A History of Wales* (London: Penguin Books, 2007), 53.
3. Anne Hagen, *A Second Handbook of Anglo-Saxon Food and Drink* (Norfolk: Anglo Saxon Books, 1999), 177.
4. Hagen, *A Second Handbook of Anglo-Saxon Food and Drink*, 179.
5. Bald-ick (ed), *A History of the English Church and People*, 26.
6. Ibid, 38–39.
7. Ibid, 56.
8. Ibid, 24.
9. G.N. Garmonsway, *The Anglo-Saxon Chronicle* (London: J.M. Dent Sons Ltd., 1953), XVII.

CHAPTER 9

Post-Roman Britain

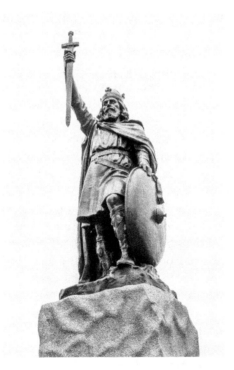

Statue of Alfred the Great, Winchester.

The date for the last of several withdrawals of Roman troops is generally accepted as 407. Roman troops had earlier strengthened defences in Wales against the Irish, but in 405 with their numbers very low, or possibly by then non-existent in that region, the Irish chieftain Nial plundered the western coast and Irish colonists settled in western Wales.[1] An accumulation of pressures with a divided Empire from 395, and Alaric, the Visigoth leader in Italy threatening Rome, Vandals and others penetrated into Gaul as far as Spain in 407 and Constantine fearing attack on Britain left with his troops to make a pre-emptive strike across the channel.[2] In Britain on the southern coast, forts had already sprung up against the threat of Saxon invasion.

The last appeal of several to Rome for defensive aid fell on deaf ears. Vortigern, High King came to power in 426. His influence extended from Wales over southern Britain and he emerges as an important ruler at a council of leaders held about 428.[3] The Anglo-Saxon Parker Chronicle records him bringing in Hengest and his brother Horsa, to lead Angles and Saxons from Germany as mercenaries to fight the Picts, who were raiding from Scotland.[4] Vortigern was also suggested to have been responsible for moving the Votadini people from the banks of the Forth, with their leader, Cunedda, driving out the Irish and establishing the original kingdom of Gwynedd covering the banks of the Menai Straits and coast in the direction of Conway.[5] This would have strengthened North Wales against attack from Irish pirates who were carrying off their prisoners to be slaves at this time. One of those Britons who had been captured from the West Country and taken as an enslaved person was later to be known as Saint Patrick. Escaping Ireland he travelled to Gaul, returning to Britain in 415 where he found the Roman system of government intact.[6]

It does not appear that Britain wanted to leave the Roman Empire, although there are differing opinions among historians, as no doubt there were also amongst the people who lived through that uncertain period. How long the Roman ways lasted is debatable. Some veterans who had settled could have stayed on and we are told by Tacitus writing late in the first century that the sons of Celtic rulers were educated in Roman ways. Local elite will have occupied posts as justices and civic officials.[7] The Roman army had been here with Roman administration in towns for over 300 years, such a system would not collapse overnight. However, without new coinage from Rome to pay troops, bartering would replace coins, and businesses which had supplied the garrisons were inevitably lost. With Saxon advances, life changed.[8] A great deal of debate has centred on the fate of abandoned towns, and disappearance of Romano-British culture.[9]

That Christianity had been one of the religions followed by members of the legions is evidenced by finds near Hadrian's Wall. The Church in Britain had been established in some areas and when Bishop Germanus, later Saint Germanus of Auxerre, travelled to Verulamiam (St. Alban's) in 429 at their request, he recorded evidence of civilised Roman ways.[10] Archaeology supports some of the old life surviving until 450 in Cirencester, Silchester, and St. Albans before it was destroyed by raiding Saxons.[11]

The Parker manuscript of the Chronicle begins in the year 494 with the Norsemen Cerdic and Cynric landing in Britain with five ships. During the next six years the account tells us they conquered the kingdom of Wessex from the Welsh.[12] Over centuries Jutes, Angles, and Saxons settled in Britain. The medicine of the Celts remained a hidden undercurrent with two other systems dominating. The Anglo-Saxon ways with herbs are brought by settlers and the Greek and Roman medicine is re-introduced by the Church. Significant conversion to Christianity is credited to Saint Augustine who arrived with the mission of converting King Aethelbert of Kent, who already had a Christian wife, in 597.[13] His success meant the establishment of the first monastery.

Christianity continued to spread into one kingdom and another, as in Kent, sometimes with the Queen having already been converted with her father before marriage. She would then be encouraged to support conversion of her husband. Meanwhile, they would each have their own separate altars for worship.

Canterbury had been a large centre in pre-Roman Britain and was one of the first Roman civitas capitals.[14] British Archbishops of Canterbury were appointed there. In 655, the holy Church of the English chose Wighard on the death of his predecessor, Archbishop Deusdedit, and he travelled to Rome to be confirmed as the new Archbishop by the Pope.[15] Unfortunately, while there he and his retinue caught plague and died. This left the Pope searching for a suitable candidate. His first choice, the monk, Hadrian, an accomplished Greek and Latin scholar, felt himself unsuited to the task and his second suggestion of Theodore, a scholarly monk from Greece was adopted. It was a condition that Hadrian accompanied him in order to guard against Theodore introducing Greek customs into the Church. Two years passed as they made their way to Marseilles and travelled in the kingdom of the Franks staying at religious houses, before finally arriving in Britain.[16]

Education was to be part of the work of the Church and a school was soon established in Canterbury. According to St Aldhelm in addition to the theology and ecclesiastical law, medicine, astronomy, and arithmetic were studied there. St John of Beverley gives us further evidence in quoting Archbishop Theodore's criticism on the right period of the moon to bleed a patient safely.[17] As a Greek from Tarsus, Theodore would naturally be familiar with Greek medicine in the works of Hippocrates and Galen.

In the fourth century, the sixteen books of Galen and four of Hippocrates had been re-worked by Oribasius at the request of Emperor Julian who ordered him to bring together all that was good in Greek medicine. By adding other works, his *Medical Collections* then totalled seventy books, covering all aspects of healthcare in medicine and surgery. Later he managed to distil this down to a Synopsis for those in the country to use and this had wider availability.[18]

Another possible source for teaching medicine was the excellent work of Alexander of Tralles an eminent Byzantine physician (525–605) who after many years of travel and practice set down his twelve books on medicine. In adding his own experience to the works of Galen and Dioscorides he recorded the best practices in medicine, surgery, and pharmacology of the time. Including some 600 drugs in his therapeutics he showed sound knowledge of far eastern drugs and gave precise dosages.[19] Paulus Aeginata [625–690] plagiarised much of the work of Oribasius in his seven books on medicine. For interested readers, this work is available online.[20] These Latin sources were certainly available three centuries later when they were translated into Anglo-Saxon, as we will see in the next chapter. Few copies of Celsus seem to have been made, only two have survived from the ninth century, one from the tenth, and one from the fifteenth, all on the Continent rather than in Britain.[21] Pliny's history was known here which, while quoting numerous Greek physicians, also contains an indiscriminate spread of folklore. This was widely plundered by later writers.

Bede finished writing his history of the Church at the monastery in Jarrow, Northumbria in 731. He wrote often of bishops and kings but he also includes queens and aristocratic women who became famous in their own lifetimes. One of these was Hilda, great neice of Edwin, King of Northumbria who was to become Abbess of Whitby, a "double house" of men and women, an arrangement which was not unusual in this period. Many double houses began with an Abbess of royal blood in charge. Bede, on writing of her life, records that she was consulted by princes and kings, being known for her wisdom and at least five bishops had been educated in her monastery.

Hilda was entrusted with hosting an important synod to decide the date of Easter, since the date followed by Rome was not the same as the calculation made by the Scots. Bede writes at length of her "wonderful devotion and grace".[22] He shows her to be a shining example of Christian goodness and charity, but her main mission was education of monks and nuns and providing copies of books for the libraries of more monasteries from the busy scriptorium at Whitby. Sadly, we do not know for certain whether some of these books were medical. If she used herbs to heal the sick, he does not mention it.

Banished from Europe for their unorthodox religious views, the Syrian Nestorian Christians had fled to the Muslim world, taking Greek texts with them. So much knowledge was lost with the burning of the library at Alexandria (date and details disputed), but the Syrian texts of Hippocrates, Galen and others, survived. One of these, the *De Materia Medica* of Dioscorides was translated into Arabic at Baghdad by a Christian in about 854. A copy was also made later in the Western Caliphate of Cordoba, in Spain. Latin translations of Dioscorides were often part of a compilation of recipes from the fifth century known as the Pseudo-Apuleius.[23]

In Britain, this appears translated later into Anglo-Saxon. In the Old English Herbarium Leechbook we find Greek and Roman references are constantly made with regard to plant names and classical mythology also referred to. The oldest Anglo-Saxon manuscript, the three Books of Bald were either written or copied in the scriptorium, which had been set up in the capital, Winchester, by Alfred the

Great. In this work from about 950, there is a greater concentration on English plants and folklore. We will look at these and the Lacnunga in detail in the next chapter.

In 871, Alfred, later called the Great, came to the throne. He had not expected to be King for he had three older brothers, which meant he had been able to turn to books and learning as a child. When he inherited the throne on the death of his brother it was a time of constant peril, with nine battles against the Danes that year and constant warfare continued for years.[24] Victorious, he ruled Wessex, West Mercia, and Kent, while Danelaw applied from the Thames to the Tees. With so many pressures it seems a miracle that during his reign he managed to support education.

He encouraged the record of the history of England in the Anglo-Saxon Chronicles, which had been written at monasteries around the country. In some years, their descriptions of constant destruction, looting of monasteries, loss of life, and many famines are painful to read. They also give dates for accession of kings, appointments of bishops, sighting of comets and eclipses of the sun and moon, plague and murrain of animals. Although brief, they give a coherent history of the whole period up until the twelfth century, recording the battle of Hastings and Norman rule beginning with William the Conqueror.

King Alfred had earlier made pilgrimage to Jerusalem. Pilgrimages as penance or to give thanks were an expected feature of Christian life, so much so that the Anglo-Saxon Chronicles record years when pilgrimages were not made to Rome and Alfred only sent letters with couriers. Prescriptions were sometimes included in correspondence. A letter to Alfred from the Patriarch of Jerusalem, Helias, concerned medicines from Syria, with the purges scammony, and aloes, gum tragacanth, galbanum, balsam, and explicit instructions on taking theriac.[25] Theriac was an ancient mixture almost as complex as Mithridatium, considered to be an effective antidote to venoms of all kinds, whether animal or disease. From the classical period, it was later used to treat the plague. The importance attributed to Theriac as a treatment will be discussed a little later in history. For now it is enough to be aware that medicinal plants such as those above and important antidotes were known and possibly even available through travelling on pilgrimage, gifts sent between churches and possibly trade at this period.

In 986, Abbo of Fleury accepted an invitation from the Archbishops of York and Canterbury to settle in England at Ramsey Abbey. Clearly, he made the Abbey a place of true scholarship, as he brought wider knowledge from the Continent. His importance to our story rests on the standard of his teaching. For the monk Byrhtferth, this inspired him to become deeply interested in science. Byrhtferth later wrote a manual on science including astronomy, mathematics, and the signs of the zodiac.[26] Astrology is an aspect of medicine which we have not yet explored but will become increasingly relevant over the next several hundred years. Illustrations of the zodiac man available in the fourteenth century are witness to the importance of medical astrology. These show the figure of a man with the signs of the zodiac overlaid on or around his figure to indicate which part of the body each sign rules. They are placed with the ram over the head for Aries, the bull of Taurus at the throat and so on down to the fish of Pisces over the feet.[27]

It is not the intention of this chapter to include all the teaching on medicine available in England during the medieval period, simply sufficient to show that many sources were accessible for the educated reader who would be either a cleric or a member of the nobility.

One much read collection of recipes, *Macer Floridus de Viribus Herbarum*, stands out from the Middle English period. It has been dated to between 849 and 1112. John Harvey expresses the belief that it was actually written early in the eleventh century by a French physician, Odo Magdunensis.[28] The published version by Gösta Frisk has been brought together after consulting multiple surviving documents and the original was translated into many languages. English translations appear to date from just before or about 1400, but since lines from the Macer appear in the Regimen Sanitatis Salerno it is placed before it here.[29] The words 'Macer Floridus' were added later to the title.

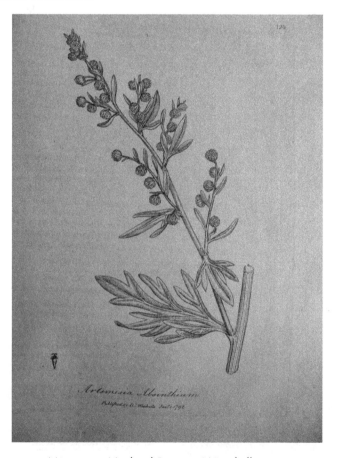

Mugwort, *Medical Botany*, Woodville.

The Macer begins with mugwort, which is given importance in the Anglo-Saxon Leechbooks in the Nine Herbs Charm. After giving the common name it is noted that the plant is also known as "Arthemisia" for the Greek goddess Diana who first found its virtues, and that the herb is especially suited to treating womens' sicknesses.[30] The ten recipes that follow illustrate a wide range of treatment methods. These include as drinks in water or wine, bathing, suffumigation, with chicken fat in an emplaster, added to wine must (freshly pressed juice of grapes containing yeast from the skins), to make a fermented medicinal wine and one which is more a charm, with the root hung around the neck against venom.

The way in which these will have been made remains exactly the same since ancient times. Suffumigation might be carried out by pouring boiling water on the herb and directing the steam into the vagina. Fire provides heat for making recipes and herbs are often pounded with a pestle in a mortar to varying degrees before being heated in a liquid often in an earthen vessel. The storage vessels discussed by Dioscorides will also be the same. In the Roman period stone stamps would have been used to impress the names of recipes and the ingredients into the soft ointment. These are not found from later periods, however. Where we are left often in the dark is in the absence of detailed instructions on amounts. Often this tells us that the recipe was intended for use by someone already experienced in medicine.

Conditions treated range from obstructed menstruation, urinary stone, stomach problems, and evil wrought by opium, to the bites of wild beasts. We will be looking at these and preparation methods in detail in the chapter on Pharmacy in the Medieval period. With each herb, either the Latin or Greek, sometimes both names are given after the common name. Then a botanical note may be added to aid identification, this is especially done as before where there is more than one species of the plant. In Macer, each herb is classified by its energetics or actions within the body of the patient. These fall into the familiar four categories from Hippocrates and Galen, hot, dry, cold, and moist. With herbs these are paired together so that a plant can be considered hot and dry or hot and moist, or any other combination. Sometimes it is even more complicated with a herb being heating to one level and yet also cooling to another.[31] One part of the plant may be perceived as in a different class to another as the action is different. A more detailed explanation may be helpful, and we can learn even more when it comes to the explanations of Culpeper.

Actions of the Herbs

Hot and dry herbs are many and as with the other temperaments they are divided into four degrees of heat or dryness. The first degree has the gentlest action on the body and the fourth the most severe. Herbs that are hot and dry in the first degree may be regarded as opening the pores of the skin to expel moisture, in modern terms it is diaphoretic. Chamomile is an example given in Macer.[32] Fennel is referred to as hot and dry in the second degree, which means it thins fluids for easier passage and will be diuretic.[33] Hyssop, hot and dry in the third degree increases the heat of digestion.[34] The fourth degree applies to the hottest and most drying herbs to be used with care, such as mustard, which is described as burning the skin and drawing out the viscous humours causing disease.[35]

Cold and dry herbs are again classified in degrees. The most powerful, hemlock, and henbane are cooling to the point of death which in modern terms is narcotic.[36,37] Sorrel is cold and drying in the third degree, as is greater plantain.[38,39] Presumably since lesser plantain, is not as strong in its action it should be considered as cold and drying in the second degree.[40]

Cold and moist is a term applied to fewer herbs, an example being orache, which, while cold in the first degree is moist in the second, dissolving hardness in the body.[41] Violet is described as right cold and moist in the fourth degree and is awarded the status of "virtue and myzt" in medicine. It cools "unkind heat" and treats epilepsy.[42]

Hot and moist is a comparatively rare classification, Galen did not partner hot and moist as the heat should produce drying. I can only find this hinted at under one of our chosen herbs in this text, elecampane. Horsehelne is the common name at this period. Macer gives it as being moist and cold in the first degree and hot in the second.[43] The taste is certainly hot and quite biting. This leads us into considering how the entries on our chosen herbs agree or differ with those of Dioscorides. His name does appear in the text, as well as those of Asclepius, Pythagoras, Constantine, and Galen.

Elecampane was also known as henula or horsehelne, meaning healing for horses. Leeches (herbalists) called the plant helenium. The shape is well known and so not described. Can we understand that it is moist and cold in the first degree and hot in the second? Dioscorides gave us little help, simply using it against venom of serpents. He did, however, comment on the sharp taste. We also found the digestive application in Columella. Now we can add to our knowledge, the first use is as an emmenagogue and the second as a diuretic. Seeing that the powdered root in honey is given for coughs, including for whooping cough and asthma brings us to an indication familiar today. In asthma, there is often hard phlegm that needs to be thinned and the area relaxed and opened for expectoration. Elecampane softens the hardness and opens the chest giving a warm feeling and encouraging release of the cold phlegm.

The pounded herb in a plaster is to be applied for sciatica, a use which is to be noted as we will not find it again. The leaves are soaked in pyment, which is a sweetened, spiced wine, and applied over the kidneys for pain and nephritic disease.[44] The juice of elecampane mixed with rue juice as a decoction is taken as a drink for those that are broken. This may be for fractures or have a less obvious meaning.[45]

We find that with plantain once again the two kinds are listed, the greater and the less. The lesser plantain is no longer named *lagopus* but now has become known as *lanceolata*, as it has a leaf shaped like a spear. Further, we are told that plantain is cold and dry in the third degree, following the classification of Greek and Roman medicine. It is stated that the greater plantain, in Greek, *arnoglossa*, is more powerful and has more virtues. Then follow seventeen uses for greater plantain beginning with the recommendation that it will dry moist wounds and a recipe with honey, salt, and vinegar is given. The drying property is also continued within the body as it stops internal bleeding. It is further applied with sheep's milk for cooling burns. More uses follow for treating dog-bites, dropsy, cleaning festering areas, and as a mouthwash or ear drops. The juice of plantain is often used. It is also recommended to treat coughs. In all, there are eighteen uses for greater plantain.[46]

The lesser ribwort has fewer uses, with treating swellings in the nostrils, or on the eyes, swellings of the parotid gland and for wounds. The juice is applied to sore eyes on soft wool, or it may be drunk to relieve the quartan fever, that is, a fever which returns on the fourth day. Ribwort stamped or pounded with wine or vinegar is applied for the foot ache, bladder sickness, and for dislocations of the body. It may also be mixed with swine's grease to make a plaster.[47] Use for dislocations is interesting as this is not a treatment we recognise with the plant today, which is limited to application for sprains, but the similarity as an anti-inflammatory can be appreciated.

With henbane, we are given both the Greek and Latin names and the warning that the herb is right cold, meaning cold in the fourth degree. A classification given to narcotic herbs, such as opium, that can cool the body to the extent the patient dies, according to the dose. It is recorded that leeches will not work with the henbane which has a black flower. This agrees with Dioscorides. The white flowered henbane is the best for medicine. The first use is for ache in the woman's breast, for which she must drink the juice. This repeats earlier advice. In fact, we can recognise the indications of pain from various causes in the genitals, eyes, ears, this time from worms, and feet from Dioscorides. For podagra, possibly gout or another foot complaint, the leaves and flowers are ground and applied if it is a hot condition. Dioscorides gave us the root chewed for toothache and here for toothache the root is sodden in vinegar and then held a long time in the mouth. This, we are told will quieten severe pain. Henbane is especially effective with toothache.

The green or fresh seed was ground small in the medieval period and used to cool inflammation that had produced hot, thick mucus. This is a much shorter list of conditions than before and may indicate a greater use of the juice. At the end of the entry, we are again warned that this herb and her plasters do much good, but if the herb is eaten it will cause woodnesse, a term meaning madness. The earlier warning was about eating the herb, but now this is extended as we read that the juice can have a similar effect when applied to a wound wherever it is on the body.

This observation might tie in with possibly increased use of the juice rather than the seed.[48]

Liquorice is described as the sweetest of herbs, not too moist nor too cold unless in the smallest measure. This we are led to appreciate is at the other end of the scale from powerful henbane—liquorice being good for all causes and with no harm. It is thoroughly recommended as an expectorant for hard coughs and helps sore throats, loss of voice, and moistens the lungs. It is described as being sodden in water until it is soft before pressing and drying into a liquorice stick and is then called chylum. This preparation is especially recommended for the lungs. It is also pointed out that there is no spice so good for the stomach. The writer is entirely taken with liquorice writing it does not torment as aloe does. I presume this refers to the gentler laxative effect than aloes.[49]

For ginger this author is almost silent, saying in a single sentence that its medicinal virtue is the same as that of pepper.[50] Disappointingly, he leaves it at that. Galingale and zeduale (Zedoary), close relations of ginger, have more detail. Pepper, since ginger is likened to it, we see is classed as hot and dry in the third degree, which is not quite the hottest, but has considerable heating effect, aiding the digestion.[51]

Betony has the Greek name *castreon*. Thirty-six uses are given, which is a huge leap forward from Dioscorides. We have to remember that Betony was adopted by the Romans from the Celts, so that traditional uses lie more with them. However, even with the wine recipe, it was indicated that it was good for many ills.[52] A couple of the recipes in Macer are ascribed to Pliny, not surprisingly this includes the direction to lay a circle of the fresh betony around a serpent, which will be powerless to cross out of it. The trapped serpent will then beat itself to death with its tail. This is a prime example of the superstitions Pliny enjoys. In later versions, the serpent was replaced by a mythical dragon. Another idea, which begins here and is not to treat illness is that eating or otherwise taking betony before drinking alcohol protects you from getting drunk. It is strange that there is no accompanying energetic classification. Since betony staunches bleeding, being stamped with salt as a plaster for all manner of wounds, it must have some drying properties. Betony is recommended here for most of the conditions we are considering, coughs, toothache, headache, treating the eyes, and fevers. It is variously mixed with oil of roses to drop into the ears, for empyema (suppuration in the lungs) the powder was sodden in honey. Betony in honey also treated less serious coughs and was laxative. The powdered leaf could be taken in wine for fevers. The diluted juice is drunk for the womb (a term then used for the stomach), the eyes, or vomiting. With the cotidian fever, understood as an ague, two ounces of plantain was mixed with one ounce of betony and the two pounded together in luke-warm water to make a drink.[53] This is an example of a recipe with some guidance on measurements. In fact, there are several under betony and these are recognisably Roman as the liquid measure is in ciatus, which corresponds to half a pint.[54]

Nettle is given the name of *Urtica* in Latin and described as hugely hot as it burns the fingers if handled. Nettle seed is taken internally with or without honey in drinks for coughs, pleurisy, and the lungs generally. Nettle leaf or seed taken in wine evidently was seen to act as an aphrodisiac as it stirred up heat. Conception was encouraged in animals by applying the juice or leaf to the female genital area. It is hard not to feel sorry for the beast. This is also recommended for a woman if very cold humours are blocking menstruation. A less painful suffumigation of myrrh and nettles would involve directing the steam into the vagina.

The decoction of nettles in oil was drunk as a laxative. Plasters of nettle and salt were applied to clean wounds and dog-bites. Using nettle leaf up the nose to stop a nose-bleed appears over and over in later recipes and we find the juice used here for the same purpose. Nettle in general is credited with drying up wicked humours, therefore it is hot and dry. The roots were pounded with vinegar to treat a swollen spleen. For podagre of the feet and all problems with the toes, the nettle could be applied as a plaster, in oil, or ointment.

With nettle we have a quality control note at the end in the instruction to gather the seed in August and dry it so that it will be "holsome" and can be profitably used.[55] There is not a great deal of reference to botanical detail unless a point needs to be made. With chamomile, the necessity of correct identification is pointed out with the instruction to compare the true plant with the stinking herb.

There are ninety-one herbs in the Macer including spices. The notes with the book are extremely helpful for anyone new to reading old text as they offer translations of many now unfamiliar words. Dating of the original manuscript of *Macer floridus de Viribus* was assisted by the mention of Walahfrid Strabo, Abbot of Reichenau and famed commentator on the Bible.

His poem *Hortulus*, written in Latin hexameters brings the medieval garden into sharp focus. I love to read his account of the labours of gardening, which anyone alive in any century immediately relates to. He writes beautifully of overcoming the initial patch of wild nettles, enriching the soil, the passing seasons and twenty-two herbs. He gives us visions of spring smiling in the leaves of the woods as it triumphs over the greed of winter, which had swallowed up the fruits of the previous year. He extols the healing powers of rue expelling noxious poisons, and recommends wormwood, which he writes "resembles the Mother of Herbs", a reference perhaps to mugwort also portrayed as the oldest of herbs in the Anglo Saxon Nine Herbs Charm in the Lacnunga.[56] With horehound, Walahfrid regards the scent as sweet, the taste bitter, and the greatest usefulness as an antidote to poisoning from aconite. Betony clearly has the same high value to him suggested in other texts for he writes, "Whatever your fancy, the wonderful powers Which this herb has will supply all your needs".[57]

Beauty appears in his garden in the shape of the lily, which he likens to glistening snow with a scent of sweetest frankincense, which, he would of course have been familiar with. The rose has similar praise being in his view the best fragrance, and he gives the lily and the rose as symbols of the Church's greatest treasures, the rose for the blood of martyrs and the lily a shining sign of faith.[58]

We find many correspondences in different works on the continent of Europe with the English. This is not surprising, as there were strong links between the established churches and monasteries here and their mother houses across the sea. The Anglo-Saxon Chronicles list many Viking raids. The Vikings regularly targeted rich Abbeys and churches because of the treasures they held and taking these, burned their books. As the surviving monks tried to restore their libraries, they appealed for replacement works from their mother houses. There was then, consistent traffic within the Orders.

In this chapter we have concentrated on those lines of contact, which proved valuable in keeping classical medicine alive in Britain through very turbulent times. The doctrine of Galen in medical treatment and application of the energetics of herbs has been our guide within the texts examined. I have translated the role of the leech as herbalist, and we can see that some leeches are using this knowledge, which, thanks to the re-workings of men like Oribasius and Paul of Aegina and channels of communication through the Church, were available in Britain.

References

1. John Davies, *A History of Wales* (London: Penguin Books, 2007), 41.
2. Michael Wood, *In Search of the Dark Ages* (London: BBC, 1981), 41.
3. Daithi o Hogain, *The Celts A History* (Woodbridge: The Boydell Press, 2002), 214.
4. G.N. Garmonsway, *The Anglo-Saxon Chronicle* (London: J.M. Dent Sons Ltd., 1953), 12.
5. Davies, *A History of Wales*, 50.
6. Wood, *In Search of the Dark Ages*, 42.
7. H.H. Scullard, *Roman Britain* (London: Thames and Hudson, 2002), 176.
8. Scullard, *Roman Britain*, 177.
9. J. Wacher, *The Towns of Roman Britain* (London: Batsford Ltd, 1979), 412–3.
10. Robert Baldick et al., (ed), *Bede A History of the English Church and People* (London: Penguin Classics, 1968), 58.
11. Scullard, *Roman Britain*, 178.
12. Garmonsway, *The Anglo-Saxon Chronicle*, 2.
13. Baldick et al., *Bede A History of the English Church and People*, 68–69.
14. J. Wacher, *The Towns of Roman Britain*, 178.
15. Baldick et al., *Bede A History of the English Church and People*, 203.
16. Ibid, 206.
17. C.H. Talbot, *Medicine in Medieval England* (London: Oldbourne, 1967), 11.
18. Talbot, *Medicine in Medieval England*, 11.
19. Scarborough, John "The Life and Times of Alexander of Tralles" *Expedition Magazine* 39, 2 (1997): *Expedition Magazine*. Penn Museum, 1997 Web. 20 Jun 2023. www.penn.museum/sites/expedition/?s=the+life+and+times+of+alexander+of+tralles.
20. Francis Adams, The medical works of Paulus Aeginata, the Greek physician translated into English: Vol. I, 1834. https://wellcomecollection.org/works/xe48qeu8. accessed May 2023.

21. Talbot, *Medicine in Medieval England*, 13.
22. Garmonsway, *The Anglo-Saxon Chronicle*, 24.
23. C.J.S. Thompson, The Mystery and Art of the Apothecary (Philadelphia: J.B. Lippincott & Co., 1929), 133.
24. Garmonsway, *The Anglo-Saxon Chronicle*, 72.
25. C.H. LaWall, *Four Thousand Years of Pharmacy* (Philadelphia: Lippincott Co., 1927), 125.
26. Talbot, *Medicine in Medieval England*, 23.
27. Carole Rawcliffe, *Medicine & Society in Later Medieval England* (Stroud: Sutton Publishing, 1997), 87.
28. John Harvey, *Mediaeval Gardens* (London: B.T. Batsford, 1981), 52.
29. Harvey, *Mediaeval Gardens*, 54.
30. Gösta Frisk (ed), *Macer Floridus de Viribus Herbarum* (Cambrifge, Mass: Harvard University Press, 1949), 57–59.
31. Ibid, 96.
32. Ibid, 143.
33. Ibid, 88.
34. Ibid, 98.
35. Ibid, 116.
36. Ibid, 133.
37. Ibid, 173.
38. Ibid, 146.
39. Ibid, 69.
40. Ibid, 72.
41. Ibid, 126.
42. Ibid, 76.
43. Ibid, 96.
44. Maggie Black, *The Medieval Cookbook* (London: British Museum Press, 1996), 121.
45. Gösta Frisk (ed), *Macer Floridus de Viribus Herbarum*, 96–97.
46. Ibid, 69–72.
47. Ibid, 72–73.
48. Ibid, 173–174.
49. Ibid, 192.
50. Ibid, 179.
51. Ibid,176.
52. Julius Moderatus Columella, *Of Husbandry in Twelve Books* (London: A. Millar, 1745), 552.
53. Gösta Frisk (ed), *Macer Floridus de Viribus Herbarum*, 105–109.
54. Ibid, 246.
55. Ibid, 66.
56. R. Payne (trans), *Walahfrid Strabo Hortulus* (Pennsylvania: Hunt Botanical Library, 1966), 41.
57. Payne (trans), *Walahfrid Strabo Hortulus*, 57.
58. Ibid, 63.

CHAPTER 10

Anglo-Saxon Leechbooks

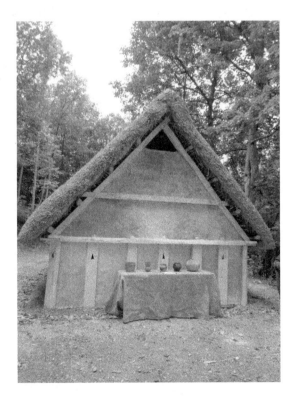

Anglo-Saxon House, Courtesy Weald and Downland Living Museum.

A s we have already seen, there is a degree of literacy in the newly established kingdom of England. The support for education from King Alfred the Great has resulted in translations of classical works into the Anglo-Saxon language. This era is, perhaps, where we come to appreciate most what a difference a change in language can make, for it has the power to open up works on medicine to a wider public.

The common theme even before the written history of Britain and on through the centuries has been a mix of races in the population, each wave of settlers or invaders bringing their own beliefs and practices. The Anglo-Saxon Leechbooks give us evidence not only of very different beliefs about the causes of disease from those followed by Greek and Roman medicine, but also of the mix of Pagan and Christian belief. Earlier, in Roman Britain, we saw that religious shrines to Roman and Gallic gods were present at the same time as Christian observance. Christianity was being spread by preaching and conviction among the more educated. Almost a thousand years later we see that a different attitude from the Church of overlaying pagan practice and mythology with Christian wording and festivals shows in the mix of Pagan and Christian medical ritual. That both are recorded alongside each other, sometimes even in the same recipe, enlightens us about the stages of partial conversion in common thought. Parts of England were still largely Pagan for the Church had been literally under fire.

For our appreciation of the content of the Leechbooks they have again been translated. Although fragments of the language survive within English, Anglo-Saxon sounds Germanic and foreign to us now. As with the medicine of previous cultures, we must beware of the vagaries of translation along with particular problems in identifying plants correctly. There have been several translations beginning with that of Oswald Cockayne in the nineteenth century, entitled rather impressively as *Leechdoms, Wortcunning and Starcraft of Early England*. An original edition of this book was the first translation I consulted, carefully copying recipes from the pages in pencil in the library, for it was considered too valuable a book for me to take home. Reprints are now widely available.[1]

For this book, I am mainly using Steven Pollington's translation, which covers the *Lacnunga, Old English Herbarium*, and the third *Book of Bald*.[2] I am then able to make comparisons of three Leechbooks with Cockayne's translation. However, this omits Books I and II of Bald that offer many sections and prescriptions, which Cockayne has identified as translations from Alexander of Tralles, Marcellus of Bordeaux, Oribasius, Galen, and Pliny.

Authority and experience ring out in these passages, there are very detailed descriptions of symptoms and diet is given first importance as treatment. There is also the enlightened advice in Book I that when applying strong leechdoms (medicinal remedies) the physical strength of the patient must be borne in mind. It is pointed out that treating a man used to hard labour is very different to treating a woman, or child.[3]

Aside from classical medicine there are recipes that speak of Saxon practitioners. A complex drink to be taken for nine days is headed "Oxa taught *us* this leechdom".[4]

Another prescription in Book II for treating lung disease reads "Dun taught it".[5] These references have been suggested to infer a school of medicine. In Book I, as in the *Lacnunga* and other *Books of Bald*, there are references to flying venom or poison as causing disease, and in response to this, prayers and an incantation described in the contents list as in Gaelic or Erse are the treatment.[6] The term elf shot is also used about a horse and explained in the glossary as a Scottish phrase relating to distension of the stomach of the animal caused in this instance by over-eating.[7]

Cockayne and Pollington added much background information on the period, magic, myth, and medicine. Another translation of the *Old English Herbarium* has been published since by Anne van Arsdall, challenging the earlier translations. Each translator believes their work is correct, since I am not skilled in the Anglo-Saxon language, I take an approach based on my knowledge and experience with herbs. I have been making selected recipes from the Pollington translation for over twenty years in conditions similar to those of the period during museum workshops. Where I note likely repeatable recipes using herbs which have the actions indicated I make them, and if they work, then they are in all probability correctly interpreted.

The book contains three separate manuscripts. We do not have all the material from Bald's Leechbooks, which is the oldest work; only the headings survive from the section on gynaecology, which is a great loss. Talbot points to accounts of surgery, which are an improvement on those of Celsus, and states that the Leechbooks embody some of the best medical literature available in the West.[8]

Looking at the seventy-three recipes in Pollington's translation of Bald, these range from the plainly practical and sensible, such as giving sweetened horehound for a cough, or applying ribwort to a dog bite with the addition of rue, an antibacterial herb often applied historically for pain. The instruction to use comfrey juice and warm cow's milk to wet your hands, hopefully washing them at the same time, before pushing a prolapsed bowel back into place and stitching it there with silk also strikes of good sense.

Giving the patient comfrey afterwards to speed healing would have been thoroughly approved until the recent concern over pyrrolizidine alkaloid content. In Bald, there is a reassurance that these remedies are, indeed, meant for practitioner use, where in one instance it gives the instruction that if the patient cannot keep the herbal porridge down it would be better not to attend as the patient is likely to die.[9]

In an age where hardship and famine had forced the poor to be very aware of all manner of wild foods and foraging and herbs were part of everyday life, there was much greater familiarity with plants than in modern times. Herb teas were made into wort drinks by fermentation with yeasts. These included wild raspberry and blackberry leaves, sweet woodruff, elder, chamomile, rose, horehound, mint, sage, and limeflower.[10] Ash keys were added as a preservative in small beer. Healthy ales included agrimony, meadowsweet, yarrow, heather, mugwort, alecost, alehoof, sweet gale, wormwood, sweet woodruff, and nettle.

Looking at Anglo-Saxon health, generally we may note the connections between predominant conditions as revealed by the archaeology and numbers of remedies for specific conditions in the medicine. After the Romans left, other influences, tastes and hardships became known. Judging by the indications in recipes the Anglo-Saxons appear to have suffered from loose and sore teeth and painful jaws. Arthritic jaw and wear from hard breads with some quern dust left in are likely to be responsible for some of these problems.[11] perhaps leading to abscesses. Also, in bad years, malnutrition and scurvy play a part. There are fifteen remedies for boils and blotches that also relate to diet. Skin problems from vitamin deficiencies, scabies (not always as we understand the cause), fleas, and lice are evident. There was infestation also with roundworms from salted pork and we see many recipes to treat all of these conditions, particularly worms.

Thinking of the frequently treated illnesses we are following through history, as noted in the chapter on Roman occupation and classical recipes that we examined in Celsus and Scribonius, those for eyes dominate. With all the indications of involvement of classical recipes it might be expected that eye remedies would be in line with Roman ideas. Certainly, all the main eye herbs are represented, but there is an absence of saffron, myrrh, and frankincense. Those listed are herbs readily obtainable in England with betony, agrimony, greater celandine, elderflower, fennel, and rue all present. In the Leechbooks, these are made into salves or washes. Toothache sufferers may have found themselves reliant on charms or prayers for their relief as found in the Lacnunga.[12] Flowers of nightshade too were given to eat. Cinquefoil is listed for a sore mouth or tongue, but toothache is not specified. Henbane is still used for the pain of toothache, also garlic, yarrow, betony, and rosemary, referred to as bothen, for a hollow tooth.[13] Elecampane was to be chewed to fasten loose teeth. In other recipes, cornflower, wood chervil, spearwort, and eating the flowers of nightshade appear. In Bald, there is also the instruction to chew pepper often.[14]

With headaches, there are many possible causes and we can guess at some of them just by knowing the actions of the herbs used. We predictably find betony and waybroad (greater plantain), specified for headaches. Betony in particular has always been associated with treating the head, and the first of twenty-two uses given for waybroad in the *Old English Herbarium* is headache.[15] Greater celandine and rue, suggest the eyes may be a cause of the problem.[16] Our native Mother of Thyme would work well with pain from congestion with a cold and has two references for headache.[17]

For coughs, taking in smoke from a ball of swail, sulphur, and incense through a horn, might be an effective way to treat the lungs. Brews for lung disease also contain effective herbs, such as elecampane and horehound. A tried and tested recipe is in the Lacnunga, "Against a cough, and narrowness: boil sage and fennel in sweetened ale and sip it hot; do likewise as often as it is needful".[18] Workshop participants found this very acceptable.

Also in the Lacnunga, there is a recipe against a cough which has four causes relating specifically to an imbalance in heat, cold, wetness, or dryness which appears to refer to the humours.[19] This one reference highlights the idea that some recipes in the Lacnunga also have classical sources. In the recipe a mashwort of wheat malt is made and boarfern, bishopwort (water betony or vervain), hindhealth, (possibly water agrimony), pennyroyal, and periwinkle added. The end note to forgo sour foods and salty, reinforces that this is a humoral prescription; therefore, we should look at the herbs in that light.

Gout appears from mentions in the texts to have been prevalent in this period, but some of these recipes may be referring to foot symptoms from lead poisoning as salt was extracted in lead containers and salted goods were sometimes kept in them.[20] These containers may, or may not have been a problem. One cure suggested is knee holly, or Butcher's broom as it is better known, in a drink.[21] Joint pain for the Anglo-Saxons, whether of the feet or elsewhere might require treatment with one or more of the following—nettle, colchicum, waybroad, marshmallow, or elderberry. There was archaeological evidence of general arthritis, from living and sleeping in damp conditions and undertaking hard manual labour.[22]

In the case of burns, treatments are surprising by modern ideas and we find dill flowers bound on and greater celandine is mixed with goat's grease and applied.[23] Not an idea that would have occurred to me when the juice is sufficiently caustic in itself to be applied to warts. Also in the *Old English Herbarium*, a plant called ancusa from Persia, has a glowing report for efficacy when the root is boiled in oil and wax added to make a plaster or poultice.[24]

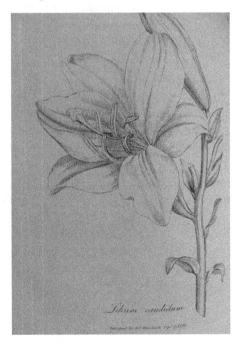

Madonna lily, *Medical Botany*, Woodville.

In Bald, we find a division is made between being burned by fire or scalded with hot liquid. For a burn from the fire, dog rose, lily, and speedwell are boiled in butter and smeared on. If, however, it is a scald, elm bark with lily root is boiled in milk and the liquid smeared on.[25] The strong tannins from the bark would be reduced by binding with protein in the milk, which would stop this application being too astringent. Herbs also mentioned are mistletoe and mandrake, the second perhaps for pain control. There is an elaborate recipe with mother of thyme, vervain, roses, silver filings, wax. and animal greases in the *Old English Herbarium*, which would be an impressive application for the wealthy patient.[26]

Fevers are many and varied, we find treatments for typhus and possibly malaria in the Leechbooks—the climate was at a peak high for temperature and these were rife, particularly in marshy areas. Waybroad has great recommendation as a treatment, along with ribwort which is specified in the *Old English Herbarium* for a fever on the fourth day.[27] Hounds' tongue has the same specification and we find delphinium for fever.

Some of the applications for boils and ringworm should work, but, as ever, there are herbs we are unsure of in translation and some completely unidentifiable. Reducing a boil is one of the twenty-nine uses of betony. In the *Old English Herbarium*, *Buoptalmon*, possibly meaning ox-eye daisy, was recommended for evil boils.[28] The root of Fox's foot (identity unknown) is intriguingly mixed with flour, vinegar, wine and fox's grease and applied on a cloth to strange boils.[29] There are many skin conditions such as impetigo and scabies, blotches, and pimples that appear in recipes. Leprosy was more of an umbrella term than necessarily a definite diagnosis. We find crowfoot in the *Old English Herbarium* for carbuncles, which is a gathering of boils.[30]

Coriander is applied for ringworm.[31] Sage is given for an itchy bottom, which was probably from internal worms. Other parasites resulting from poor diet and living conditions would be roundworms from eating salted pork, the larvae of these causing breathing problems and coughs as they crawl up through the lungs. There are numerous recipes against worms in all parts of the body. Waybread juice was favoured for internal worms.[32]

Special instructions of interest include warming either hen's fat to obtain the oil in an oyster shell and dripping it into the ears, or coriander juice and woman's milk treated in the same way. There are treatments of steam baths or bathings, with a hot stone lain on herbs with water poured over, reminding us of a northern European sauna approach. As already mentioned, taking in smoke from a ball of swail, sulphur, and incense through a horn for a cough might be an effective way to treat the lungs. Brews for lung disease also contain effective herbs, such as elecampane and horehound.

Of those recipes in drinks by far the most are taken in ale, a third of that number in water, and several in milk variously specified as from a cow, goat, or woman. Cures were not always so simple, however. In a case of palsy of the mouth, it is clear everything possible is being tried to apply sufficient heat to restore the muscular control of the patient who has clearly had a stroke.[33] After applying powdered coriander in milk to the cheek and dripping it into the ear, a complex bath of barks and herbs is prepared for a steam bathing to be carried out for as long as the patient can endure it. If that does not work even an anthill is boiled and the water applied to stimulate a response. There is also a drink and then letting blood with specific instructions. That it would all be unsuccessful is not the point, the care and thought that has gone into the treatment is considerable.

Another instance is in treating an enlarged body, presumably dropsy. A drink containing both diuretics and agrimony for the liver is accompanied by a porridge which includes elecampane for the digestion with other herbs, before giving a bathing.[34] The only undesirable part of this well thought out prescription is the inclusion of *thung*, which is generally taken to mean a poisonous substance, in a smear with more elecampane and dock to rub on.

Only ten recipes use animal parts, which were not simple fats. There are many herbs where identification is uncertain and elements which we cannot understand or find disgusting, but there are also diuretics given for the bladder, astringent herbs for diarrhoea, and clearly effective antibacterials and pain relief from henbane that would have worked. There are few exact measurements beyond third quantities, spoonfuls, or handfuls, except for libcorn seeds, which are always numbered.

With charms, magic, Christian ritual, and recipes including the magical numbers of three and nine, there are some impressive and elaborate examples. In recipe seventy-one, however, the *pater noster*, which is said three times once the recipe comes to the boil, and nine times after it is taken off the heat to stand, could simply be a timing mechanism.[35]

To gain some idea of the intention behind certain recipes in any of the Leechbooks, we should look first at some that illustrate the beliefs of causes of disease. They include humans being elfshot, flying venoms, a hint of humoral medicine and more generally not only evil from without, but, in line with the doctrine of the Christian church, evil from within the patient.

If we can imagine ourselves back into an age when stories of devils, gods, elves, charms, and magical powers were told in the firelight, we may more easily appreciate how in your mind the darkness takes on evil powers. When a family member was suddenly taken ill or suffered sharp pain, a natural response might be to describe it as feeling as if they had been shot by an arrow. The arrow would, of course have come from the bow of a wicked elf and, if physical proof were needed, they might recall tiny flint arrowheads turned up occasionally by ploughing.

Evidently there were different kinds of wicked elves causing disease. We find a recipe to treat water-elf sickness. "If someone should be in water-elf sickness then his fingernails will be pale, and eyes watery and he will look downwards. Do this for him as a leechdom: boarthroat, hassock, the lower part of iris, yewberry, lupin, elecampane, a sprig of marshmallow, fen mint, dill, lily, attorlothe, pennyroyal, horehound, dock, dwarf elder, felter, wormwood, strawberry leaf, comfrey; pour out with ale, add holy water".[36] This is followed by a charm to sing three times, and it is from this charm against injuries that burn, burst, spread, and throb and leave scars, that Pollington surmises it may be referring to chickenpox or measles.

We are not actually told whether this is to be drunk as well as being poured over the wound or eruption on the skin, but often in the Leechbooks both a drink and a salve are used to heal difficult wounds. An herbalist today would also treat both internally and externally. This applies whether this wound is a skin condition manifesting due to a systemic condition, or a straightforward wound in the body.

As to the contribution of the herbs, at first glance it seems a random list of nineteen herbs but looking at their identities, these were certainly not just anything to hand. Of this great list of herbs comfrey heals and soothes internally. The elecampane, boarthroat (carline thistle), and horehound are strongly antibacterial, the iris at a lesser level, while the pennyroyal is antiseptic and cooling. They have all been used on wounds as well as internally against bacteria, the water mint also might be cooling when there is burning pain and wormwood too was commonly used as an external pain killer in the past. The lily, marshmallow, and wild strawberry would soothe as anti-inflammatories.

Felter is translated by Cockayne as lesser centaury, a bitter stimulant herb and I have noted the presence of felter with pennyroyal, thyme, and wormwood in a drink to combat inflammation in the *Lacnunga*.[37] Translators have been unable to identify hassock and atterlothe, although Pollington's literal translation is "poison hater" which would bring it into line with the antibacterials.[38] The yewberry, which would be harmless if the seed is removed, has had a use on wounds. Aside from the lupin, dill and dwarf elder we now have an understandable prescription for an inflamed, possibly open skin condition with herbs to stimulate healing, act as antibacterials, anti-inflammatories, analgesics and in the case of lupin and dill, fight the elfish source of the problem by magic. These two herbs also appear in a salve for the elvish race and another prescription for elf sickness. I suspect the dwarf elder may have a similar role.

Again in Pollington's translation of the third book of Bald we have, "Make a salve for the elvish race, and nightgoers, and the people with whom the devil has intercourse, take ewehumble (hop), wormwood, bishopwort, lupin, ashthroat (vervain), henbane, harewort (cudweed), whortleberry shoots, cropleek, garlic, hedgerive, (cleavers), corn cockle, fennel, put these plants into a vessel, set it under an altar, sing nine masses over it, boil in butter and in sheep's grease, add a lot of holy salt, strain through a cloth, throw the plants into running water. If any evil temptation should befall one, or an elf, or a nightgoer, let him smear his face with this salve, and put it on his eyes, and where his body may be sore, and smoke him, and make the sign over him often, his case will soon be better".[39]

Note this recipe is also for protection from temptation to do evil, as not only outside evil, but also evil done by the patient was believed to bring on sickness.

The plants are a mix of narcotic and potentially toxic herbs, which can at a lesser dose be mood and mind altering. Perhaps this is understandable in a prescription against nightmares. We also have anti-viral herbs and cleansers believed powerful against witchcraft and disease—garlic and onion, wormwood and fennel. Hedge-rive or cleavers is also a deeply protective plant as it stimulates the lymphatic system. Once again, we have lupin as a protector, another potentially toxic plant.

The manuscript of the Lacnunga, which is in the British Library in London, dates from around 1000 AD and was written by two scribes. Pollington muses that it may have been a commonplace book of jottings, as it is not organised and contains many errors. It has perhaps the strongest range of contrasts in illustrating perceived causes of illnesses and responses, ranging from polypharmacy, through simple effective remedies to magical charms and complex Christian prayer and ritual. The numbers three and nine appear twenty-seven times but may not all have a magical connotation. With twenty-nine Christian prayers and seventeen other charms, the Lacnunga is rich in this approach to healing.

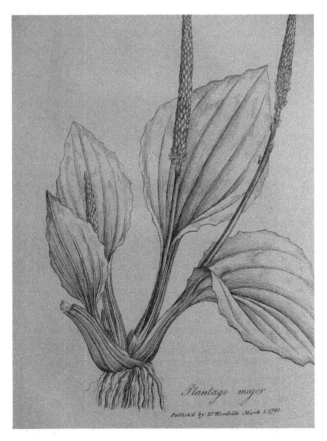

Greater plantain, *Medical Botany*, Woodville.

There are long, complex recipes that defy imagination—the most famous piece of all is the Nine Herbs Charm in the Lacnunga.[40] Listening to it recited in Anglo-Saxon is to be transported into this period of history. Understanding the selection of herbs for such an elaborate remedy has to take into account it is a charm. Mugwort oldest of herbs and waybroad as the mother of herbs seem right to our knowledge, waybroad, known to us as *Plantago major* was tremendously important during this period. Fennel and nettle are also picked out for special attention in other recipes. With crab apple legend enters the recipe and atterlothe we cannot translate. The nine poisons against which the herbs have power have colours from red, through blue, yellow, and green to purple and sound almost like the progress of really bad bruising.

A number of different flying venoms were believed to cause various contagious diseases. Pollington's translation of the charm gives the nine herbs power over nine different coloured poisons, which might fly from any corner of the earth. Although he uses the word 'infections', he points out that he is not doing so with "any implications of precise medical terminology".[41] Cockayne uses the terms flying vile things and "loathed ones".[42] The nine herbs in question are not known for their anti-infective properties, but it is after all, a charm. Sometimes we have to accept we do not have the knowledge of that period to put something into the proper context for understanding.

In the Lacnunga eighteen, we have a salve for flying venom and a sudden eruption. If maythe does refer to chamomile, then it is a mix of anti-inflammatory herbs with waybroad (greater plantain), water dock root and pellitory of the wall.[43] The quantities of the herbs are each a handful. Cockayne has not translated hammerwort in this recipe, which is number six in his translation, yet Pollington has given one possible translation for the herb as pellitory of the wall.[44,45] This is a diuretic, and to a modern herbalist it might seem an understandable application when mixed with an eggshell full of honey and clean butter for treating skin eruptions. Butter salves are satisfying to make, keep well in wooden boxes, and would have been made in spring or early summer, preferably after the animals producing milk for the butter had eaten new grass.

Looking at the recipes again, with some conditions there are helpful herbs being used. With bladder stones, we find a number of diuretic and well supported herbs, cough herbs are effective and centaury stands out as an empiric remedy possibly for treating a cough due to reflux, but that could be my modern imagination. Nevertheless, someone could have found that it just worked in certain situations. There are many options with cough herbs, and it is up to the practitioner to know which will be right for the individual patient.

One recipe we have made several times as a successful remedy, which is repeated in later collections of recipes reads, "against a cough: take drops of honey and wild celery's seed, and dill's seed; pound the seeds small, mix with the drops thickly, and pepper it heavily; take three spoons full having fasted overnight".[46] The lung pottage in which hyssop is boiled in butter, with radish, elecampane, and a portion of barley meal for a long time; is another tried and tested, tasty recipe.[47]

All four haemorrhoid remedies would work, as would all of the recipes for lungs, but pepper in eye recipes sounds painful. In a sleeping drink we have a combination of radish, hemlock, wormwood, and henbane pounded, taken in ale. This is left to stand overnight before drinking, and alarmingly no quantities are given either of herbs or dosage.[48] Another where henbane seed and mint juice are smeared on the head is a good deal safer.[49] The sleeping remedies would be effective, but strangely when it comes to toothache reliance is not always on the familiar henbane, which works brilliantly, but on charms! When it comes to treating poison, we find horehound, which we read about in Walahfrid Strabo's poem.

Of 194 recipes in my analysis, several are for treating animals, including cattle, sheep, pigs, and horses, only ten contain animal ingredients other than simple fats. Twenty-five drinks are in ale or beer, with Welsh ale mentioned twice. Twelve are decoctions or infusions in water with eleven in wine or with wine specified as first choice. Milk is from a goat, hind or woman, and again edible recipes are included. With the five for the eyes, there are twenty-three salves. Measures are rarely given except libcorn and peppercorns are numbered, an ounce appears, and ten pennyweight, also a sester of ale, otherwise it is predictably bowlful, eggshellful, etc. Herbs are pounded to dust, there is often the instruction to wring herbs or infusions through a cloth, and an eye salve is kept in a horn. There are more making stone bathings, using a whetstone in one case and cold water is also heated with a hot iron.

The most ingenious instructions are to give anaesthesia by seating the patient in cold water to numb the backside before lancing an eruption, and a salve in number forty-nine for inflammation containing antibacterials and pain relief where the pounded herbs in butter are left in a bronze vat until the mix turns blue before straining and applying.[50,51] Some womens' problems are addressed, such as morning sickness, pain of womens' teats, and being unable to bear a child.

The *Old English Herbarium* contains clear material from classical sources and is ordered in such a way as to suggest it was meant to be used professionally. Pollington identifies that this has been the case from notes made later in the margins. Each chapter concerns one herb which is named in Latin and gives numbered uses of that herb. This material comes from a series of documents, the first chapter on betony has been identified as having been a separate work and much comes from the Latin Herbarium of Pseudo-Apuleius, which in turn was made up of several other works. The book names 159 plants in 185 recipes.

The numbered uses range from a simple "CXXVI Herb fenuculus that is fennel. 1. For coughing and shortness of breath. 2. For pain of the bladder"—both uses still followed today—to betony with twenty-nine uses. These range from treating the eyes and ears, to foot disease and from protection against nightmares to dog bites, all of which detail covers almost three pages of the book[52]—this is contrary to the limited knowledge and use of betony in modern herbal medicine. My experience in practice using betony as a herbalist, however, was very positive with many of the historical uses. This included using betony with cowslip and thyme to cure a patient of nightmares that had given her such a deep fear of sleeping that she had been an insomniac for several years.

This introductory list of contents is followed by each of the herbs in more detail, often including actual recipes. Some of these have measurements of ingredients, particularly for internal remedies, but many others do not. Again, some measurements are problematic in themselves, as when faced with two pennies weight, or how much is as much as you can take with two fingers? Others such as fifty grains, tremisses weights, or pounds and ounces are exact. Peppercorns, ivy seeds, and corns of coriander seeds are numbered. An oil jar of pulicaris seeds has one imagining an amphora, which would be a huge amount—I presume there was a smaller oil jar. Wooden vessels are stated for pounding ingredients, while cornflower juice is kept in a ram's horn for winter use. Orris root is dried by hanging it in a linen cloth in the shade and feathers and wool are used to apply preparations gently.

Greek and Roman names for plants are given regularly with some English translations. There are references to Homer and Esculapius as well as gods and goddesses with legends accompanying the plants. Twenty-six recipes are magical and six have special instructions including timings linked to the phase of the moon. Ashthroat, known to us as vervain, is to be taken on Midsummer Day and hellebore root to be taken around midsummer. It is reassuring to see that there are cautions when giving hellebore, always mixing with food, according to the quality of the disease. There is also a note with a treatment for itch and pain in the genitals that if the patient is a woman then the same should be made up for her and applied by a midwife.[53] This text may have been available to such women since we find also the use of *dictamnum* for stimulating loss of a stillborn child.[54]

When it comes to heart pain, as with the recipe in the *Lacnunga* the reader hopes it has nothing to do with the physical heart or the patient may die. One recipe stands out as an ingenious way to judge the presence of infection—the herb ashthroat and wheaten corn are laid against a festering dog bite and absorb the moisture they are drawing away. When soaked, the corn is put before a hen and the treatment is continued until the hen is happy to eat it.[55]

The number of drinks given in wine is a much higher proportion than in the other books with seventy to just over forty prepared in water, ten in beer or ale and seven in vinegar. There is only a single mention of goat's milk. Herb juices are used a great deal either drunk alone, in wine or vinegar. They were also applied again in wine or vinegar, some, such as cleavers, betony, and henbane, were dripped into the ear. Rose juice has several mentions. There are more poultices than salves, with many herbs also applied in oil, honey or wine.

Reading the recipes from all three manuscripts, there is plentiful evidence of two of the three Anglo-Saxon methods of healing, that of spell medicine using charms and herbal medicine either in herbal recipes to apply or drink, or sometimes as dietary advice, and in pottages. Of the third, healing by hand, or surgery, there is less, but it does exist in other documents. When the vitality of a person appeared to be sucked out of them leaving them in an unhealthy state, these negative qualities, which now predominated would be removed from the body by purging, emetics, or bleeding, reminding us of classical medicine.

Just as diet was an important part of Roman medicine, we also find dietary recipes and restrictions, as with fasting before taking the remedy. The number of herbs used medicinally runs into several hundred and in the Lacnunga and Book of Bald this includes the barks of a dozen trees, which largely continue in use through the medieval period.

Although herbs introduced by the Romans are evident, some of which were still readily available, a great many could be picked from the countryside in Britain. Names for the herbs are evocative and beautiful and often illustrate the connection people felt for plants. My favourites are aethelfarthingwort for chickweed, ashthroat for vervain, ewehumble for hop, harespeckle for viper's bugloss, and wolf's comb, which clearly is teasel. Those herbs in my analysis showing most use in the *Lacnunga, Old English Herbarium* and the third *Book of Bald* are betony, waybroad, rue, wormwood, and fennel.

In Pollington's translation, wormwood (*Artemisia* spp.) appears in thirty-two recipes, mostly in the Lacnunga or Bald, for pains, in pottages for lung disease, in a sleeping drink, and a Holy salve. There is definitely a protective theme as wormwood also appears in a drink against temptations, salve against the elvish race, elf sickness, water-elf sickness, and the devil and madness.

Rue also appears in the Book of Bald to protect against the devil, madness, and elf sickness and the same Holy Salve. For a dog bite, it is boiled in butter with ribwort and applied.[56] In the *Lacnunga*, rue treats heart pain, inflammation, and much more. Again, pain is a common indicator. "Against headache: rue and pennyroyal and beet's root and woodruff, take as much of each as you may pick up with your forefinger and thumb; pound them small, and melt butter and take off all the scum, and put it into a clean pan and boil the plants well in it, and wring them through a cloth; add oil if you can get it; and smear his head with it wherever it aches".[57]

Fennel is in sixteen recipes in the Lacnunga—most importantly it is in the nine herbs charm.[58] It is included in a general panacea, a drink against evil, and in several salves, including a Holy Salve. Again in Bald, the implication is that it is working against evil in a recipe for devil sickness and madness.[59]

From the times of famine towards the end of the millennium life expectancy is correspondingly low. Judging from cemetery evidence, there is a tendency for women to have an average earlier death rate, more dying between twenty and thirty years old, than between thirty and forty-five.[60] Few people of either sex lived to be over fifty. The bread winner would, of course, have first serving of any food. Hunger was such at times that infanticide was legal if being left to live the child would die of starvation. Children might also be sold into slavery where they would at least be fed.

In the monasteries, food could be consistent and generally better than for the poor feeding themselves, although there was still quite an emphasis on bread as the staple. Only the rich could afford aged cheese, the poor ate new cheese, referred to as green, which might have been curdled with thistle or teasel flowers, lady's bedstraw, or nettle.[61]

For those better off, their bread might be sweetened with honey and spiced with poppy, cumin, caraway, or sweet cicely seeds on feast days. Cumin may possibly refer to native black cumin. A culinary herb list might also include herbs such as chervil, dill, fennel, celery, parsley, mint, garlic and onions of all kinds. Also in the cookery in rich households, we find mustard seed, sage, rue, tansy, radish, savory, pennyroyal, and sweet gale. In the diet of the rich fruit and flowers were popular, and colourings and garnishes were important. The combination of flowers with meats dates to pre-Norman times. Elderflower and haw blossom might be partnered with white meats and red rose petals with red meats.[62] These three flowers are effective both in savouries and delicious sweet desserts as practical experiment has proved. Other herbs in sauces are dittany, tarragon, basil, parsley, sage, costmary, thyme, garlic, lovage, coriander, bay, cumin, fennel, rosehips, elderberries, and mulberries.

With the aid of the Leechbook recipes we have also explored diet and general health in this period. Examination in detail enables a wide picture of life at the time to be appreciated through the inter-relationships between living conditions, good diet or malnutrition, and the prevalence of certain diseases. Where recipes can be traced to specific sources, this gives an insight into travel and communication. The choice of herbs and whether the balance is heavier on those growing in Britain or imported tells us also about trade. In addition, a letter from the Patriarch of Jerusalem to King Alfred on the subject of exotic herbs and preparations included in Bald has reminded us of the strong bonds that survived across sea and land.

References

1. Oswald Cockayne, *Leechdoms, Wortcunning and Starcraft in Early England* (London: Longman, Roberts, and Green, 1864–66).
2. Stephen Pollington, *Leechcraft* (Norfolk: Anglo-Saxon Books, 2000).
3. Cockayne, *Leechdoms, Wortcunning and Starcraft in Early England*, Vol. 2, 85.
4. Ibid, 121.
5. Ibid, 293.
6. Ibid, 11.
7. Ibid, 157 & 401.
8. C.H. Talbot, *Medicine in Medieval England* (London: Oldbourne, 1967), 19.
9. Pollington, *Leechcraft*, Bald Leechbook, (22), 389.

10. Anne Hagen, *A Second Handbook of Anglo-Saxon Food and Drink* (Norfolk: Anglo Saxon Books, 1999), 236.
11. Hagen, *A Second Handbook of Anglo-Saxon Food and Drink*, 362.
12. Pollington, *Leechcraft, Lacnunga*, (22), 191, (166), 237.
13. Pollington, *Leechcraft*, Bald III, (4), 385.
14. Ibid, (4), 385.
15. Pollington, *Leechcraft, Old English Herbarium*, (II), 249.
16. Ibid, (LXXV), 261.
17. Ibid, (101), 335.
18. Pollington, *Leechcraft, Lacnunga*, (107), 223.
19. Ibid, (180), 243.
20. Anne Hagen, *A Handbook of Anglo-Saxon Food* (Norfolk: Anglo-Saxon Books, 1998), 45.
21. Pollington, *Leechcraft, Old English Herbarium*, (59), 315.
22. Hagen, *A Second Handbook of Anglo-Saxon Food and Drink*, 12.
23. Pollington, *Leechcraft, Old English Herbarium*, (75), 321.
24. Ibid, (168), 367.
25. Pollington, *Leechcraft*, Bald III, (29), 391.
26. Pollington, *Leechcraft, Old English Herbarium*, (101), 335.
27. Ibid, (98), 333.
28. Ibid, (CXLI), 273.
29. Ibid, (47), 311.
30. Ibid, (9), 293.
31. Ibid, (104), 337.
32. Ibid, (10), 285.
33. Pollington, *Leechcraft*, Bald's Leechbook, (47), 399.
34. Ibid, (26), 391.
35. Ibid, (68), 407.
36. Ibid, (63), 405.
37. Ibid, Lacnunga, (74), 213.
38. Pollington, *Leechcraft*, 98.
39. Pollington, *Leechcraft*, Bald, (61), 401.
40. Pollington, *Leechcraft, Lacnunga*, (79), 215.
41. Ibid, 215.
42. Cockayne, *Leechdoms, Wortcunning and Starcraft in Early England* (Cambridge: Cambridge University Press, 2012), Lacnunga 33.
43. Pollington, *Leechcraft, Lacnunga*, (18), 189.
44. Cockayne, *Leechdoms, Wortcunning and Starcraft in Early England*, Lacnunga, 7.
45. Pollington, *Leechcraft*, 126.
46. Pollington, *Leechcraft, Lacnunga*, (11), 187.
47. Ibid, (60), 201.
48. Ibid, (62), 201.
49. Ibid, (157), 233.
50. Ibid, (98), 223.
51. Ibid, (49), 199.

52. Pollington, *Leechcraft, Old English Herbarium*, (1), 281–285.
53. Ibid, (123), 343.
54. Ibid, (63), 317.
55. Ibid, (4), 289.
56. Pollington, *Leechcraft, Bald*, (34), 393.
57. Pollington, *Leechcraft, Lacnunga*, (17), 189.
58. Pollington, *Leechcraft, Lacnunga*, (79), 215.
59. Pollington, *Leechcraft*, Bald, (64), 405.
60. Ann Hagen, *A Handbook of Anglo-Saxon Food* (Norfolk: Anglo-Saxon Books, 1998), 135.
61. Hagen, *A Handbook of Anglo-Saxon Food*, 29.
62. Ibid, 64.

SECTION V

HERBS AND INFLUENCE FROM SALERNO
AND BEYOND | 8TH CENTURY—1443

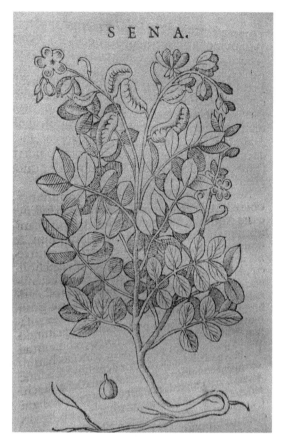

Sena, *Opera de Medicamentorum*, Mesue.

Key Figures

Geber (c721–815), Mesue (780–857), Serapion (802–849), Al Rhazi, (Rhazes) (c864–925), Albucasis (936–1013), Avicenna (980–1037), Ibn Botlān (died c1068), William of Normandy, reigned 1066–1087, Constantine the African (c1020–1087), Nicolai of Salerno, (dates unknown), Trotula, (dates unknown), Ibn al-Baytar (1197–1248), John of Gaddesden (1280–1361), Physicians of Myddfai.

Key Texts

Liber Continens, Rhazes.
Liber al Mansorum, Rhazes.
A Treatise On The Smallpox And Measles, Rhazes.
Canon of Medicine, Avicenna.
Trotula.

Antidotarium of Niccolo Salernitano, Nicolai of Salerno.
The Tacuinem Sanitatis (originally Taqwim as-Ṣiḥḥa), Ibn Botlān.
Syriac Book of Medicines.
Rosa Anglica, John of Gaddesden.
Chaucer's *Canterbury Tales*, Geoffrey Chaucer.
Red Book of Hergest.
Fourteenth Century Manuscripts.
XVth Century Leechbook.

Roles of Women in Medicine

A number of references confirm that women practised as empiric physicians in Salerno.[1] In the fourteenth and fifteenth centuries in Europe, midwives were licensed after being examined by a physician as to their competence.[2] In England women could style themselves physician or leech, be midwives and herb gatherers without examinations. Wives and daughters were expected to contribute to the trade of their husband or father,[3] and the widow of an apothecary could continue his business.[4]

Quality Control

In the Arab world, pharmacies were regulated and inspected, pharmacists took examinations to qualify for a licence.[5] In England, some imported drugs were required to be garbled at the ports before being landed. This method of testing for adulteration is recorded as being enforced and the perpetrator fined in 1456.[6]

Herb Energetics

Avicenna's Canon explains herbal energetics in detail.[7] In Europe the health guide, *Tacuinum Sanitatis* refers to the energetic status of the herbs, and classifies actions of the emotions, diet, and environmental influences.[8]

Travel and Trade

The first Crusade to re-take Jerusalem began in 1095 and with an already established fine reputation the hospital in the convenient port of Salerno became the base hospital for returning Christians.[9] Further campaigns continued throughout this period. There would no longer be safe passage granted to pilgrims as it had been in the days of Alfred the Great. Those who fought in the Crusades in Syria and Palestine returned with knowledge of new plant medicines and tastes, such as oranges from Jaffa, and sugar. This would stimulate demand for these to be imported.

Introduction

While Bede was writing his history in the monastery at Jarrow in the eighth century, the Arabs, having earlier conquered most of the Middle East, had colonised Spain. First the Abbasid Caliphate, established in Baghdad in 750 and then the western Caliphate of Cordoba in 929 became centres of civilisation and learning with vast libraries, hospitals and dispensaries. These were the main centres for development of herbal medicine.[10]

European practice and the first pharmacopoeias in the West owe much to the knowledge of Arabic pharmacy. In the western Caliphate, Avenzoar wrote on syrups and electuaries, while Avicenna introduced pills coated with gold and silver leaf to enhance their effect.[11] Mesue (780–857) was another highly knowledgeable eminent physician in the service of Haroun Al Raschid, Caliph of Bagdad. Serapion (802–849) also wrote on pharmacy and both appear as authorities in the *Opera de Medicamentorum*, which we will consider in a future chapter on the Pharmacopoeia.

Rhazes and Avicenna lived in the period of Persian Renaissance. Medical texts were originally written in one of several languages, Greek, Syriac, Persian, and Indian. When the Arabs had conquered Egypt centuries before, classical Greek philosophy was already established at the medical school of Alexandria and before this school closed one of the last teachers took his knowledge to Baghdad.[12] Openness of the Islamic culture towards knowledge from any source meant there were many combinations of translations. As in the West, talented physicians received patronage at the courts of princes and the Caliphs vied each other to have the best. Avicenna found himself an unwilling pawn in their rivalry.

Norman rule in England meant the end of the constant battles between Vikings and Saxons and once the time of adjustment to the new monarchy was over, England flourished and grew economically. This in turn led to a rise in population so that just before the Black Death numbers were high. When the Black Death arrived in 1348, it appears to have taken more of the older members of society and children. Average life expectancy was twenty-nine and a half years for a woman and twenty eight for a man. Many plague victims were older. Recovery of society was initially swift, as tenancies were re-allocated to the next generation but the plague returned less ferociously in 1361, taking the new generation. With plague again in 1368–9, 1371, 1375, and 1390, by the end of the century the population had declined considerably.[13]

The Hundred Years War with France meant sporadic battles on French soil from 1337 onwards. Ladies in large households were therefore often left in charge of running them. They needed knowledge of many skills, and were making remedies for the sick in their household. With foreign trade increasing, Southampton was a major port for incoming spices. Cloves, cinnamon, and galingale came from the East Indies, while more cinnamon and the finest ginger were from India. Sugar arrived in loaf form from Sicily with candied peel and comfits for the rich. Demand for sugar was raised after the return of Crusaders who had experienced sucking sugar cane in Tripoli.[14] Almonds, pomegranates, figs, oranges, and lemons came from Southern Spain.

This section closes with an in-depth study of several texts in order to try to establish how much Arabic influence is evident in medicinal recipes here, how the herbs we are following are being used, and how conditions are treated, now that a millennium has passed since the Romans left Britain.

References

1. Monica Green, *The Trotula* (Philadelphia: University of Pennsylvania Press, 2002), 48.
2. Carole Rawcliffe, *Medicine & Society in Later Medieval England* (Stroud: Sutton Publishing, 1997), 198.
3. Henrietta Leyser, *Medieval Women* (London: Phoenix, 1996), 163.
4. Leyser, *Medieval Women* 178.
5. Basher Saad & Omar Said , *Greco-Arab & Islamic Herbal Medicine* (New Jersey: John Wiley & Sons, 2011), 7.
6. C.J.S. Thompson, *The Mystery and Art of the Apothecary* (Philadelphia: Lippincott Co., 1929), 93.
7. Laleh Bakhtiar, (adapt), *Avicenna Canon of Medicine* (Great Books of the Islamic World inc., 1999), 220–221.
8. L.C. Arano, *The Medieval Health Handbook.Tacuinum Sanitatis.* (New York: George Braziller, 1976).
9. Charles LaWall, *Four Thousand Years of Pharmacy.* (Philadelphia: Lippincott Company, 1927), 130.
10. Saad & Said, *Greco-Arab & Islamic Herbal Medicine* 7.
11. La Wall, *Four Thousand Years of Pharmacy*, 107.
12. Soheil M. Afnan, *Avicenna* (Kuala Lumpur: The Other Press, 2009), xv.
13. Francis Pryor, *Britain in the Middle Ages* (London: Harper Collins Publishers, 2006), 231–232.
14. Margaret Wade Labarge, *A Baronial Household of the Thirteenth Century* (London: Eyre & Spottiswoode, 1965), 96.

CHAPTER 11

Arabic Medicine and Pharmacy | 750–1037

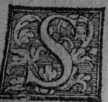

largius sumptum parit.

MESVES.

YRVPVS Glycyrrhizæ tuſ=ſim antiquam iuuat, thoracem & pulmones expurgat. Reci pit glycyrrhizæ vncias duas, a-dianti albi vnciam vnam, hyſſo pi ſicci vnc. dimidiam, horas vigintiquatuor macera aquæ lib.quatuor,coque ad dimidias, expreſſum percoque cum mellis,ſaccha.peni-diorum ana vnc.octo, aquæ roſarum vnc.ſex.

CHRISTOPHORVS.

Yrupus de liquiritia ſecundum hãc deſcrip. confert principaliter paſſionibus pectoris & pulmonis, & maxime tuſſi antiquæ factæ ... matica quæ non eſt multæ

Liquorice Syrup, *Opera de Medicamentorum,* Mesue.

U nder Arabic rule huge contributions in the field of medicine were made. Their pharmacy in particular was highly developed from the eighth century onwards as the many valuable herbs growing in arid environments were studied. The East was the habitat of the trees and shrubs that supplied the then known world with aromatic gums and valuable spices such as olibanum, myrrh, cinnamon, and cassia. We also owe increased use of senna, rhubarb, tamarind, musk, camphor, nutmegs, cloves, saffron, and liquorice to Arabic influence.[1] Arabia Felix, now Dhofar in Oman, had commanded the main trade route of the spice merchants east to west, which also brought them into touch with the Orient.[2]

In the sixth century, Khusraw Andsharwin (who ruled the Sāsānian empire from 531 to 579) protected the Nestorian Christians from persecution after the schism, which split the Eastern Church into three. Their centres were at Edessa and Gundishāpūr in southern Persia where there was a medico-philosophical school. The Nestorian Christians translated Aristotle, Hippocrates, and Galen into Syriac. Later some of their number travelled to Baghdad and translated works either from Syriac into Arabic or from Greek into Arabic.[3] Andsharwin also sent his physician Burzuya to India. He returned with Indian physicians and books on Indian medicine to enrich the knowledge of Persia.[4] There is no space here to explore Sanskrit sources in Arabic medicine, in particular those used by Rhazes, however, there is an excellent work available for further study.[5]

The first known date of a pharmacy shop in Baghdad is 762. The work of pharmacists was monitored by the State and they were obliged to pass exams to qualify for a licence.[6] The language of the pharmaceutical manuals was Arabic, but as many physicians were Persian or Syriac Persian names for drugs and diseases became used in Arabic from early times.[7] Hospitals were established in both Caliphates. The first in the sense of a modern hospital was founded by Caliph Harun al Raschid in Baghdad in AD 805.[8] The great hospital of Al-Mansúr had male and female wards open to all who were sick. There were dedicated wards for fever patients, eye patients, sufferers from dysentery and like conditions and for those undergoing surgery. The mentally ill had separate chambers. Other rooms were kitchens, stores, lecture rooms, and a dispensary.[9]

The Arabians combined Greek and Jewish medicine with Egyptian practice in pharmacy. Apothecaries were divided into those who sold simple medicines for agreed prices and the more professional compounders who dispensed prescriptions for physicians.[10] Prescriptions were made up of a base ingredient with adjuvants, synergists, and succedanea. Adjuvants should be interpreted as helpful support for the main ingredient; synergists would be more medicinal substances that worked well together to bring about a desired action; and succedanea are substances seen as interchangeable with others, if appropriate. The Arabs combined Greek and Jewish medicine with Egyptian practice in pharmacy and added the astrology and occult lore of both Egypt and India. They are believed to have taken the Egyptian word for the black Nile valley soil 'khem' and applied this to chemistry. With their prefix 'al' this becomes alchemy—the black art.[11]

Jabir ibn Hayyan known in the West as Geber is an almost mythical figure, his dates are uncertain, (c721–815). Most of the Latin treatises attributed to him are thought to be spurious, but some in Arabic are regarded with more respect. He was the only Arabian who had studied medicine in Baghdad to write exclusively about chemistry.[12] His researches were concentrated on alchemy involving distillation, which he detailed. Such descriptions as his sublimation of sulphur, and producing salammoniac from sublimation of common salt, in his treatise on furnaces, led to him being recognised as founding modern chemistry.[13]

His treatise *Of the Invention of Verity, or Perfection* details the six properties of things from which the medicine is extracted and the seven properties of the medicine, as he searched for the secrets of the stone and the elixir of the philosophers.[14] Constantly concerned with purification, Geber takes the bodies to be perfected through a series of regimens, relating these to the planets, while using a great deal of language that is totally obscure to the ordinary person.[15] His importance lies in being reputed to have discovered sulphuric and nitric acids as oil of vitriol and aqua fortis, as well as aqua regia.[16] Relevance of these substances in medicine will be apparent when we come to the pharmacopoeia.

In the early ninth century the Caliph al-Māmūn wrote to the Byzantine Emperor asking for copies of Greek books and was rewarded with a positive reply. He kept scholars and translators in luxury at his court and geographers were sent to explore countries conquered by Islam.[17] Many of the physicians, surgeons, and pharmacists associated with the Islamic world were not Arabs. Almost all those who translated works from Greek into Arabic were Christian. Thanks to the open welcome given to scientists from all cultures, some in the Western Caliphate were from Spain and there were also Jews, such as Avenzoar of Seville, and Maimonides from Cordoba who translated the Canon of Avicenna into Hebrew. He became court physician to Saladin in Egypt and refused an offer from Richard the Lionheart to come to England as his personal physician. His talents seem to have been more those of a philosopher than practical physician and his lasting legacy was an oath and prayer ranking with that of Hippocrates in setting the way for modern medical ethics.[18]

A record of almost all that had been written or translated between the four main languages appeared in *Kitab al-Fihrist* written in 987. This would be an amazing source book from then onwards.[19] Although the large number of translations of the same documents into different languages clearly offers many pitfalls, it did mean that they could be compared one with another later. The great Arab surgeon and physician Albucasis (936–1013) while best known for his work on surgery, introducing new instruments and methods of surgery, also wrote *The Book of Simples*, an important source of knowledge for European medicine, as it listed works written and translated in Baghdad, demonstrating the full appreciation of the Greek writings on medicine and philosophy there.[20] In Tabriz the medical community lived in the street of the healers close to the hospital. Fifty skilful physicians from India, China, Egypt, Syria and elsewhere are recorded as well as bone-setters, students, and oculists.[21]

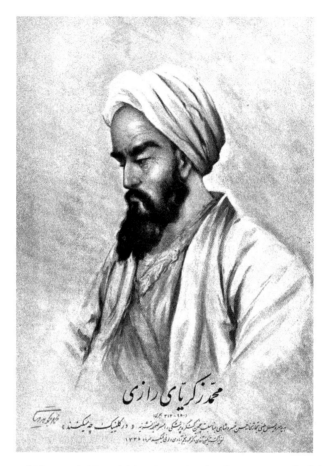

محمد زکریای رازی

Portrait of Rhazes (al-Razi) (AD 865–925), Physician and Alchemist
who Lived in Baghdad.

The two Arab physicians who are best known in Europe are Abu Bakr Muhammad
Ibn Zakariya al-Razi (c864–925), or Rhazes as he is also known in the West, and
Ibn Sina known as Avicenna, often described as prince of physicians. Both were
highly accomplished, but in different ways. Rhazes in his youth was a musician
and poet. He became a mature student of medicine choosing this path after visiting
a house for the sick and being much affected by what he had seen.[22] He was influenced in his thoughts by the Greek Democritus and the atomists. Rhazes wrote a
book on the five eternal substances, God, Soul, Matter, Space and Time and unlike
Avicenna repudiated the elaborate cycles of emanation from God with potential
for existence. Much worse was his denial that there was a need for prophets, saying a man could work on his own salvation. This deeply offended Muslim society
around him and he was denounced as a heretic.[23]

To extend his study he travelled in Persia, Egypt, Syria, and Palestine and also visited the Western Caliphate in Spain, adding to his knowledge. On his return to Rey in 918 the Caliph asked him to set up a new hospital. The attractive story that he hung meat at various sites to find the healthiest by testing how long the meat took to rot, is supported by the Saudi Annals of Medicine.[24]

Rhazes took an individual view on many matters. He had been deeply interested in alchemy and wrote twelve treatises on the subject.[25] His wide experience and sympathy f or the suffering of others, coupled with a scientific approach to chemistry, led him to suggest that new medicines should be tested on monkeys before being given to patients. Depending largely on his clinical experience when teaching, he found sufficient differences to conclusions reached by Galen on humours to write *Shukuk ala Jalinus, Doubts about Galen*. Rhazes also had progressive views on mental health. Rather than seeing the cause of mental illness as coming from a supernatural source, he looked for damage to the brain and nerves, or deprivation and suffering earlier in life. Rhazes established an area for treating psychiatric patients in the hospital and contributed to knowledge on neuroanatomy of the cranial and spinal nerves.[26]

His work on paediatrics was ground breaking.[27] He had a special interest in infectious diseases, with his treatise on the differences between smallpox and measles still being considered an important work by the famous Dr. Mead who wrote a preface to a translation of this work seven hundred years later in 1747. He refers to Rhazes as "the greatest physician of the age he lived in".[28] The Treatise on Smallpox and Measles is a good illustration of his mastery of detailed observation and care in medicine. He clearly had deep understanding of Galenic theory when using it to explain why children are more affected by these diseases than adults. He also quotes lines from Galen's works *On Pulses* and *On the Use of the Members*, describing putrefaction of blood, which he believed caused such inflammation and heat that blisters broke out on the body.

Rhazes gives a long list of early indications of the diseases, then stating "… inquietude, nausea, and anxiety are more frequent in the Measles, than in the Small-Pox; while on the other hand the pain in the back is more peculiar to the Small-Pox".[29] He classifies measles as coming from bilious blood, producing more a state of nausea and anxiety.

His detail on drinks and foods during the illness is exacting. No physician could want for more instruction as it comes to care of the eyes when pustules break out in the tunica sclerotica, the cornea or tunica uvea. The same level of care is seen with the inside of the nose and particularly the throat as there could be risk of suffocation from pustules there.[30] He recommends if there is heat to give a linctus of the mucilage of fleawort seed, gourd seed, peeled almonds, and white sugar-candy.[31] In short, the treatise gives treatments for every stage of the diseases, including removing scars afterwards.

With growing knowledge of infections expressed in the works of both Rhazes and Avicenna, quarantine became an accepted practice. Rhazes also believed, as had the ancient Greeks, Hippocrates amongst them, that the quality of the patient's surroundings, through altering their mood, also affected the course of the disease. He recommended the therapeutic value of listening to music and congenial company.

He is best known for writing the largest of his works *Al-Hawi fi al-Tibb*, known in Europe as *Liber Continens*. As he writes about each disease, he cites the Greek, Syrian, Arabic, Persian, and Indian authors before giving his own experience.[32] As a whole, it has been judged to be a collection of his observations and opinions, which may never have been meant for publication. Nevertheless, it has held respect even when compared with the systematic *Canon of Medicine* written by Avicenna. A shorter handbook on medicine, *Liber ad Almansorem* published during his lifetime, was among over two hundred works written by him.

Avicenna has been viewed by some as the greater philosopher of the two men. He seems to have looked down on Rhazes, saying derisively he would be better testing urine samples than expressing views on philosophy. Avicenna was known to have a violent temper when arguing with other philosophers on such matters. The praise for him in the following years has all been for his writing rather than his personality.[33] It seems his choleric humours could surface when the situation provoked him. He is described as a physically attractive man who remained unmarried and enjoyed entertaining; loving women, wine, and song. He also had an incredible drive for study and writing which he mostly had to fit around service to Caliphs.[34] Later in life having served one Amir until his death he refused to accompany the new Amir to war and went into hiding in the house of a druggist fearing reprisal. There he is described by his friend Juzjani as writing fifty leaves a day on *The Book of Healing*.[35]

His substantial *al-Qāṇūn fi'l-tibb*, known to us as *The Canon of Medicine*, echoes much of Galen's work on humoral medicine, while adding his own experience and occasionally questioning Galen's interpretations. Galen prided himself on not teaching anything he had not tested for himself. Avicenna followed him adding his own evidence-based medicine.

Studying the translation of the first book of his *Canon of Medicine* requires concentration. The reward is added insights from Avicenna's brilliant mind and his experience. By the end, it is easy to feel he must have said everything about the knowledge of the period, but this is only a précis that he expands on in other writings, which he refers to occasionally. Such collections of concise knowledge as this with added personal experience followed the earlier pandects, which listed medicine starting at the head and ending with the feet.[36] Texts of this older form are still found in medieval collections in the West several centuries later.[37]

Avicenna will have had Hunayn's translation of Dioscorides *De Materia Medica* from a century before available to him when he wrote this. Thorough as ever, Avicenna included tests for quality as well as succedanea, supportive synergists, and adjuvants.

Herbs on our shortlist to follow through the centuries—betony, elecampane, ginger, liquorice, and henbane—are included in the 797 drugs detailed in the first book of the Canon.[38] Betony is used in one of the occasional mentions of herbs as a local application for hands and feet exposed to severe cold.[39] Ginger is recommended in a supportive role with a purgative,[40] and henbane predictably as a strong pain killer.[41]

Avicenna began writing from the age of twenty-one with a compendium and a text on jurisprudence. Of Persian family, he is said not to have mastered the Arabic language until he was embarrassed by a courtier who pointed out a mistake he had made. After that he studied Arabic for two years before writing a book to show his mastery and having it presented to his critic.[42] Avicenna writes on medicine as any philosopher would, beginning by defining the subject. He points out that the practice of medicine actually refers to the knowledge gained by a physician which allows him to form his own opinion on how to treat a patient. Placing the highest value on ascertaining the causes both of health and disease in the physical body, he directs attention to the organs and their vital energies, the fluid humours and to the elements as primary constituents of the body. Rather than looking at medicine as entirely about disease, he gives the first aim as to preserve health.[43]

These are concepts we have already discovered with Hippocrates and Galen, and Avicenna totally agrees when he says that the four elements, varieties of temperament, humours, drives and vital forces should be accepted without proof along with the four causes.[44] Beyond this basis, reason should be applied to considerations of the symptoms of diseases, their causes and treatment. He explains that the temperaments result from the intermingling of minute particles of the elements, earth, water, fire and air producing dryness, moisture, heat, and cold. As the balance of these constantly changes within the body, this either supports health or leads to disease. This is illustrated by descriptions of eight equable balances or temperaments and then simple and compound imbalances.[45]

Individual organs of the body may also have hot or cold temperaments and as we may recall, all of this is affected by age, gender, and environment. With anatomy comes the explanation that the tissues are created out of the coarser particles of the humours while the breath is produced from the finer particles of the humours, and out of heat and dryness. The three types of drives responsible for physiology, emanating from the temperament, he presents as the vital, natural, and animal. Aristotle regarded the heart as the source of all the drives. Avicenna states that the vital drive preserves the breath, the rational drive physicians following Galen place in the brain, the reproductive drive in the organs, and the animal drive consisting of perception and sensation relates to the five senses and senses from memory and imagination to common sense and instinct.[46]

In addition to Greek thought on medicine, Avicenna had also consulted the works of recent physicians[47] and addresses matters of controversy between physicians themselves and physicians and philosophers. He states that they generally agree that the brain and the liver receive their heat and power of life from the heart, but they cannot agree as to how these interacted with other parts of the body. The questions of whether organs received the drives and passed them on and some parts of the body, such as bones needed to receive a drive in order to have life, involve philosophy as well as medicine.[48]

The origin of the temperaments and drives, indeed, of life, is God and is made manifest as an emanation. This is of prime importance—he states, "The beginning of the breath is as a divine emanation from potentiality to actuality proceeding without intermission or stint until the form … is completed and perfected".[49] That first breath, Avicenna writes, is viewed by philosophers as coming from the heart before passing to the brain where it receives a temperament enabling it to receive the drives of sensation and movement, then on to the liver where it receives the drives for nutrition and generation from the generative glands.[50] The intermingling of the humours produces not only an overall temperament for the patient, but also individual temperaments for the organs and parts of the body such as flesh and bones. With emotions, which are understood to be connected with the breath of the heart, he points out that each one, joy or sadness, tends to create its own type of breath and the more often that emotion is experienced the more this is strengthened.[51] He certainly had reason to understand sadness and regret, possibly more so considering the number of times he was forced by circumstances to leave welcoming places such as Gurgān where he had been happy.

Emotions are seen as affecting the motion of the humours within the body and psychology is given importance. Avicenna notes that to physicians the soul is the power which gives understanding and voluntary movement. This is different to the definition of soul by philosophers.[52] Other of Avicenna's writings explore the metaphysics on the soul supporting the view of Aristotle that the soul has parts and acts through these with the body. Since the rational soul in the brain produced intellect, he used this in his proof of the existence of God.[53]

Appropriate medicines for stimulating, nourishing, and strengthening the breath such as aromatics, amber, lapis lazuli, and wine, are briefly discussed. To prevent the breath from dissipating, the plum-like fruit, myrobalan is suggested. The temperature of the breath may need to be modified and cooling may be achieved using camphor or rosewater, or more heat added with doronicum.[54] This is a root which the 1751 *History of Medicine* says was first used by the Arabs and was then identified as leopard's bane, but doubt is expressed as to whether that was the plant meant in Arabia.[55]

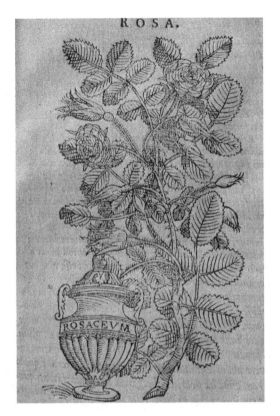

Rose, *Opera de Medicamentorum*, Mesue.

Avicenna makes it clear that the humoral state of the patient is not the only consideration when it comes to the causes of disease and symptoms. He informs his students that disease may be an abnormal state either in the structure of the body or in the temperament. A symptom, he writes, may additionally be a sign indicating the essential nature of the disease to the physician or it may also be the disease itself, rather than being the effect of disease. Referring to Galen's classifications of health, disease, and an intermediate state, he looks at simple disorders of temperament affecting only a simple organ or tissue of the body. Following this with complex diseases where a number of morbid states emerge from one disease.[56]

His writing on the seasons is of interest since it links with our earlier discussion in the last chapter and is a continuing theme. Physicians differed on the definition of each season from astronomers who divided the zodiac into quarters, starting from the vernal equinox for each, physicians defined spring as when leaves opened on the trees and lighter clothing might be worn, ending in early June. He overrules generally accepted Hippocratic belief and agrees with Galen by writing that spring should not be regarded as hot and moist, but as well balanced. The proof he says rests with physicists, but physicians should view it so.[57]

Avicenna covers interesting observations such as the body not being as sensitive to cold in spring as it is in autumn, due to the preceding temperature. The idea that changing seasons affect bodily health, particularly in chronic disease will already be well understood by readers who are experienced practitioners. Specific forms of disease which relate to the effects of the season were recognised and advice given for avoiding prevalent disease. Spring was considered to stir up humours that have lain dormant over winter and so patients suffering chronic phlegmatic diseases such as those involving joint pains, may find them increased. Avicenna warns not to eat too many hotly seasoned dishes or take vigorous physical or mental activity to excess, which would worsen the situation.[58] Such instructions are the origin of the advice on health issued from the Medical School of Salerno, later translated, along with descriptions of the humoral types, by the godson of Queen Elizabeth I, Sir John Harington.

The point is well made that seasons and climate vary in different parts of the world. Also, that people of different nations in hot or cold climates therefore have tendencies towards certain temperaments. The student physician is encouraged to study their own climate before treating patients. Avicenna combines incidental mutations of climate, physics, meteorology and astronomy in a fascinating discussion on the effects of heavenly and terrestrial factors in producing likely diseases and abnormal physical states. In short, every aspect of the whole patient and their lifestyle recommended for study by Hippocrates is covered in depth. Naturally this includes exercise, sleep, influence of psychological factors, and food and drink. All exercise, he states, heats. Sleep strengthens the drives and lack of it oxidises the humours, producing hot diseases. Too much sleep, on the other hand, dulls the mental faculty and the nerves and produces cold diseases.[59]

Avicenna treated with diet, exercise, and lifestyle changes where he could, when that did not work then he would prefer to use simples rather than the complex pharmacy available around him. On food, he sets straight the idea that heating or cooling foods could transfer their temperature to the body tissues. He points out that both cold lettuce and hot garlic can be transformed through the four stages of digestion—in the stomach, and then the liver and on into the blood and become assimilated in the last stage into the tissues without changing the nature of the tissue or blood. Temperature refers to the temperature of the food or drugs, when compared to the physical patient's body. It does not describe the literal action on the body.[60]

Medicines are described as having potentialities and in these, not surprisingly they correspond with those terms of degrees of action we have already seen expressed in Macer in the last chapter. However, more detail can now be added for our better understanding. Avicenna explains that first degree drugs have a slight action that is barely felt unless they are taken repeatedly. Second degree drugs are slightly more potent but again somewhat indirect in their actions and need high doses for real effect. Third degree drugs act directly to affect normal functioning. While in the fourth degree are drugs capable of causing real damage, or even death, such as the effects of poisonous substances.[61] Avicenna's definitions should be kept in mind when considering the actions of herbs and necessary dosage.

A general discussion of the causes of pain and the list of fourteen distinct types of pain is instructive for recording detail when taking case histories. We tend to think only of dull or sharp, stabbing and throbbing pain today, identifying also pain from tension. Avicenna adds boring, compressing, heavy, tearing, pricking, incisive, and irritant.[62] Agents to relieve pain are divided into resolvents that remove the cause, narcotics inducing sleep, and analgesics which produce cold, dulling the senses. The study of pain and its effects on the bodily drives, the functions of the organs and dispersion of the vital force is acutely observed.[63]

Classification as the reader will have gathered is important to Avicenna and he applies it to distinctions between the disease itself and secondary effects. Diagnostic signs when giving a physical examination include awareness by the physician of their own body temperature and whether it is naturally hot or cold, since this will affect their judgment of the temperature of the patient. Observational skills are highly important during physical examination of a patient as signs of their dominant humour can be judged by the amount of flesh, complexion, colour, and condition of hair and eyes.[64]

When it comes to the pulse, the possible combinations of regular and irregular factors are overwhelming. The pulse is taken using three fingers in order to judge the length, breadth, and thickness. The impact of the beat against the practitioner's finger in the three areas is something still looked upon by Western herbalists as meaningful, as well as the rhythm and balance. This ancient art of pulse diagnosis offers so much more than a number on a screen. Beginning with a calm patient who is not hungry, the text gives ten main features to be observed and these features are then expanded and expanded upon.[65] This includes considering the effects of bathing, exercise, food, drink, sleep, and emotions on the pulse.

The examination of urine has a similar fine detail in observations, which, it may be noted with satisfaction, Avicenna states do not include tasting or feeling the substance as he knows some suggest, as "that would be both impractical and undesirable."[66] Naturally pre-determined conditions for the state of the sample, how long it is left to stand, age and sex of the patient and their dominant temperament all enter the criteria and considerations for diagnosis.

Health and its implications for longevity are an ongoing theme as we look at history and Avicenna wisely advises guiding ourselves towards enjoying our natural span of life by paying attention to what helps us to maintain equilibrium. This will foster our nutritive and sensitive drives. He lists seven matters for special care. These relate predictably to diet, evacuation, breathing wholesome air, safeguarding inner heat and nutrition, guarding against outer influences and following a moderate lifestyle in terms of balancing exercise, rest, and sleep.[67]

We will come back to these seven instructions with other writers, and some regimens given here concerning childbirth, travelling, and relating to treating pestilential air, in order to compare Avicenna's views with instructions from that period. If patients are to remain healthy after treatments then careful choice and management of drugs has to be considered. This entails respecting the strength of the patient and the particular organ involved. Avicenna preferred using simpler, gentler methods first in non-critical situations. There is guidance on not using potent drugs to treat vital organs such as the brain, liver, and heart, for fear of causing serious damage. If the physician does not understand the disease, then he is cautioned to withhold treatment and leave the situation to nature.[68] Here I am reminded of an aphorism of Hippocrates "Life is short, the Art long, opportunity fleeting, experiment treacherous, judgment difficult".[69]

In the same spirit of safe guarding, we find rules for deciding whether venesection is required and exactly how and when a vein should be opened. It was not to be done with a patient under fourteen years or during pregnancy. A particular contra-indication would be a weak heart, brain, liver, or sensory organ. Sometimes specific drugs were to be partnered with purging a selected humour as with scammony purging bilious humour.[70] Humours were seen as being drawn out from the vessels or into adjoining organs, which case required extra instructions to avoid problems. Enemas, emesis, cupping and application of leeches are also described. The correct leeches to use for treating ulcers were to come from healthy water and it is stated "The Indians have specified which leeches are venomous".[71]

Unlike Rhazes he does not regularly cite authors from other civilizations. So, the comment on the leeches is the closest to such a reference I have found in this first volume. Juzjani wrote that in twenty-five years of their friendship he never saw Avicenna read a whole book. He was only interested in what the author said on matters he was still finding difficult and judged them on that. There are definite parallels to be drawn between Galen and Avicenna as men but they lived in very different environments.

In Avicenna's case he had lived almost a nomadic life in part due to the power struggles which saw places where he had happily settled, attacked, forcing him to move and at others fleeing situations where he refused to comply with what was expected of him. In the case of escaping the demand of Sultan Mahmud to join his court, it was perhaps due to fear of punishment for his unorthodox views and family connections. On that occasion, copies of a portrait of him were circulated to assist his arrest.[72] Bitter at the trials he had undergone, he indulged in excesses even when his health was breaking down and an overdose of his treatment given by a slave who had robbed him, damaged his already ulcerated gut further. Travelling with the Amir, he finally gave up treating himself, acknowledging his time had come and soon after arriving at Hamadhān in 1037 he died, aged fifty-eight.[73]

Avicenna had lived as he had wished with more breadth to his life than length, and left a considerable legacy to posterity. This surely justifies the high status of his work as a source of knowledge in Universities around Europe for centuries after his death.[73] His works, including small texts number about 250. The Canon of Medicine is still being studied and applied in Unani t'ibb medicine in Britain today. Through discovering the physicians and their written works, and the system of quality control in hygiene, preparation of drugs, and patient care in the Islamic world, it becomes possible to imagine the huge potential for influence on Western thought and development.

References

1. C.J.S. Thompson, *The Mystery and Art of the Apothecary* (Philadelphia: Lippincott Co., 1929), 82.
2. J. Innes Miller, *The Spice Trade of the Roman Empire* (Oxford: Oxford University Press, 1998), 13.
3. Soheil M. Afnan, *Avicenna His Life and Work*s (Kuala Lumpur: The Other Press, 2009), XV.
4. E.G. Browne, *Arabian Medicine* (A Series of Lectures) (Reprint. Cambridge Press: 1921), 21.
5. Oliver Kahl, *The Sanskrit, Syriac and Persian Sources in the Comprehensive Book of Rhazes.* (Leiden: Brill, 2015).
6. Bashar Saad and Omar Said, *Greco-Arab & Islamic Herbal Medicine* (New Jersey: John Wiley & Sons, 2011), 9.
7. Afnan, *Avicenna His Life and Works*, 15.
8. Saad and Said, *Greco-Arab & Islamic Herbal Medicine*, 23.
9. E.G. Browne, *Arabian Medicine*, 101–102.
10. Thompson, *The Mystery and Art of the Apothecary*, 82.
11. Charles LaWall, *Four Thousand Years of Pharmacy* (London: J.B. Lippincott, 1926), 94–95.
12. LaWall, *Four Thousand Years of Pharmacy*, 102.
13. Geber, *Geber's Best Writings on Alchemy*, (*Of Furnaces*), (Montana: Kessinger Publishing, 2010), 19.
14. Geber, *Geber's Best Writings on Alchemy*, (*Of the Invention of Verity*), 5–6.
15. Geber, (Of Furnaces), 27–31.
16. LaWall, *Four Thousand Years of Pharmacy*, 100.
17. Afnan, *Avicenna His Life and Work*s, XII.
18. LaWall, *Four Thousand Years of Pharmacy*, 111–112.
19. Afnan, *Avicenna His Life and Works*, XVI.
20. Ibid, XVI.
21. Browne, *Arabian Medicine*, 108–109.
22. Ibid, 45.
23. Afnan, *Avicenna His Life and Works*, XXXIII.
24. Amr, Samir S., and Abdulghani Tbakhi. "Abu Bakr Muhammad Ibn Zakariya Al Razi (Rhazes): Philosopher, Physician and Alchemist." *Annals of Saudi Medicine* 27, no. 4 (2007): 305–7. https://doi.org/10.5144/0256-4947.2007.305.
25. Browne, *Arabian Medicine*, 45.
26. Amr, Samir S., and Abdulghani Tbakhi. "Abu Bakr Muhammad Ibn Zakariya Al Razi (Rhazes): Philosopher, Physician and Alchemist." *Annals of Saudi Medicine* 27, no. 4 (2007): 305–7. https://doi.org/10.5144/0256-4947.2007.305.
27. G. Bos & M. McVaugh (eds), *Al-Razi, On the Treatment of Small Children* (De curis puerorum) (Leiden: Brill, 2015).
28. W.A. Greenhill (trans), *Rhazes. A Treatise on The Small-pox And Measles.* (London: The Sydenham Society, 1843), 13.
29. Greenhill, *Rhazes. A Treatise on The Small-pox And Measles*, 34.
30. Ibid, 53.
31. Ibid, 54.

32. Afnan, *Avicenna His Life and Works*, 165.
33. Ibid, 39.
34. Afnan, *Avicenna His Life and Works*, 30.
35. Ibid, 31.
36. Ibid, 166.
37. Johannes Mesue, *Opera de Medicamentorum*. Supplements, (Venice, 1581)
38. L. Bakhtiar (adapt), *The Canon of Medicine. Avicenna* (Great Books of the Islamic World Inc., 1999), LXXXIX/XC.
39. Bakhtiar, *The Canon of Medicine. Avicenna*, 451.
40. Ibid, 497.
41. Ibid, 544.
42. Afnan, *Avicenna His Life and Works*, 34.
43. Bakhtiar, *The Canon of Medicine. Avicenna*, 13.
44. Ibid, 13.
45. Ibid, 18–24.
46. Ibid, 132.
47. Ibid, 49.
48. Ibid, 49–50.
49. Ibid, 144.
50. Ibid, 144.
51. Ibid, 153.
52. Ibid, 141.
53. Afnan, *Avicenna*, 102.
54. Bakhtiar, *Canon of Medicine Avicenna*, 157.
55. Sir J. Hill, *History of Medicine* (London, 1751), 625.
56. Bakhtiar, *Canon of Medicine Avicenna*, 176.
57. Ibid, 188.
58. Ibid, 197.
59. Ibid, 217.
60. Ibid, 220, 221.
61. Ibid, 221, 223.
62. Ibid, 249–251.
63. Ibid, 246–252.
64. Ibid, 266–271.
65. Ibid, 289, 287–315.
66. Ibid, 319.
67. Ibid, 358.
68. Ibid, 468.
69. W.H.S. Jones (trans), Hippocrates Vol. IV. 99.
70. Bakhtiar, *Canon of Medicine Avicenna*, 484.
71. Ibid, 524.
72. Afnan, *Avicenna His Life and Works*, 71.
73. Ibid, 36.

CHAPTER 12

Norman Influence, Physicians, and Surgeons | 1066–1443

SECVNDVM NICOLAVM.
Pilulę fine quibus effe nolo
Pilulę aureæ
Pilulæ ftypticę
Pilulę de fpeciebus benedictæ
Pilulæ de hiera logodion
    SECVNDVM GALENVM.
Pilulę de hiera picra cum agari.
Pilulę de hiera fimplici Gal.
    SECVNDVM RASIM.
Pilulę cochię
Pilulę foetidę
Pilulę iliacæ
    SECVNDVM AVICEN.
Pilulę de fumo terrę
Pilulę affaiaret
    SECVNDVM RVFFVM.
Pilulę communes ex aloe, croco, &
    myrrha, ex inuentione Ruffi, vel Gal.
    fecundum aliquos, & funt optimę có
    tra peftem.
    DE TROCHISCIS SE-
        cundum Mefuem.

Recipes from Salerno and Arabic Sources. *Opera de Medicamentorum*, Mesue.

153

After the battle of Hastings in 1066, William of Normandy set about making the kingdom his own. Initially this involved putting down rebellion as it arose and building castles to maintain power centres, with three required in London and two in York.[1] Changes were largely in the upper layers of society and administration. The extent of removal of thegns who had previously been powerful overlords is revealed in the Domesday Book, commissioned at Christmas 1085. This shows that only eight percent of land in England remained owned by people with English names. The rest belonged to Normans, the Crown, or the Church.[2]

The Anglo-Saxon written language is replaced by Norman French, and William brought with him his most learned physicians, respected both for their practical abilities and their literary works. Among them was Faricius of Arezzo who later became Abbot of Abingdon where he increased the library of the Abbey by ordering copies of books on physic in Latin. Monasteries flourished under Norman rule and more Continental Religious Orders came to Britain.[3]

Ten years after William conquered England, the Norman Duke Robert took the port of Salerno, building an impressive castle there, raising the status of the town. The already established medical school was to become a leading centre. The geographical position of Salerno on the Amalfi coast meant it was already a busy port, well placed for voyagers from Africa and the East. From 1095, it became the base hospital for the Crusaders.[4] The first document referring to the Salerno Medical School is in the articles of Federico II, published in Melfi in 1231, but activities of the school are recorded from three centuries earlier. According to La Wall, Salerno was the first educational institution of a university type.[5]

The Benedictine Abbeys of San Benedetto in Salerno and Montecassino with their infirmaries played an influential part. The translations of Constantine the African made in the Abbey at Montecassino in the twelfth century encouraged the understanding of knowledge from Greek, Latin, Jewish, and Arabic sources, for which the school became famous.

In the case of Jewish medicine, this had a particular emphasis on preventive hygiene as we see in the Bible. In Leviticus chapter eleven, we find the rules concerning foods and those animals to be regarded as unclean. Anyone carrying an unclean carcase is instructed to wash his clothes. Contaminated food containers must be washed and so on. Disease is threatened for those who do not obey the commandments in both Leviticus chapter twenty-six and Deuteronomy chapter twenty-eight.

The Essenes, a monastic community dedicated to godliness and cleanliness sometimes associated with Jesus, influenced Christian medicine.[6] The central text of Judaism, the Talmud, names physicians and surgeons, mentioning rooms walled with marble for cleanliness where operations took place. There was general acceptance that over-eating and drinking, sexual excess, blood, contaminated water, animals and insects were responsible for disease. Flies were seen as transmitters of infection. Taking such precautions as not drinking uncovered water, and avoiding overcrowding during epidemics, reveal the level of early understanding.[7]

We can appreciate from considering the lives and testimonies of Dioscorides and other physicians that travel broadened experience and increased knowledge both of plants and the effects of the environment on people. The migrations of the Jews, spending time in Babylon and Egypt surely contributed to their study of medicine. I have already mentioned highly respected Jewish physicians such as Avenzoar and Maimonides, for them medicine was a spiritual vocation. Migrations also encouraged linguistic ability for translation, Jewish scholars being proficient in Hebrew, Arabic, and Latin, as well as, occasionally in Greek. It should not be thought that there was no exclusively Jewish school, for one was founded in the sixth century by Asaph Judaeus, who wrote the oldest known medical work in Hebrew based on Hebrew traditions but also containing knowledge from Babylonian, Persian, Egyptian, and Greek sources.[8]

We know works produced at Salerno, particularly those from the twelfth century, from the few surviving in Britain. Copies of Constantine's *Pantegni*, (a translation from the Arabic which is thought to be the *Maliki* originally written by Haly Abbas) and Constantine's Pantegni, *a Passionarius Galieni* were in Exeter, Battle and Canterbury and a variety of manuscripts were in the libraries of Westminster, Exeter, Bury St Edmunds, Durham, and Lanercost Priory. The comprehensive collection of Salernitan texts at Lanercost may have been copies made between 1177–1194.[9] These bear witness to the earliest use of Salernitan texts in England.

Constantine the African was born in Carthage and studied medicine in Baghdad, Cairo, and India.[10] He had travelled far and wide, including Persia, Egypt, Syria, Africa, and the Western Caliphate of Spain, before becoming a Benedictine monk. He arrived in Salerno around 1072 and died just before the end of the century. Among the thirty-seven books he translated from several languages, perhaps the most important was one mentioned above, The *Kitab al-maliki* or *Royal Book of Haly Abbas* on surgery. This became known as the Bamberg Surgery and was the first surgical treatise in medieval Europe and the first to mention an inhaled anaesthetic.[11] His *Liber Graduum* was quoted by a monk at St. Albans in the mid-twelfth century. Four monks, including Warin who would later become Abbot and all of whom had studied at Salerno, entered the Abbey on the same day and it has been presumed they took their medical books with them.[12]

A number of other influential texts are associated with Salerno. The one which has caused most controversy on the gender of the author in relatively recent times has been that of Trocta, or Trotula on womens' health. With her in-depth studies of available source documents Monica Green has identified three different texts within the material. Each she believes is written by a different author. With two, Green has identified them as written by men, including one on cosmetics and a main text on Conditions of Women. While the third, Treatments for Women, was brought together with the first two texts at a later date. If not written by a woman, Green judges this text contains remedies prescribed by a woman.[13] Reluctance by male scholars to accept all three texts, previously seen as by one author as the work of a female physician has provoked ongoing discussion.

The work has been stated in Italy to have been written by Trotula, wife of Giovanni Plateario il Vecchio during the mid-eleventh century.[14] Identification with an actual person has been hotly contested by academics from other countries. Looking back at the role of women as both midwives and physicians who specialised in "women's problems" in earlier periods, what we can say is that it is known female physicians were associated with Salerno. It is therefore not unlikely a treatise on women's problems both general and in pregnancy through to childbirth was written by one of them.

A number of other authors on medicine were associated with Salerno over the centuries. Archbishop of Salerno from 1058 to 1085, Alfano I wrote two medical works, one on humours and the other on the pulse. *De Pulsibus* enlarges on the work of Galen using the pulse not only in diagnosing the disease the patient is suffering from, but also their physical condition and temperament, and when in critical condition whether they were likely to live or die.[15]

For the average person it was sufficient to understand how to distinguish when one of the four humours was too powerful, in the case of the sanguine humour it would give a short, soft pulse. With too much choler the opposite could be felt in a hard and fast pulse. It would be hard too for the overly melancholic, but slowed and softened in an excess phlegmatic state.[16]

Avicenna had already detailed the main features of measuring the pulse in terms of its length, breadth, and thickness, interpreting the amount of diastole and rating the feel of the pulse as it meets with the practitioner's fingers. He instructs the practitioner to note the length of pauses between beats, how equal each beat is to the last, how long the movement lasts, how full the blood vessel feels, regularity, equality of rhythm and duration of pauses, and how hot or cold the pulse feels to the touch.[17]

Putting a complex art simply, certain features Avicenna associates with each temperament. These are, of course, affected by factors such as age, season, having eaten, emotional states, and so on. In those of a hot temperament, the pulse is likely to be large with a feeling of resistance against the fingers of the practitioner. With a cold temperament, the pulse is small and slow and the beat may be infrequent. With a moist temperament the pulse feels soft and will be wide, whereas a dry temperament gives a hard and wiry pulse.[18]

The pulse is taken on both wrists as the two sides may show different aspects of the patient, with the condition of the blood vessel walls accounting for the difference. With someone in good general health while their vital force is strong this will add to the resistance felt. Interpretation of the pulse is a potentially vast subject based on a great deal of experience and clinical observations.

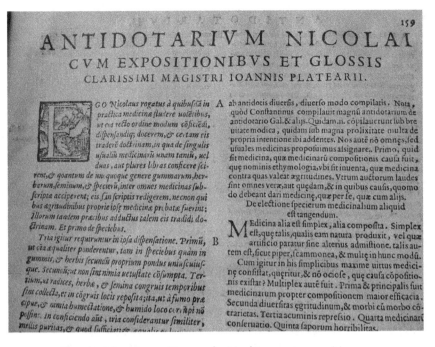

The Antidotarium, *Opera de Medicamentorum*, Mesue.

Copies of the Antidotarium of Niccolo Salernitano found their way to Britain where one has survived in Durham from the early twelfth century. Various medical manuscripts, including the Antidotarium also belonged to Lanercost Priory. I was delighted to find on first reading through my copy of a compilation on pharmacy, the *Opera de Medicamentorum* printed in Venice in 1581 that his Antidotarium had been included as a supplement.[19] The original manuscript of the Antidotarium has been dated to just after the translations of Constantine the African as it contains medicinal substances such as tamarind and muscat nut from the Arabic pharmacy. It is a practical pharmaceutical textbook and was used at the Salerno medical school. Within it is the spongia soporifera, which we find appearing in a slightly altered form in Britain as an inhaled anaesthetic in the fourteenth century. This death-defying prescription contained opium, henbane, mandrake, hemlock, blackberry, lettuce, and ivy.[20]

A museum for the medical school greets visitors today and on visiting Salerno some years ago I was interested to find a copy of the *Antidotarium of Niccolo* on display with other documents. There are varying spellings of the name of Niccolo and there have also been discussions as to whether the true identity of the author of the Antidotarium was actually Nicolaus Praepositus, a French physician who wrote in about 1500. In the pages following I will use Nicolai of Salerno.[21] For most visitors, however, the pages from the *Tacuinem de Sanitatis* are the star exhibits. Beautifully illustrated and evocative of the medieval age the Tacuinem offers advice on healthy living according to Galenic ideals. It is, however, not an exact copy of Galen's text and it shows the Arabic interpretation on the humours. The tabular form indicated by the title—Tacuinum is derived from the Arabic taqwim, translated as meaning tables—and main concepts can be traced back to the 'Taqwin As-Ṣiḥḥa', by Ibn Botlân an Arabian physician who trained in Baghdad and travelled widely, visiting Constantinople and Egypt and practising as a physician in Mossul, Diyarbekir, and Aleppo. He wrote widely on health, finally retiring to a monastery in Antioch in the eleventh century.[22] It is delightful to follow the illustrations of the Tacuinem as they range from the effects of individual herbs, through foods, clothing, wind directions and seasons of the year, to emotions. In each case the temperament, heating, drying properties, etc., of the item are given along with their best form, usefulness, possible dangers to health, and ways to neutralise those dangers.

The piece on anger is quite revealing of the understanding of the human condition behind the advices. It is described as the boiling of the blood. It is stated this can be useful in restoring colour to pale cheeks, but also might lead to symptoms of a stroke with paralysis and "torment of the mouth" Anger, the reader is warned, is particularly dangerous to those who make illicit decisions, but it can be neutralised using philosophy.[23] For another instance the herb, sage, is classified as warm in the first degree, and dry in the second. It is recommended to treat the nerves and paralysis. The danger of use appears surprisingly to be that it may remove the colour from dark hair.[24] Quite opposite to the role sage has been given in more recent cosmetic recipes.

In response to requests for guidance on health, The Regimen Sanitatis Salerni correlates directly with the Tacuinem. The six factors for daily preservation of health are described and include diet, mobility, sleep regime, and moderating desires, and emotions. These were all understood to work towards the correct regulation of elimination or retention of the humours. Symptoms of disease states are also classified with inflammation clearly demonstrating a hot condition, cold as lack of stimulation in body systems, dryness was seen in weak states, and damp by the discharge of body fluids. The right herbs, diet, and general approach to life needed to be chosen to balance the diagnosed condition of the patient.

The Regimen Sanitatis Salerni was translated into Irish in the fifteenth century due to the interest taken by Irish physicians in European medicine.[25] The Regimen was the most famous document to emerge from the school at Salerno as far as the layman was concerned. Initially a book of instruction written in Latin, it was translated into English in the reign of Elizabeth I by her godson, Sir John Harington and published in 1607.[26] His achievements in translation were rather overshadowed as it was written while he was banished from court after sharing bawdy stories with the Queen's ladies. However, during his exile he invented the flushing toilet, which impressed her majesty sufficiently for her to order one and allow him to return. His poetry about his toilet called Ajax then resulted in him being banished again.

The Regimen gives simple advice beginning with the instruction to use three physicians, "first Doctor Quiet, Next Doctor Merry-man, and Doctor Dyet".[27] The verses lay out the humoral theory in picturesque and easily understood ways. It states that all four states of the humours are present in everyone, sanguine, choleric, melancholic, and phlegmatic. These corresponded to the order of the four seasons and the health advice is given for each period. In this way, warmth and moisture are associated with spring, when bathing, sweating, and purging are recommended to cleanse the body. In summer when the drying heat of choler is strongest, the recommendation by some, the text says, is to have cooling and moist foods to counteract the heat. Autumn is judged as being a colder version of spring, presumably with similar regimen and then in winter the cold can be balanced by increasing wine and spices.[28]

The idea of tailoring regimen to the season is first found in the Hippocratic Corpus, where gradual change is recommended.[29] In the Regimen the verses continue with the character traits and certain physical signs and symptoms likely to reveal when one of the humours is dominant. The rhyming descriptions of appearances, virtues, and vices of each type are entertaining and physical detail on pulse and urine are interwoven along with accounts of the patients' dreams.

In the verses referring to herbs in diet and for medicine we find the nettle accused of stinking yet proving useful when the seed is taken in honey to treat colic.[30] Elecampane is recommended as strengthening the digestion, acting as a mild laxative, cheering the heart and soothing grief.[31] The toothache remedy we so often find is there, with the description of using the smoke from burning henbane and onion seed, funnelled into the hollow tooth[32] and "Lycoras" (liquorice) is portrayed as a herb liked by the brain.[30,33]

It was more usual at this time for English physicians to have trained abroad, in Montpellier, Paris, or Bologna. By 1137, Montpellier, close to Spain, also appears to have had a fully developed faculty of medicine. From 1220 the medical school there included teaching Arab medicine, using books by Avicenna, Rhazes, and Al Mansouri and ten other books on Arab-Islamic medicine. Among Englishmen who studied at Montpellier and returned with fruits of Arabic science was Adelard of Bath who translated many important Arabic and Greek scientific works on astrology, astronomy, philosophy, mathematics, and alchemy into Latin. Robert of Chester who translated *The Book of the Composition of Alchemy* from Arabic making it the first book on alchemy available in Europe in 1144 also studied at Montpellier.[34]

By comparison, Oxford University had a small faculty of medicine mentioned for the first time in 1303. John of Gaddesden may have begun the medicine course in that year. Training as a physician at Oxford University and being able to practise in the City required firstly four years for a Master of Arts degree, which at the time consisted of seven subjects: grammar, rhetoric, logic, arithmetic, music, geometry, astronomy, and natural, moral, and metaphysical philosophies. After this grounding in being able to dispute a case and knowledge of the natural sciences, a further six years of medicine involved study of theory and practical medicine entirely from two books.[35] There does not seem to have been any link with a hospital, for instance, where patients might be seen. Even had there been, there were so many restrictions on who might gain treatment in hospitals, either of St Bartholomew's or of St John the Baptist, which was more simply a religious establishment, that there would have been little benefit. At St John's, those with leprosy, the paralytic, insane, sufferers from dropsy (retaining water from whatever cause), fistulas, incurable diseases, epileptics, and lascivious pregnant women, were not admitted.[36]

John of Gaddesden, who was born c1280 graduated from Oxford and wrote his treatise, the *Rosa Anglica*, he tells us in the preface, in the seventh year of his lecture.[37] In his work he sets down names and definitions of diseases, their incidence and cause, prognosis, and a great variety of treatments which are intended both for the rich and poor. His sources show his education as they are Greek, Arabic, and Jewish as well as Bernard of Gordon who taught in Montpellier and Gilbertus Anglicus, a scholar of Salerno, physician to the Chancellor of Richard I, who wrote *The Practica*.[38] Bernard, Gilbert, and John are all mentioned in Chaucer's Canterbury Tales.[39]

Not surprisingly, with so many years of training, there was only a small number of academically highly qualified physicians, with their knowledge of the Naturals, the pathological Contra-Naturals, and Non-Naturals, including environment, motion, nourishment, sleep, evacuation, and mental equilibrium. Added information came from the complex examination of the pulse, any blood drawn and other bodily evacuations. Astronomy was an additional part of training in Europe where the physician carried tables of the planets, eclipses, phlebotomy, and urine analysis offering twenty-seven types, on his belt to aid diagnosis.[40] The doctrine of correlating the signs of the zodiac and the parts of the body was available in Western Europe from the twelfth century onwards. We see this in the diagrams of the zodiac man. A clear distinction was made between astrology with a history in medicine going back to Hippocrates and given credible scientific support by *Introductorium in Astronomiam* written by Abu Ma'shar who died in 887,[41] and soothsaying, (predicting the future), which was forbidden by the Bible.

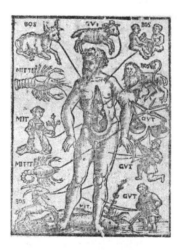

Zodiac Man, Woodcut from the Almanacs of Petrus Slovacius,
Published by Johan Scharffenberg, Breslau, 1580.

Astrology came to the fore in attempts to explain the outbreak of the plague. It had clearly been of importance to find the cause of such disaster from the outset. When Philip VI of France asked the cause of the Black Death in October 1348 the faculty of medicine at the University of Paris blamed the plague mainly on a conjunction of Saturn, Jupiter, and Mars in the House of Aquarius at 1pm on the 20th March 1345. It was explained that a conjunction of Mars and Jupiter meant great pestilence in the air, while that of Saturn and Jupiter meant the death of many peoples.[42] It was therefore seen by many, including the Church, as punishment sent by God. In 1405, the Universities of Paris and Bologna stipulated that all medical students should study astrology for four years as part of their training. This was not the case in England.

Physicians could also be surgeons, but lay surgeons were not educated at University. They seem to have been required by some authorities to have served a six-year apprenticeship; however, this was rarely enforced in England as it was in Europe. There does not seem to be any precise information as to when the practice of six years apprenticeships began but it has been identified as required from the 1435 regulations, although there remains uncertainty.[43] Statutes on training were laid down in Oxford as early as 1350 but had no general jurisdiction or enforcement. In York between 1350 and 1449, a variety of medical men were admitted to the freedom of the city. Among them were those referred to as medicus, leche, fisicus, triacler, surgener, clericus, who was a doctor of medicine, and a tuthdragher.[44]

Surgeons also prescribed herbs for their patients. John Arderne (1307–1392) had not attended University but learnt much working in the battlefields of Flanders and Spain. He used styptics and five different narcotic pain-killing prescriptions.[45] Formularies of European surgeons contain valuable records—William of Saliceto wrote the great Chirurgia in 1277, which dominated Italian surgery. His pupil Lanfranchi of Milan later wrote his own Chirurgia, which, together with the Antidotary and Pharmacopoeia of Henri de Mondeville, provided much fascinating and instructive material interpreted by a retired surgeon and Professor of Surgery. The text explains terms commonly used, such as incarnatives, for instance leaves of pomegranate and lily which were applied to promote generation of granulation tissue in a wound.[46]

Plantain also appears in this role in the formularies of both Lanfranchi and Henri de Mondeville. Both the greater form and ribwort were used and all plantains were described as cool and dry in the third degree. Plantain was further classified as a potent repercussive and as such was applied to inflamed, swollen areas to reduce the fluids or humours, allowing the wound to be sutured. The herb also promoted the coagulation of blood and was looked upon as a detergent cleanser, unnecessary on a fresh, clean wound but used to remove pus or dry scabs.[47] **Henbane** was also classed as a repercussive by Henri de Mondeville and cool and dry in the third degree.[48]

If the patient could not tolerate the use of a repercussive on a swollen, painful wound then unless there was severe pain a resolutive would be applied to draw out the humours causing the problem. Resolutives are heating and these would be made into a decoction and used to bathe the wound. **Elecampane** is listed under synonyms for resolutives, being warm and dry in the second degree.[49]

Nettle seed appears in Lanfranchi's formulary as a resolutive. Henri de Mondeville does not specify the seed, but uses nettle as a simple, that is, alone.[50] He also places nettle in a long list of ingredients used in corrosive or escharotic compound applications. Corrosives had varying degrees of action ranging from weak to the very strong, such as quick-lime used on gangrene and often included herbs to temper the main purpose.[51]

There are many classes of herbs and other ingredients for wound applications, caring for wounds was an important and complex skill for the herbal practitioner of the past, largely lost today for lack of practice. Other classes of medications were maturatives, applied topically to bring inflamed matter to a head for release, cicatrizers, used to bring the edges of a wound together, and soothing emollients. Resins, such as mastic and frankincense, minerals, and metals were also included in the many compounds made using the simples.

Anaesthetics are a natural accompaniment to surgery, if at all possible. Theodoric's Chirurgia includes a recipe for the soporific sponge which was boiled with a mix of narcotic herbs, among them henbane, opium, mandrake and more until they were absorbed. The sponge could then be soaked in hot water later before applying it to the nostrils of the patient.[52] In the Syriac text of a *Book of Medicines*, there is also a sleep-producing plaster, made with opium and henbane seed, which is attributed to Asclepiades.[53] A book of native medicines accompanies the text and is a stark contrast with a mix of recipes often containing animal ingredients. This is followed by divination and a description of the sicknesses that attack men under each sign of the zodiac.[54]

Other medics who prepared herbal treatments for patients included apothecaries, midwives, treaclers, herbalists, and "wise-women", who might further call themselves a leech or even medicus. The treacler specialised in making mixtures which were originally antidotes to poisons. As time passed treacle also referred to thick compounds used as panaceas to remedy any kind of poison or vile humours in the body system.[55] Apothecaries mentioned in Chaucer were regarded as sellers of remedies, in the same way as spicers, but with no access to physicians for a large part of the population, in all likelihood they treated patients at times.[56] We may add to that list ladies who might treat members of their own large household and nursed them.

In this chapter we have traced the links between Norman rule and increased ties with the Continent through the monastic orders continuing in the roles of spreading medical knowledge through copying documents on physic. They also care for the sick and it would be predominantly if not always clerics who studied medicine at the Universities. The first stone-built hospital dates to around 1080 soon after Norman rule. While Crusaders experienced use of certain spices, fruits, and other goods, sparking increased demand for them in England, medical knowledge came largely through English physicians training on the Continent and returning to practice. Astrology became a necessary part of medical training in other countries, it was not officially adopted in training at Oxford or Cambridge. Following the plague, the guilds of physicians, surgeons, and merchants grew more important and wealthier, building their company halls. The structure of agricultural society also changed with peasant workers moving from directly owned manorial farms.[57]

References

1. Francis Pryor, *Britain in the Middle Ages* (London: Harper Press, 2006), 208.
2. Pryor, *Britain in the Middle Ages*, 230.
3. C.H. Talbot, *Medicine in Medieval England* (London: Oldbourne, 1967), 46.
4. Charles LaWall, *Four Thousand Years of Pharmacy* (Philadelphia: Lippincott Company, 1927), 130.
5. LaWall, *Four Thousand Years of Pharmacy*, 131.
6. Magnus Magnusson, *BC The Archaeology of the Bible Lands* (London: The Bodley Head Ltd., 1977), 225.
7. Vaisrub, Samuel. "Ancient Jewish History—Medicine." (In the Bible, Status of the Physician) Medicine. Accessed April 22, 2023. https://www.jewishvirtuallibrary.org/medicine.
8. Vaisrub, Samuel. "Ancient Jewish History—Medicine." (In the Byzantine Era) Medicine. Accessed April 22, 2023. https://www.jewishvirtuallibrary.org/medicine.
9. Talbot, *Medicine in Medieval England*, 46–47.
10. H.P. Cholmeley, *John of Gaddesden and the Rosa Medicinae* (Oxford: The Clarendon Press, 1912), 168.
11. Leonard Rosenman, *A Medieval Surgical Pharmacopoeia and Formulary* (San Francisco: Rosenman, 1999), 119.
12. Talbot, *Medicine in Medieval England*, 47–48.
13. Monica Green, (ed, trans), *The Trotula* (Philadelphia: University of Pennsylvania Press. 2001), 51.
14. G.B. Spazzapan, *Il Cinquantesimo libro sulla storia di Salerno il meglio e di più'*. (Istituto Grafico Editoriale Italiano, 1992), 76.
15. M. Pasca et al., *Salerno School of Medicine* (Regione Campania: Assessorato al Turismo, 1990), Alfano I.
16. Sir John Harington, *The School of Salernum* (Salerno: Ente Provinciale per il. Turismo, 1957), 79–82.
17. L. Bakhtiar (adapt), *The Canon of Medicine. Avicenna* (Great Books of the Islamic World Inc., 1999), 289.
18. Bakhtiar (adapt), *The Canon of Medicine. Avicenna*, 303–4.
19. Joannes Mesue *Opera de Medicamentorum* (Venice, 1581), 159–191.
20. Mesue *Opera de Medicamentorum* Supplement, Antidotarium Nicolai, 185.
21. G. Urdang, *Pharmacopoeia Londinensis* of 1618 (Wisconsin: Madison State Historical Society, 1944), 7.
22. L.C. Arano, *The Medieval Health Handbook. Tacuinum Sanitatis* (New York: George Braziller), 11.

23. Arano, *The Medieval Health Handbook. Tacuinum Sanitatis*, plate 176.
24. Ibid, plate 224.
25. Rosarie Kingston, *Ireland's Hidden Medicine* (Lewes: Aeon Books, 2021), 44.
26. Harington, *The School of Salernum*, 18.
27. Ibid, 22.
28. Ibid, 70.
29. W.H.S. Jones, (trans), *Hippocrates Volume IV* (London: Harvard University Press, 1931), Reg. III. Chapter LXVIII. 377.
30. Harington, *The School of Salernum*, 58.
31. Ibid, 60.
32. Ibid, 66.
33. Ibid, 48.
34. Talbot, *Medicine in Medieval England*, 57.
35. H.P. Cholmeley, *John of Gaddesden and the Rosa Medicinae* (Oxford: Clarendon Press, 1912), 20–21.
36. Nicholas Orme & Margaret Webster, *The English Hospital 1070–1570* (London: Yale University Press, 1995), 58.
37. Cholmeley, *John of Gaddesden and the Rosa Medicinae*, 25.
38. Ibid, 172.
39. N. Coghill, (trans), *Chaucer—The Canterbury Tales* (Middlesex: Penguin Classics. Penguin Books, 1975), 31.
40. Talbot, *Medicine in Medieval England*, 125–126.
41. Carole Rawcliffe, *Medicine & Society in Later Medieval England* (Stroud: Sutton Publishing Ltd., 1995), 86.
42. Rawcliffe, *Medicine & Society in Later Medieval England*, 82.
43. Huling Ussery, *Chaucer's Physician* (New Orleans: Tulane University, 1971), 11.
44. Ussery, *Chaucer's Physician*, 20.
45. Rawcliffe, *Medicine & Society in Later Medieval England*, 77.
46. Rosenman, *A Medieval Surgical Pharmacopoeia And Formulary*, 81.
47. Ibid, 72.
48. Ibid, 84.
49. Ibid, 70.
50. Ibid, 72, 79.
51. Ibid, 83.
52. Ibid, 118.
53. E.A. Wallis Budge, *Syrian Anatomy, Pathology, And Therapeutics* Vol. I. (Alpha Editions, 2020), LXXVII.
54. Budge, *Syrian Anatomy, Pathology, and Therapeutics*, CXVIII.
55. Ussery, *Chaucer's Physician*, 26.
56. Ibid, 25.
57. Pryor, *Britain in the Middle Ages*, 255.

CHAPTER 13

Pharmacy in the Later Medieval Period | c1300–1500

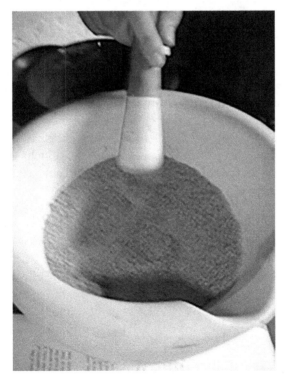

Pounding Herbs in a Mortar.

In this chapter, I will be asking some important questions about the state of pharmacy mainly in the fourteenth and fifteenth centuries. This will involve using comparisons with specific recipes, but also looking at use of accompanying rituals, charms, and prayers, modes of administration, ingredients and whether these reveal Arabic influence and so on. Having looked at the roles of the herbs we are following and treatments for specific conditions, the search for forgotten herbal applications that could be useful today closes the chapter.

The conclusions arise from analysis of recipes in three sources. The first, *Medical Works of the Fourteenth Century*[1] includes two similar Middle English manuscripts; MS A from a commonplace book used in a large household, recording items of broad interest written before 1400, and a second manuscript, MS B (Harleian 2378) containing fewer recipes and thought to be from the fourteenth century.[2] Professor Skeat's accompanying analysis of the Middle English language in Manuscript A shows a transitional state from Anglo Saxon. He judges the scribe to be of Norman birth, conversant with Anglo-French and English, probably from Hampshire, Surrey, or Sussex.[3] This gives us some insight into the literate class some generations on from the coming of the Normans. The date 1464 appears at the end of this manuscript, which contains recipes clearly copied from one or more earlier sources.

The second main source, *A Leechbook of the XVth Century*[4] contained over a thousand recipes and was used by the English leech, in this case an educated practitioner, who had not had University training. It appears to be a handbook for an inexperienced, perhaps newly professional leech or healer, I say this because towards the end are instructions for writing quantities of drugs on the bill and for making red or green wax to seal it.[5] It would be fascinating to know who received those bills. Instructions on using the urine of both partners to find out whether the man or woman is responsible for infertility, is marked by Dawson who edited the collection in the twentieth century, as a practice originating in ancient Egypt, also found in other recipe collections.[6]

Sources of recipes are sometimes acknowledged and include, not surprisingly recipes attributed to some well-known physicians and surgeons. There is a recipe from the work of Henri de Mondeville (1260–1320) for treating cancrous sores.[7] Henri was referred to in the last chapter as of Norman birth and trained at Montpellier. Originally an army surgeon, he was later surgeon at the royal court, with a successful civilian practice.[8] An early teacher from Montpellier, Gordianus, otherwise known as Bernard of Gordon, author of the *Lily of Medicine*, who has also already appeared in the preceding pages is referenced in a recipe for treating scales.[9]

This very practical guide includes general instructions that every herbalist needs to know, such as gathering all parts of herbs with reference to their maturity, the weather, and specific days or months. Wild gathering is generally considered preferable. It is emphasised that where a particular day is specified this is the time when the plant has the greatest virtue.[10] Rosemary flowers are to be gathered in May. Unlike leaves and flowers which are to be dried in shade, moist roots such as galingale are set firstly in the sun for three days, to avoid rotting; while for best quality cucumber seed, the fruit was deliberately left to rot in moist conditions.

How long some dried herbs will keep is noted, water calamint is given as not longer than a year, fennel root dried in spring for a year, and lily for two years. The harvesting season begins in March with violets and fennel root and ends with the fern, hartstongue, in November.[11] Again, I have made many of these recipes successfully over the years, after being interested by their possible efficacy. In 2010, I tutored a practical day of making such recipes as a post-graduate course for the National Institute of Medical Herbalists. At the end of the day there was a general discussion on whether such recipes could be incorporated into modern practice and a number of them were chosen as suitable to give as effective remedies today.

The third source, Medieval Welsh Medical Texts[12] is a translation and commentary on the four earliest Welsh manuscript sources available, thought to date largely to the fourteenth century. The reference to the physicians of Myddfai, Rhiwallon and his sons is now seen by Diana Luft in her translation as applying to a small part of the collection which immediately follows.[13] This she likens to a similar introductory piece relating to Galen and Hippocrates.[14]

In comprehensive notes accompanying the translations Luft identifies a number of sources for the collection. These include the *Macer Floridus de Viribus* and the Anglo-Saxon *Bald's Leechbook* both already familiar to readers from earlier chapters.[15,16] Some recipes can be found in a large and important treasury of Welsh culture, the *Red Book of Hergest* also containing poetry, and the famous ancient legends of *the Mabinogion*.[17] It was written between 1382 and 1405. Others are from the Middle English *Agnus Castus*, which we will explore further when we come to 1525 when it provides material repeated almost word for word in the first printed herbal in England.[18,19]

Some Welsh recipe texts support the classification of use by a physician with mention of cautery and blood-letting. There are complex recipes and occasional use of spices, gum resins, orpiment, arnament, and copperas. Arnament also appears in recipes in the Commonplace book. The explanation of written measurements as in the Welsh translation of the recipe God's Grace reminds us of a similar explanation in the Leechbook.[20,21] However, these texts do not have guidance for gathering herbs or provide a complete manual.

The lack of guidance in the majority of recipes as to amounts of ingredients underlines intended use by a sufficiently experienced leech or physician. Concern centres on specifying the number of days of treatment with further detail on dosage, diet, and methods of administration. As in the Leechbook, there is occasional explanation of types of a condition, such as the four hernias. Watery and windy hernias, described as incurable and treatable hernias of the bowels or testicles.[22]

Methods of Preparation

Ingredients are pounded, simmered, stewed in skillets, or boiled (sometimes in brass pans), meanwhile being stirred with a slice, or skimmed with a feather. Herbs are burnt on a glowing hot tile-stone or iron hotplate, roasted inside an egg or onion in the embers, even fried at the end to be applied hot, as in the case of some plasters.

Liquors might be cooled by pouring through a colander, and strained through canvas or a hair sieve, or wrung through a linen cloth.

In the Welsh manuscripts, recipes in water are almost always boiled whether in a skillet or a clay pot. Occasionally they are fried, usually in a skillet, or baked in embers or within an onion. A thin white-hot stone is used in the recipe to burn henbane seeds for toothache, a recipe common to many collections.[23] Herbs are pounded on a mortar stone or in a mortar, sometimes being ground to powders for application, adding to foods such as porridge, or taking in a drink. Most recipes requiring straining are put through a linen cloth, in one a newly washed linen cloth is specified and there is a single mention of straining through canvas.

The measurements across the sources may be an eggshell-full, or more particularly, the quantity of a goose's or pigeon's egg. They range from the greatness of half a walnut, down to pellets the size of vetch or a grain. There might be as much as will stand on a groat or crown in the English recipes or the weight of coinage is used, with a farthing-weight and a varying number of pennyweights. A pennyweight and a pennyweight-and-a-half also appear in the Welsh manuscripts. In the Welsh translation of the famous recipe for God's Grace, the manner of writing the symbols for the weights given is explained, together with their relationships to each other.[24] Weights are also explained in the Leechbook. The dram is equal to sixty grains and the scruple to twenty. Knowing a pennyweight was then equal to a scruple and there are eight drams to one ounce allows us to use this measurement.

A pennyweight is precise but we also see a very variable handful or pinch in many recipes, along with as much as will fit between the tips of three fingers. Saucers, pots and inevitably spoons are also used as measures. In liquids, a pottle equalled two quarts and gallons are occasionally given of liquid, as well as in the Welsh recipes where pounds of wine and juice are also referred to.[25]

Timing is often absent from the instructions, although in all of the sources it might be directed to seethe or boil a mixture until it was reduced by half or two thirds, as in cookery. In one remedy the herb is wrapped in cabbage leaves and laid under hot ashes for half a mile way.[26] This to us, novel instruction, translates as the time it takes to walk half a mile at a brisk pace, which would be ten minutes.

Much used complex mixtures have directions to seethe while saying a specific Psalm. In the entret or plaster, Gratia Dei it is given as the *Miserere mei Deus* times three.[27] This might well be a timing mechanism. In the Welsh texts the Paternoster is mentioned twice, once while gathering a herb, which might be more about the time of day to gather, as prayer would be a daily practice.[28]

Where water forms a main base for drinks sometimes use of fountain water or spring water is specified. Head-washes and medicinal baths appear and the patient may be asked to drink or eat a recipe while in a bath or even to be bled while there. For drinks, wine is very often specified, or sometimes ale or beer. Herbs might also be steeped in vinegar to be drunk or applied. There is much less use of vinegar in the Welsh texts, although there is a recipe for making it.

Juices of fruits or green herbs were often included in complex recipes and were obtained by pounding to extract the juice or by heating with a little water. Juices of fruits might be combined with honey to make what was termed rob. This is not very different to syrup and the honey not only made them palatable but aided preservation, plus adding its own qualities.

Juices of wormwood, rue, and other, milder herbs are included in many mixtures. Red fennel and eyebright juices were used cold to soothe infected eyes. Red mint juice was dropped warm into aching ears, presumably from a quill as with eye drops. Ash juice or sap, obtained by heating a small branch appears in all sources for the ears as well as houseleek juice in the Welsh texts. Plantain juice is included in cough and bronchial remedies, for the eyes, and as a healing ingredient for wound applications. Yarrow juice was used in the Leechbooks for the eyes, mixed with egg-white, while rue, fennel, greater celandine, and ground ivy juices appear in an eye wash and drops in other texts.

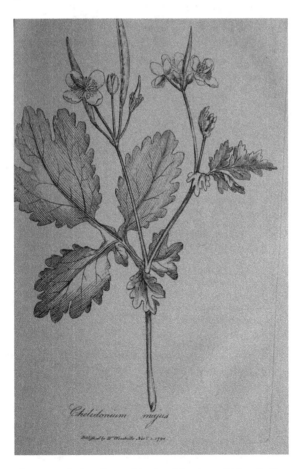

Greater Celandine. *Medical Botany*, Woodville.

A juice may also find its way into syrup, such as one for scab, leprosy, and itch. We should remember that leprosy was a broad term for disfiguring skin disease and did not always refer to leprosy as we understand it. This syrup was made with juices of fumitory and scabious with added distilled water of borage.[29] Syrups could be made with sugar or honey.

Distilled aromatic waters are in the minority in the recipes. In Manuscript B, a precious water to clear a man's eye is given containing numerous herbs.[30] Of these, fennel, eyebright and betony are still used today to treat the eyes. There were more aromatic water recipes which Professor Henslow has unfortunately omitted from the text. The same recipe is repeated in our second source, the Leechbook.[31] Following another recipe for complex eye water, in the Leechbook there is a list of eight simple waters and their uses, followed by aqua vitae, a spirit distilled from wine, and two others. Distilling is described as done in a still in two recipes and an alembic (two vessels joined by a tube), in a third. We will look in more detail at the uses of the individual waters in the chapter on the stillroom. They do not appear in the Welsh texts.

Dependence on ingredients from the apothecary is shown in the first sources with gum resins. Frankincense is most used appearing in eleven remedies with mastic next and myrrh in only three. Distilled aromatic waters used are of rose and madder. Leechbook recipes include dragon's blood, a red powder from the tree *Pterocarpus draco*.[32] In others brimstone, gum resins, unslaked lime, orpiment (yellow arsenic), and preparations from metals, verdigris, and litharge of lead, gold or silver, and red lead appear.

Litharge of silver or gold were actually yellowish-red or lighter coloured substances obtained in hard, scaly, crystalline masses by calcinations of lead nitrate and other lead salts. Litharge came from the copper works where lead was used to purify the copper. It was soluble in oil and very drying to the skin, making it considered a good base for ointments and plasters. To prepare it for use, the litharge had first to be pounded and washed repeatedly with water, then dried.[33]

Has the Use of the Herbs We are Following Through Time Changed?

Our first two herbs, betony and plantain, continue in popularity more especially in the Welsh texts as discussed below, with a wide range of uses.

Betony retains nineteen of the thirty six uses given in the Anglo-Saxon period. These are represented in recipes within the three collections. The Commonplace book and Leechbook show the emphasis on wounds and in all three sources recipes for the head and eyes are more frequent than for other problems and continue the former pattern. Treatment of vomiting, particularly when blood is vomited, seems to be an accepted application, while fevers and problems with the urinary system are well represented. Two mentions amongst other uses stand out—one for delusions, which perhaps continues the theme of protection from evil and nightmares, and the other for drunkenness.[34,35]

Plantain is slightly divided between ribwort and greater plantain, yet many recipes could refer to either. The number specifying ribwort is small compared to greater plantain and wounds are the common application. The treatment for glandular swellings continues, but now with greater plantain. The Leechbook contains the most recipes for greater plantain with twenty-nine, the majority are for treating wounds. Venomous wounds with snake bites and dog bites are in both the Welsh collection and the Leechbook. Use for dropsy is again mentioned and now diuretic properties are extended to treating festered gout with smallage and wormwood.[36]

Nettle was used much as we saw it in the surgeon's formularies with wounds and halting bleeding in recipes in all three sources. Use of the seeds against cold continues and in the Welsh collection nettle is given for urinary gravel.

Henbane appears in all three for treating toothache with variations of the familiar theme and in anaesthetics, both of which find further comment below. The herb is included in wound treatments and use is widened by a few recipes in the Leechbook, treating the liver, one for a boil, and interestingly one recipe to stop the patient weeping.[37] It does not say whether they are crying with pain or for another reason.

Elecampane only appears in the largest collection and there some former uses prevail with the highest number of recipes for coughs, then for the stomach and one for migraine. The herb is also used on the skin and, as in Macer, is applied for pain in the hip.[38] Properties as a diuretic and emmenagogue have not been followed here.

Ginger does not appear in the Welsh collection but in the other two as with elecampane, coughs and remedies for digestion come to the fore, with a single recipe for migraine from the Leechbook. This is a promising recipe.[39] Ginger is also used in its stimulatory capacity for the brain in a recipe for headache from cold.[40]

Liquorice appears in all three collections, again with the emphasis on coughs and stomach treatments in the Commonplace and Leechbooks. This is a continuation from the earlier period. A further appreciation is surfacing in the Commonplace book recipes using liquorice for the heart.[41]

Detailed Analysis

Questions to be answered are:

Has herbal medicine greatly changed since 1066?

Dietary treatment has strong precedents in both Anglo Saxon and classical medicine. Some recipes in the first two sources cure by diet, for instance giving a pottage of senvey (the seed is used to make mustard), and eating only barley bread for the palsy.[42] Thirteen remedies are to be eaten as foods. Diet also enters Leechbook recipes and there is specific information on bitter, sweet, roasted and raw foods.[43] In the Welsh recipes we find powdered herbs given in stew, which is reminiscent of herb pottages in the Anglo-Saxon period.[44] Dietary instructions and foods enter the recipes with breads made from specific flours of barley, rye, or wheat and many containing honey.

Variations of Anglo-Saxon recipes remain evident. A popular remedy will be altered slightly according to the experience and availability of ingredients of the person recording it. In the Lacnunga we read, "Against a cough: take drops of honey and wild celery's seed, and dill's seed; pound the seeds small, mix with the drops thickly, and pepper it heavily; take three spoons full having fasted over-night".[45] The result is basically an electuary.

In the fifteenth century Leechbook, the recipe has been adapted for a specific kind of cough. The main herbal combination is the same but in this the pepper is omitted and the honey changed to wine. "For the dry cough. Take anete (dill), smallage seed, of each equally much; and make powder of these and temper with wine, and seethe them well till they begin to wax thick; and afterwards keep it in a box or in another clean vessel, and use it first and last. *Probatum est*".[46]

In the Commonplace book, the Leechbook, and the Welsh texts, we have a recipe that continues to appear over the centuries for removing worms from the teeth, so curing toothache.[47,48,49] In these versions, the **seeds of henbane** and leek are heated on a very hot tile and a pipe is used to take the smoke from the burning seeds into the patient's mouth. A similar treatment appears in the Syrian medicine, when seeds of henbane, leek and onion are made into pills using fat and these are burned on hot coals for the patient to inhale the smoke.[50]

The Leechbook contains two more variations, in the first the herbs are heated with flour to produce the "breath" that will slay the worms.[51] In the second, henbane and leek seeds are more imaginatively mixed with incense and a "pipe of latten" used to convey the smoke.[52] Later writers comment on quacks using this method to defraud people under the influence of the henbane.

Polypharmacy, as seen in the treatment for water-elf sickness in Bald (see page X), remains and in a few recipes involves many herbs. The famous wound drink 'Save' contained over fifty herbs—comfrey, betony, rosemary, smallage, and wormwood amongst them in an elaborate preparation. It has been immortalised by mention in Chaucer's Knight's Tale, or so I thought. Checking for a modernised quote revealed how easily information is lost in translation. While converting the text into modern language, the editor had replaced the original lines, "Fermacyes of herbes, and eek save They dronken, for they wolde here lymes have"[53] with "Herb pharmacies and sage to make them trim; They drank them off, hoping to save a limb."[54] Replacing 'save' with a more familiar wound herb, sage, meant the meaning along with valuable information was lost.

The Anglo-Saxon sleeping drink containing hemlock and henbane is now further developed into the anaesthetic dwale, which appears in Manuscript B. This contains the gall of a pig the same sex as the patient; hemlock juice, wild catmint, lettuce, poppy, henbane, and ale vinegar, which is all boiled and then kept in a glass bottle. Three spoonfuls of this recipe are added to a bottle of good wine or ale and mixed well. The patient is sat near a good fire and told to drink the medicine until he falls asleep. With the operation over, his temples and cheeks are washed with vinegar and salt to waken him.[55] The Leechbook contains two versions of the recipe.[56]

Dangerous as these prescriptions appear to be, we know from the archaeology of the large medieval hospital at Soutra Aisle in Midlothian that such recipes were used. In the cellar of the hospital traces of a mix of black henbane, hemlock, and opium poppy were found. The find was testament to use with patients by Augustinian monks from the friary adjoining. The site of the buildings covering over an acre was clearly important in the period prior to 1460, situated close to the main route between England and Edinburgh.[57]

In the Welsh texts we have an anaesthetic recipe with a full complement of opium, poppy, mandrake, ivy, lettuce (wild), hemlock, and blackberries in Book five,[58] and Luft suggests in her notes that that particular version most resembles one from the Antidotarium of Nicolai, an influential manuscript which was mentioned in the last chapter.[59]

Use of animal parts in medicine is largely restricted to fats in the Anglo-Saxon Leechbooks we have looked at. *Medicina de Quadrupedibus* thoroughly covered the subject and might have been a companion volume. In our first sources, other than as fats and greases in applications, mentions are largely for gall or dung. Blood or bile in recipes is rare. Seventeen different fats are specified from domestic and wild animals, birds, and eels in the whole analysis. There are several animal recipes in the Welsh recipes, some involving cruelty and reducing a toad or other small animal to ash in a pot appears also in the Leechbook.

There we also find ants' horses (ants' eggs), perhaps for their acidity, goat's hoof, hartshorn, snail shells, oysters, the white roe of a red herring, and so on. Ants and snails were used in the Anglo-Saxon period too. Some physicians have taken delight in using animal parts, but they do not appear in the bulk of the recipes I have reviewed for the less affluent patients.

Is the medicine appreciably based on knowledge of surviving classical medicine?

Manuscript B (Harleian 2378), begins with the instructions of Hippocrates on observing the moon and stars with regard to effects on the condition and predominant humours of the patient. There is a note that when the moon is full, blood, brain, marrow, and other humours will be at their fullest power—these being moist and hot, or moist and cold. Several pages of astrological tables present in the original have been omitted, passing straight to recipes.[60]

There is also a long quotation purportedly from Galen in Manuscript A with advice on diet, and perilous days to bleed the patient for each month.[61] Similar quotations are common in medical manuscripts of this period. Warnings on activities including blood-letting on evil days appear in the Leechbook.[62] These vary on dates of peril from other versions. Galen's recipes are also referred to, for instance in the white colyrium for the eyes.[63] Material presented as straight from Hippocrates, or the completely unlikely Asclepius may be a later addition.

Galen and Hippocrates are referred to in each of the sources as authorities, and there are slightly garbled references in the practice, but we do not find reference to Dioscorides in any of these sources as we did very plainly in the Olde English Herbarium. Oribasius, Alexander of Tralles and the work of Paulus Aeginata are all clearly distinguished as sources of Bald's leechbooks, which in turn appears to be a source of some of the Welsh recipes.

Many correspondences to recipes from the works of Continental surgeons and other sources of the later medieval period are pointed out by the editors in the further notes to our sources. It may be fair to say there is a distinct presence of classical medicine forming a backdrop to empirical recipes.

What proportion of recipes are empirical herbal preparations as opposed to those dependent on superstition and psychology through added charms, ritual, or prayer?

The proportion of charms and elaborate ritual is very small when we consider these texts beside the Anglo Saxon Leechbooks. The social and cultural changes have been such since Norman rule that the emphasis is different. Medicine appears to have moved on to a certain extent with glimpses of the past that have been retained. An example is found in one recipe title which Professor Henslow has not interpreted, labelling it as having an obscure meaning, but it has connotations of the Anglo-Saxon period—this is "elf cake".[64] Interestingly the powdered root of gladene or yellow flag is to be taken in the common Anglo-Saxon way in meat and drink for nine days and nine nights. A magical number feels right for treating the elfshot. There is also a recipe on the same page as that above for anyone of either sex suggestively "blisted with wicked spirits".[65]

In Irish folk medicine, there is plentiful evidence for use of charms to cure specific conditions.[66] In England, wart charmers were still practising in my childhood. No doubt charms remained to a greater extent with the cunning woman and possibly the midwife. In our first source, we noted the only charms were to be used during childbirth. Midwives would later be obliged to swear to licensing bishops that they would not use them, or encourage the patient to use them.[67] Use of charms, particularly with pagan wordings is a factor in the formation of a picture of the lone woman healer as a witch.

Has use of herbs in herbal medicine greatly changed in response to Arabic pharmacy since the Anglo-Saxon period?

Arabic pharmacy brought us greater use of distilled waters, sugar, and syrups, as well as spices and increased use of senna, rhubarb, tamarinds, musk, camphor, nutmegs, cloves, saffron, fennel, and liquorice.[68] In the Commonplace texts apart from liquorice there is only the odd mention of saffron, senna, and rhubarb and one of cloves. With the exception of fennel, these have only one or two mentions in the Welsh texts, if any. In the Leechbook, liquorice is quite frequently used, senna, rhubarb, and cloves less so, with just a few instances of use of saffron. There is a direct reference in the recipe for a precious distilled water to be used against poison and pestilence in the Leechbook. It is to this water being called Imperial because all emperors and "great lords among the Saracens use to drink it".[69] Distilled waters appear in the first two of our sources but are not apparent in the Welsh texts.

Arabic pharmacy used conserves, recommending sugar for the chest. Early crusaders experienced the delights of sugar in Tripoli and encouraged importation from Damascus. There are numerous references to rose and violet sugar in the Wardrobe Account of Edward I.[70] A recipe for making Penydes twisted sugar sticks like those of barley sugar in more recent times, is given in Manuscript B of our first source.[71]

In the Leechbook under gathering of roses, there is a reminder to make sugar rosets and syrup with the fresh herb. Violet sugar and syrup is also emphasised. Sugar appears only once in the Welsh texts, when a large amount is used in syrup with scabious juice and egg-white.[72] As we consider the Pharmacopoeias In a later chapter there will be considerably more evidence of change.

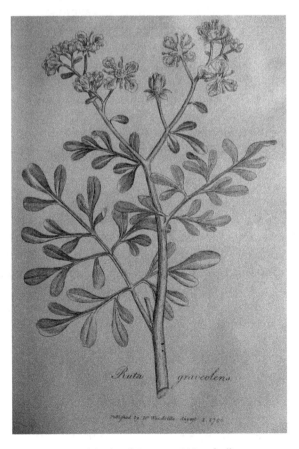

Rue, *Medical Botany*, Woodville.

Are the most used herbs of the Anglo-Saxon Leechbooks still the most used?

Our sources are in considerable agreement on the most commonly used herbs.

In Manuscript A in just under 200 recipes, the most commonly used herb is rue, appearing in twenty-five recipes, with smallage next then betony and waybroad or greater plantain closely following in frequency. Cumin, peppercorns, and fennel each score eleven. Particular attention is paid to betony with a list of the virtues in treating the stone, haematemesis, dropsy, the ear, eyes, cough, stomach, and oozing humors.[73] In manuscript B the most used herb by far is rue, appearing in twenty-eight recipes, with smallage twenty-two under that name or as ache, then fennel and betony in over twenty. Next come plantain and vervain.

In the Leechbook the herbs with most use are—rue, pepper and sage in fifty or more recipes, then betony, smallage, wormwood and waybroad (greater plantain close behind) cumin and fennel are almost as common.

In the Welsh texts, greater plantain and betony feature with thirty or over mentions and rue has just fewer, and then fennel. The top five herbs across the recipes are rue first in three sources out of four, smallage, betony, waybroad, and fennel with use of the foreign peppercorns and cumin adding heat. As with the other two sources wild celery ranks quite high and there is a prevalence of indigenous plants in the recipes.

These can be compared with earlier use in the Lacnunga, Old English Herbarium and Leechbook of Bald where just over two hundred different herbs appear in the remedies. Of these sage is included fifty one times, with rue almost as frequently used, then fennel, with betony and plantain having thirty five mentions. Greater plantain which is really important in the Old English Herbarium with twenty-two uses, scores most highly in the Leechbook and highest of all in the Welsh texts, but less so in our first sources.

Betony, significant in the Anglo-Saxon Leechbooks is present in many recipes in our first sources, and is the most important herb from the Leechbooks, also ranking almost as highly as greater plantain in the Welsh texts. Rue is the most popular or close to it in almost all our sources. Smallage scores highly in Manuscripts A and B, less so in the Leechbook and Welsh texts. Sage featured much less in the first two sources. The third and fourth herbs with most uses from the period preceding Norman and Arabic influence, yarrow and pennyroyal, now appear to be less important.

Of course, these numbers are also affected by the balance of conditions treated within the recipes, but this has not greatly changed.

Categories of Conditions that we are Following the Treatments of Throughout History

Most are well represented as seen below with eye conditions, boils, toothache, fevers, and rheumatic pain, coughs, burns, and headaches are the exceptions. In our first two manuscript sources sixteen remedies are for the eyes and about as many for the ears, with drops for each and herbal preparations to apply. There are numerous remedies for toothache. Other categories are minimally represented.

Analysis of the one thousand and seventy-one Leechbook recipes shows over two hundred and fifty herbs are used to treat a wide variety of diseases and discomforts, with the largest number of recipes being to treat eye problems. Many terms are used for various skin conditions, such as morphew (a skin blemish, sometimes thought to resemble the tight, dry skin of scleroderma), mormal (an ulcerated sore), tetters (eczema) and sausfleme (acne). There are also remedies for sores in several parts of the body—with the legs gaining most mention, palsy, gout, stomach problems, swellings, and wounds.

Within over five hundred recipes from Welsh texts the highest number deal with treating patients for worms of various kinds, and of course the term worms might be applied to insects as well. These recipes are concentrated in Books six and eight. Eye and ear applications are again high, also fevers and boils. Most of the ten toothache remedies appear in a single text, and all can be found in other earlier sources. The number of urinary remedies is unusual and there are a great many remedies for corrupt flesh. There are few for coughs or other conditions.

Looking at treatments for specific conditions we have been following, have these changed?

Eye Remedies—These remain frequent in the recipes, in the Anglo-Saxon period we noted the predominance of native British herbs, the balance has only slightly changed with fennel used most and then betony, eyebright, greater celandine and rue. Rose appears as water of roses in several official recipes attributed to authorities such as Master Peter of Spain, Galen and the school at Montpelier, in the Leechbook and plantain juice also seen in Roman medicine for eyes appears as a remedy for swollen and inflamed eyes.[74]

Toothache—As we have already seen, henbane remains in consistent use with the same recipes. Pellitory of Spain has equal place in the Leechbook, greater plantain and yarrow would have been readily available. Mastic is long gone from the scene but long pepper emerges as an imported remedy.

Coughs—Pepper appears again in a treatment for the perilous cough in the Commonplace book.[75] Across the three sources liquorice is narrowly beaten as prime herb by hyssop, with white horehound and elecampane continuing from the Anglo-Saxon recipes and sometimes two of them used together in a number of recipes. Sage from the Anglo-Saxon recipe I tested appears again in two sources and comfrey has a mention.

Joint Pain—Recipes are found in both the Welsh collection and the Leechbook. Commonly used herbs are wormwood and rue and a number of other herbs are mentioned including chamomile, henbane, nettle, and betony.

Burns—treatment in the Leechbook shows the practice of applying white lily leaves or bulbs has continued.[76] Treatment of burns is one area where it seems many possibilities were tried, those that did not involve herbs were olive oil whisked with water, and other greases. One understandable one was houseleek and three remedies in the Welsh collection use greater plantain.

Fevers—This encompasses many conditions and often treatments contain many herbs, greater plantain still features, as do wormwood, mugwort, and betony. Heating herbs such as cumin and pepper are also used in the Leechbook.

Boils—The Commonplace texts have no remedies for these but there are three using greater plantain in the Welsh collection. The Leechbook has many recipes but the only herbs repeated in these are lily root, hollyhock, and garlic.

Headaches—Betony is the most used herb, then rue, wormwood, vervain, and fennel, in that order. Typical recipes involve anointing the head, applying a plaster of the herbs or making a head wash, but there are drinks as well. In the Leechbook southernwood, honey, and vinegar are pounded and drunk while fasting. In the same source a wonderful fabric garland is made and stuffed with a mix of powdered *Ammi visnaga* from the spicer and chamomile pounded to dust, this is then seethed in wine before being squeezed almost dry and wound still hot, around the head.[77]

Is there a common use of any herb which is no longer present in modern herbal medicine and could this be beneficially re-introduced?

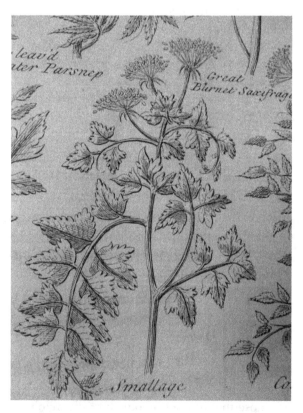

Smallage. *The British Herbal*, Hill.

In the Old English Herbarium, Apium appears for soreness of the eyes and swelling, "March which is Apium. For soreness of the eyes and for swelling take this plant which one calls 'appium' and by another name 'march' well pounded with bread, lay it to the eyes."[78] Since it is well pounded and laid to the eyes, I am presuming this recipe is using the foliage rather than seed, but again we have confirmation of the various names and from the Book of Bald inclusion in a recipe for the seed with other seeds.

In the Leechbook of the fifteenth century the number of applications of smallage to swelling from various causes drew my attention and this greatly interested me as different parts of the plant are used for different conditions, but the action required appears to be the same. The range covers the juice for swelling of a sore, also applied for swelling of a woman's teats, the root was given with fennel for swelling in the stomach, and smallage applied with other herb foliage for fractures with sudden swellings. Finally, it was recommended with breadcrumbs to be applied for all manner of swellings.[79]

Use of smallage externally for swellings was not something I had come across in modern herbal medicine and the latest I could find it was 1746. I decided to use a test ointment in my herbal practice, adhering to the historical method, it was made by heating the fresh foliage in cold pressed extra virgin olive oil, using a fire for heat and thickening the ointment with local beeswax.

Firstly I prescribed it for swelling of arthritic joints, using it for patients with rheumatoid arthritis. The resulting relief quickly brought a request for more. Then a patient with a stubborn condition, who came feeling desperate as over five weeks on from her injury, modern medicine had been ineffective at reducing the swelling of her hand. This time the result was startlingly fast, improvement being reported almost immediately. This use of course tied in with the old recipes, both recipes were made from the leaf.

In the third instance it was chronic lymphoedema, which affected under the patient's arm and across the breast, causing great discomfort, especially at night. After a battery of tests to establish this was not a return of the cancer, the patient had been left without treatment. This time I used the ointment made from the seed in a water bath for extraction, this was slower to work, but again successful.

Finding gems such as this is the bonus of detailed historical research.

References

1. G. Henslow, *Medical Works of the Fourteenth Century* (New York: Burt Franklin, 1972).
2. Henslow, *Medical Works of the Fourteenth Century*, 76.
3. Ibid, XV.
4. Warren Dawson, (ed), *A Leechbook of the XVth Century* (London: Macmillan & Co., 1934).
5. Dawson, *A Leechbook of the XVth Century*, (956–7), 295.

6. Ibid, (523), 171.
7. Ibid, (42), 29.
8. Leonard Rosenman, *A Medieval Surgical Pharmacopoeia and Formulary.* 1170–1325 (San Francisco: Rosenman, 1999), 19.
9. Dawson, *A Leechbook of the XVth Century,* (776), 243.
10. Ibid, (386), 141.
11. Ibid, 141–147.
12. Diana Luft, *Medieval Welsh Medical Texts. Vol. 1 The Recipes* (Cardiff: University of Wales Press, 2020). 82, 164.
13. Luft, *Medieval Welsh Medical Texts* Vol. 1, 82, 164.
14. Ibid, 5.
15. Gösta Frisk (ed), *Macer Floridus de Viribus Herbarum* (Cambridge, Mass: Harvard University Press, 1949).
16. Stephen Pollington, *Leechcraft* (Norfolk: Anglo-Saxon Books, 2000).
17. *The Red Book of Hergest,* Oxford, Jesus College, Manuscript 111.
18. G. Brodin, *Agnus castus.* (Upsala: Harvard University Press. 1950).
19. S.V. Larkey (ed), *An Herbal* (1525), (Scholars Facsimiles and Reprints, New York. 1941).
20. Luft, *Medieval Welsh Medical Texts,* Vol. 1, 118–120.
21. Dawson, *A Leechbook of the XVth Century,* (956), 295.
22. Luft, *Medieval Welsh Medical Texts,* Vol. 1, Book 1, No. 5, 60.
23. Ibid, Book 9. No. 41, 252.
24. Ibid, Book 5. No. 2, 118.
25. Ibid, British Library, 17. 296.
26. Dawson, *A Leechbook of the XVth Century,* (297), 115.
27. Ibid, (299), 117.
28. Luft, *Medieval Welsh Medical Texts,* Vol. 1, Book 6. No. 22, 174.
29. Dawson, *A Leechbook of the XVth Century,* (788), 247.
30. Henslow, *Medical Works of the Fourteenth Century,* (287), 117.
31. Dawson, *A Leechbook of the XVth Century,* (988), 303.
32. Ibid, (723), 229.
33. John Hill, *A History of the Materia Medica* (London: Longman, Hitch & Hawes, 1751), 21–22.
34. Dawson, *A Leechbook of the XVth Century,* (312), 123.
35. Luft, *Medieval Welsh Medical Texts,* Vol. 1, Book 6. No. 67, 186.
36. Dawson, *A Leechbook of the XVth Century,* (382), 139.
37. Ibid, (960), 295.
38. Ibid, (174), 71.
39. Ibid, (608), 195.
40. Ibid, (699), 223.
41. Henslow, *Medical Works of the Fourteenth Century,* 68.
42. Ibid, 43.
43. Dawson, *A Leechbook of the XVth Century,* (1019), 311.
44. Luft, *Medieval Welsh Medical Texts,* Vol. 1, Book 9. No. 35, 248.
45. Stephen Pollington, *Leechcraft* (Norfolk: Anglo Saxon Books, 2000), (Lacnunga II), 187.

46. Dawson, *A Leechbook of the XVth Century*, (199), 77.
47. Henslow, *Medical Works of the Fourteenth Century*, (243), 111.
48. Dawson, *A Leechbook of the XVth Century*, (33), 27.
49. Luft, *Medieval Welsh Medical Texts*, Vol. 1, Book 9. No. 41, 252.
50. E.A. Wallis Budge, *Syrian Anatomy, Pathology, And Therapeutics*, Vol. I Native Prescriptions, (Alpha Editions, 2020), XCV.
51. Dawson, *A Leechbook of the XVth Century*, (33), 27.
52. Ibid, (912), 283.
53. Henslow, *Medical Works of the Fourteenth Century*, 55.
54. Nevill Coghill, (trans), *Chaucer. The Canterbury Tales* (Middlesex: Penguin Books, 1975), 92.
55. Henslow, *Medical Works of the Fourteenth Century*, 90–91.
56. Dawson, *A Leechbook of the XVth Century*, (852 & 853), 263.
57. Wu Mingren, "The Incredible Medical Interventions of the Monks of Soutra Aisle." Ancient Origins Reconstructing the story of humanity's past, June 22, 2018. https://www.ancient-origins.net/ancient-places-europe/incredible-medical-interventions-monks-soutra-aisle-003285.
58. Luft, *Medieval Welsh Medical Texts*, Vol. 1, Book 5. No. 71, 154.
59. Ibid, 369.
60. Henslow, *Medical Works of the Fourteenth Century*, 76.
61. Ibid, 63.
62. Dawson, *A Leechbook of the XVth Century*, (1073–4), 329.
63. Ibid, (485), 161.
64. Henslow, *Medical Works of the Fourteenth Century*, 89.
65. Ibid, 89.
66. Rosarie Kingston, *Ireland's Hidden Medicine* (Lewes: Aeon Books, 2021), 22.
67. Carole Rawcliffe, *Medicine & Society in Later Medieval England* (Stroud: Sutton Publishing Ltd., 1997), 201.
68. C.J.S. Thompson, *The Mystery and Art of the Apothecary* (Philadelphia: Lippincott Co., 1929), 82.
69. Dawson, *A Leechbook of the XVth Century*, (977), 301.
70. Margaret Wade Labarge, *A Baronial Household of the Thirteenth Century* (London: Eyre and Spottiswoode, 1965), 97.
71. Henslow, *Medical Works of the Fourteenth Century*, 121.
72. Luft, *Medieval Welsh Medical Texts*, Vol. 1, Book 8. No. 33, 216.
73. Henslow, *Medical Works of the Fourteenth Century*, 70–71.
74. Dawson, *A Leechbook of the XVth Century*, (479), 159.
75. Henslow, *Medical Works of the Fourteenth Century*, 101.
76. Dawson, *A Leechbook of the XVth Century*, (666), 211.
77. Ibid, (13), 21.
78. Pollington, *Leechcraft*, (Norfolk: Anglo-Saxon Books, 2000), (120), 343.
79. Dawson, *A Leechbook of the XVth Century*, (799), 251.

SECTION VI

PROGRESS IN CHEMISTRY
AND BOTANY | 1509–1712

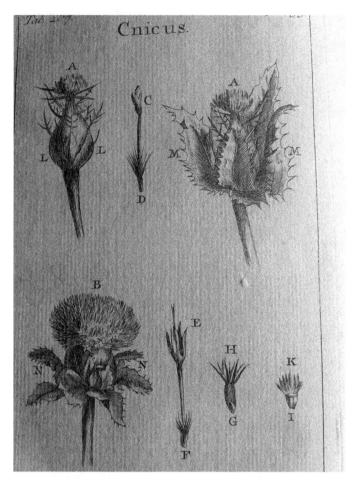

Blessed Thistle, *The Compleat Herbal*, Tournefort.

Key Figures

Thomas Linacre (c1460–1524), Luca Ghini (1490–1556), Paracelsus (1493–1541), Henry VIII (reigned 1509–1547), Richard Banckes, (dates unknown), William Turner (c1508-10–1568), Andreas Vesalius (1514–1564), Elizabeth I (reigned 1558–1603), John Gerard (1545–1612), Thomas Muffet (1553–1604), Gervase Markham (c1568–1637), Théodore Mayerne (1573–1655), James I (reigned 1603–1625), Sir Hans Sloane (1660–1753).

Key Texts

Syon Herbal, 1517, Thomas Betson.
An Herbal, 1525, Richard Banckes.

Virtuous Book of Distillation, 1527, Brunschwig.
Treatise on Surgery, 1536, Paracelsus.
Fabrica, 1543, Vesalius.
Herbalists' Charter, Act of 1543.
Of the Birth of Mankind, 1545, Richard Jonas.
The Names of Plants, 1548, Turner.
Great Herbal, 1548, Gerard.
Paragranum Astronomia Magna, 1548, Paracelus.
The English Housewife, 1615, Gervase Markham.

Roles of Women in Medicine

Midwives work as before but during this period the religious houses and infirmaries close. Responsibility for care moves to the parishes and ladies with the means to give assistance offer Christian charity with medicines. Women may now be nurses in small hospices caring for the sick or infirm. A few London hospitals reopen.[1] The Herbalists' Charter applied for anyone of either sex who has knowledge to administer herbs, and the role of women with such "cunning" continues for the poor.[2]

Quality Control

Correct identification of herbs, is aided by William Turner's book[3]—Luca Ghini's hortus siccus (or dried garden, a collection of pressed herb samples, now more commonly referred to as a herbarium) recorded herb botany both with the herb specimens and with living plants in the new botanic gardens.[4] Laws on weights and measures, who was entitled to make medicines, sell and prescribe them became a hot issue. Britain began in a small way to catch up with European legislation, although the examination of stocks of drugs was not always rigorously enforced. Training of surgeons and apothecaries became more standardized.

Herb Energetics

Detailing the energetics of herbs is the norm in herbals. Energetics dictate how long distilled Aromatic Waters may be kept and are best prescribed for patients of different temperaments.[5]

Archaeology

A wealth of archaeological finds both from cities such as London and from shipwrecks offer many insights. The barber surgeon's chest containing ointment boxes, instruments of surgery, etc., from the ship the Mary Rose is an example.[6]

Travel and Trade

Trade in spices and therefore prices paid in Europe had previously been controlled by Venetian merchants who bought them in Constantinople and sold them on, making a considerable profit. Maritime exploration led to the Portuguese sailing to the spice islands and taking control of the port of Malacca in 1511.[7] This was followed by a scramble by Spain, England, France, and Holland for lucrative discoveries in other lands and a good deal of piracy. Battles follow in the ensuing decades over who should have the right to cheat the indigenous peoples of commercially valuable herbs and spices. This pattern was repeated often as downright theft and with dire consequences for the population from foreigners introducing previously unknown diseases to an area. The threat of losing control to the enemy in the future was dealt with by setting up new plantations in other tropical areas, where they had a more secure hold. This led in turn to the need of large numbers of workers who could cope with tropical climates and transportation of enslaved people was seen as the horrifying answer.

Introduction

Already themes we will be following in the three chapters of this section are emerging under the headings above. A series of social changes coupled with the advent of printed books, exploration overseas, introduction of new plants, and regulations in medicine lead to a very different picture of herbal medicine from that seen previously. The reign of Henry VIII with his deep interest in medicine, closure of religious houses, and new regulations sets off a domino effect. Where previously the monks had laboriously made beautiful copies of individual books, William Caxton had already set up his printing press in Westminster in 1476 and this method was taking over.[8] Closure of some monasteries put a strain on nearby communities who found themselves with responsibility for the lay workers and anyone formerly looked after at the large establishments.

The wives of local landowners, particularly the ladies of manors and those in higher positions, would take up the role of charitable providers of medicine. The lives of these women as revealed in their diaries, consisted of prayers, supervising the preparation of herbs for many uses, including medicine, and other daily chores between entertaining guests.[9] In some families, generation after generation passed down their records of recipes, alongside cookery in their household books. There was great excitement at the news from voyages of discovery and the introduction of new plants from far away countries, and this became translated into a rising interest in gardening and growing unusual plants. Books on gardening appeared beside the herbals and devotional works.[10] Physic gardens for harvest lead to botanic gardens to aid identification and further botany.

Throughout the whole period there is concern over improving standards, and this is applied through regulating physicians and apothecaries.

References

1. Nicholas Orme and Margaret Webster, *The English Hospital 1070–1570* (London: Yale University Press, 1995), 161.
2. Barbara Griggs, *Green Pharmacy* (London: Jill Norman & Hobhouse Ltd., 1981), 62.
3. Britten et al, (intro), William Turner. *The Names of Herbes 1548* (London: The Ray Society, Facsimiles, 1965), 29.
4. Anna Pavord, *Searching for Order* (London: Bloomsbury, 2009), 173, 176.
5. Theophrastus von Oberstockstall, (trans), *The Virtuous Book of Distillation* (The Restorers of Alchemical Manuscripts Society Digital, 2013), Chapter XXIIII.
6. Robin Wood, The Wooden Bowl (Ammanford: Stobart Davies Ltd., 2005), 122.
7. Giles Milton, *Nathaniel's Nutmeg* (London: Sceptre, 1999), 23.
8. J.D Mackie, *The Earlier Tudors. 1485–1558* (Oxford: Clarendon Press, 1962), 239.
9. Joanna Moody, (ed), *The Private Life of an Elizabethan Lady* (Stroud: Sutton Publishing, 2001), 58.
10. Richard Mabey, (ed), *The Gardener's Labyrinth*. Thomas Hill (Oxford: Oxford University Press, 1988).

CHAPTER 14

Regulation, Paracelsus, and Chemistry | 1509–1553

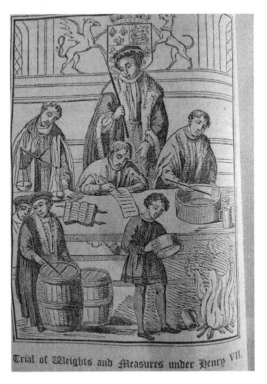

Weights and Measures, *The Every Day Book*. Hone.

Henry VIII came to the throne in 1509. His reign was to be formative in many ways. He was very interested in medicine and devised his own medicinal recipes. Some of these are contained in "A Booke of plaisters, spasmadraps, ointments, pulthes, etc. devysed by the King's Majestie, Dr. Butts, Dr. Chambre, Dr. Cromer and Dr. Augustin."[1] This text is in the British Museum. Spasmadrap is a liquid preparation applied by dipping strips of linen into it and applying on the skin.

One of his physicians, Thomas Linacre, had graduated in Padua and seen the control exercised by the Collegium of Physicians there. Another 'college', the *arte dei medicie speziali* of Florence had already compiled the first official pharmacopoeia in 1498. In Italy apothecaries had to pass exams set at Salerno in order to practice. In 1518 Linacre's influence moved Henry to found the Royal College of Physicians to regulate the practice of physic and repress unlearned and incompetent practitioners. From then on, unless graduates of Oxford or Cambridge, physicians must pass an exam set by the College in order to practice within seven miles of London. English graduates were exempt elsewhere. It had already become illegal for a woman to practice medicine in 1421 when a University education was required, but that does not seem to have been enforced.[2]

The founding of the College and first regulation of physicians led to many squabbles within the prevailing hierarchy of medicine. Physicians sued the surgeons for using herbal treatments along with surgery, both, along with barber-surgeons criticised the apothecary and all of them left a medical void for the poor. We hear little if anything about midwives in these exchanges. The act regulating physicians does not mention them. However, licensing of midwives by the Church had existed for centuries on the Continent and in England bishops could license midwives within their diocese from 1511 onwards.[3] This licence depended upon the good references of patients on their professional ability, and on their moral character. The church had a specific interest since if the baby was likely to die without a priest present the midwife had a duty to baptise the child.

The Pharmacopoeia in England was still far in the future, but the contents would be partially influenced by new ideas for medicine envisioned by an arrogant Swiss physician appointed professor at the University of Basle in 1536. Born in c1493, Aureolus Bombastus Hohenheim was also called, either by his tutor or himself, Paracelsus, meaning he was superior to the Roman writer on medicine, Celsus. He was the son of a physician serving a mining town and perhaps took some of his initial inspiration for alchemy and chemical medicine from experience in the mining school and his apprenticeship. Alternatively, it came from the tuition of Abbot Trimethius, a Benedictine monk who was a theologian and astronomer who taught the sciences.[4] The life of Paracelsus has been surrounded by speculation and accumulated myth for centuries, which means there is little except a few basic facts that may be depended upon.

He is thought to have taken his bachelor's degree in Vienna, although Basle has also been suggested.[5] He then identified Italy as the best place to go for training in medicine. He chose Ferrara in 1513 and graduated three years later.[6] He was then a pupil of a wealthy physician, Sigismund Fugger, and already researching mineralogy and chemistry as well as medicine.[7] He did not practise medicine immediately, but instead set out to travel and learn from nature, a form of learning which he valued more than academic education. Along the way for almost ten years that are factually unaccounted for, he is said to have worked as a surgeon and accumulated knowledge. Having travelled extensively across Europe, reputedly into Russia, and experienced medicine in Constantinople and possibly Egypt, working sometimes as an army surgeon, he developed his ideas.

It is perhaps on safer ground that we may say that he studied alchemy through the works of Isaac the Hollander—these texts were also later to be regarded by the Anglo-Irish philosopher and chemist Robert Boyle, as the clearest on alchemy. The work of Isaac the Hollander and his son, in turn, rested on that of Geber, who we have already considered.[8] Paracelsus taught that the operations involved in alchemy could be resolved into sublimation. He quoted Geber on this as meaning elevating dry matter by fire.[9] Paracelsus concentrated on what he understood as the three elementary constituents of all matter—salt, sulphur, and mercury. He wanted to found a new, better, simpler medicine and was utterly scathing of Galenic medicine with its complex compounds.

He refers to the need of man and animals for salt as part of their nourishment and points out that salt is used to prevent decay of flesh, and he calls salt a natural balsam in man.[10] Paracelsus instructs physicians to pay attention to the three forms of salt which he describes, sea salt, salt from springs, and mineral salts from metals or mineral ores. He notes that whether salt is liquid or dry it dries up all humours that come from the body, more especially the liquid form.[11] To Paracelsus alchemy was essential to medicine so that when he speaks of medicine the two are generally entwined. He refers to the ways in which physicians can use salt baths to treat skin diseases, and salt washes for wounds and ulcers.

On sulphur, Paracelsus points out that it has been entirely misunderstood by many writers, which provokes him to pass judgement on simpleton doctors, charlatan alchemists, and Aristotle. He refers to his long experience and points out that the physician uses only cleansed sulphur and not what is ordinarily understood by the name. We need to remember that this is the sulphur contained in all things when he states that through alchemy particular sulphurs can be separated from metals, as a nutshell is separated from the nut. He lists various sulphurs from metals and the human organs they benefit—sulphur of copper for the kidneys, and sulphur of quicksilver for the lungs.[12] He regarded all sulphurs as sleep-producing and analgesic and yet without the harmful effects of henbane and *Mandragora*.[13] Paracelsus details a preservative prescription against plague, pleurisy, and abscesses using purified sulphur, myrrh, aloes, and saffron.[14]

There is no corresponding text on the subject of mercury in the Geneva folio but an edition of the *Archidoxorum Libri Decem* was published in Latin in 1582 and this contains chemical experiments specific to mercury. Paracelsus is adamant in refuting Galen's doctrine of the humours. On the subject of hermetic medicine, he begins with "two complexions of Nature"[15] hot and cold, decrying the four terms in use, saying hot being moist is a contradiction in terms. He further states clearly that for the perfect knowledge of medicine astrology is necessary. He relates the four degrees we have previously met in the classification of herbs in this way—those plants emerging from earth are of the first degree; whatever is from the air, and here contagious diseases are listed, is of the second degree; the third degree comprises those things springing from water and here he places lead and precious stones such as topaz; from fire come crystal, and, confusingly, ice, which are in the fourth degree.[16]

Within the degrees are sixteen points so that each of these broad classes are divided again, as some substances within the degree excel each other. This is far more complex than the Galenic system, here the fourth degree of cold consists of whatever is born of fire and has the action of congealing the humours. In the Galenic system the fourth degree of cold is the most dangerous to life and this includes narcotics, regarded today generally as potentially poisonous. Narcotics in the system envisaged by Paracelsus are presented as less harmful if given in a safe dose and so are relegated to the third degree.

Animals, minerals and plants he argues should be more carefully separated than into four categories and he sets out a system with a further four points of strength within each of the four degrees for a more accurate definition. He writes that it is mistaken to place camphor, sperm of frogs, nenuphar (a water lily) and alum all together in one degree with no further division. There are points of difference.[17]

The ruling on degrees is not from the nature and proportion of the elements of fire or water, but from the predominance of salt, mercury and sulphur within them. With this in mind degrees and points within them are also applied to diseases and the stages of healing in a wound along with the applications necessary to heal it. Paracelsus also uses astrological considerations, making classification of mixtures exceedingly complex.[18]

Colours are also related to revealing the nature of plants, metals, etc. We might presume that a red object would always classify it as hot. He explains that the external colour does not always reveal its true nature. An exception to red being warm and white cold is shown in the case of the red rose since the yellow anthers in a red rose attract the heat from it, making it of a cold nature. He also applies this rule to other flowers where there is yellow within red petals. All are cold.[19] He follows this reasoning through into chemicals where his argument is even more difficult to understand.

When it comes to herbs, elecampane, ginger, and liquorice are all listed as of a warm nature but only in the first degree of heat as they spring from the earth. Henbane is given as of a cold nature, but in contrast to the Galenical fourth degree it is rated in the first degree as the plant is also of the earth. Examples of medicinal substances included under the element of air are vitriol, sulphur, topaz, and quick-silver. Water he maintains produces silver, three kinds of coral, and camphor, while from fire proceed ice, crystal, and snow.[20] Returning to the subject of herbs, when they are placed in a composition for preparations, such as roses into oil or vinegar, this can change their degree which is then raised from first to second and so on. By being separated further in spagyric medicines then they can make larger changes.[21] Spagyric preparations are those in which the substance is separated for alteration and the separate parts of the mass are individually purified and then those purified parts re-united.

On his return to Basle in 1536, Paracelsus was appointed as a professor to Basle University, but his relationship with other professors did not go well. His lectures included public attendance and were delivered in German rather than Latin, reput-edly while wearing an alchemist's leather apron rather than an academic's gown. Paracelsus presented his new approach to medicine and his lectures drew large audiences as he spoke on tumours, wounds, uroscopy, and pulse diagnosis.

From his now extensive experience he sought to combine knowledge as a phy-sician and surgeon in an unprecedented way using progressive chemical treat-ments, thus upsetting physicians, surgeons, and apothecaries whose territories he was invading. According to some sources, in a matter of months his unpopularity increased until one story tells us, on St John's Day as part of student festivities he incensed the faculty by publicly burning the works of Avicenna and Galen. He left Basle soon afterwards to travel again re-visiting the mining districts of his youth, where he wrote the first treatise on industrial disease. His written works included the *Paragranum*, which stated that medicine should be based on four pillars: natural philosophy, astronomy, alchemy, and the virtue of the physician who must be able to understand and apply the other three.[22]

Hermetic astronomy he considered within the subject of philosophy, beginning with the creation of all things by God. Paracelsus taught that man was made last out of all those things earlier brought out of nothingness. In other words, human beings have a little of all creatures, all elements, the stars and the earth within, making each one of us a microcosm of the macrocosm or universe.[23] He portrays each foetus as having four parents—mother, father, elements from the earth, and from the stars. As they come together at conception then the strongest influences prevail.[24] Pointing out that nothing would grow on earth without the influence of the stars, he names them as the source of intellect in man and of his spirit. The con-clusion is that knowledge of medicine relates to the elements and knowledge of the stars to astrology, both need to be involved in a cure.

The close relationship of the microcosm of man with the macrocosm of the universe in astrological medicine was of prime importance to him. His writings reveal that remedies required direction from the heavens in the manner in which they are prepared in order to work. In his view, the physician could not simply rely on the temperaments and humours, such as using cold medicines in treating

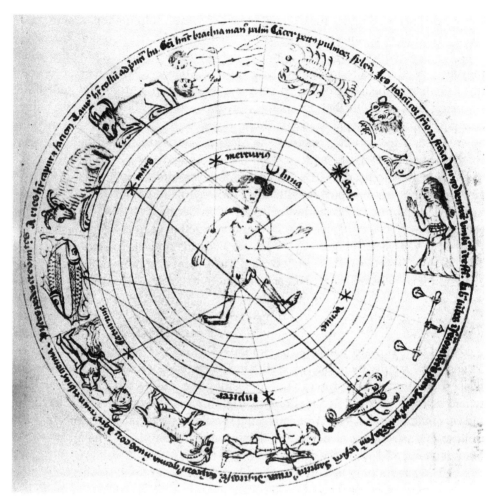

The Microcosm (man) and the Macrocosm (the World). Line Engraving
by T. de Bry, 1617.

hot conditions. When using a herb under the influence of the moon to treat the
brain, he believed the physician must know how to do so when the moon is propi-
tious, bringing about a link between the heavenly moon and the herb. The basis of
these ideas is partly shown in the medieval diagrams of the zodiac man, where each
of the organs is assigned to a zodiac sign of the heavens.[25]

Paracelsus foreshadowed homoeopathy when he wrote on the anatomy of diseases, maintaining the cause of the disease is identical with its' own anatomy or
source. He prepared treatments such as the anodyne specific, designed to act not
merely on the patient, but actually on the disease. For this he used Thebaic opium,
orange and lemon juice, cinnamon, and cloves. The ingredients were pounded and
then having been mixed were digested in glass in the sun, or set in dung for steady

heat for a month. With the ingredients digested, they were again mixed with more hermetically prepared ingredients, such as the magistery of pearls and quintessence of gold. The resulting anodyne specific was to remove diseases without affecting the body of the patient.[26]

Paracelsus stated that each disease must be cured with its own medicine, making him the proposed "father of iatrochemistry". His views on properly prepared poisons being harmless if given in tiny amounts validated something already noted historically by Eupator, King of Pontus (ruled 120–63 BC), who habitually took small doses of poisons in order to protect himself from being poisoned by larger doses. Paracelsus railed against physicians who offset the potentially poisonous effects of drugs like scammony by adding comfrey for the patient's better tolerance, pointing out that the poison had not been removed but was still in the system of the patient.[27] Poisons must be hermetically transmuted to be safe. The knowledge he gained by introducing mercury and other poisonous drugs into medicine became the basis of toxicology. Above all he encouraged seeing all knowledge in the light of nature.

Paracelsus believed the physician should also be an alchemist and here his youthful experience shows as he recommends all physicians should go to the mountains to see where the minerals grow. Travelling, meeting people of all walks of life and gaining knowledge in this way is described as he writes "He who wishes to explore Nature must tread her books with his feet".[28]

He takes us further than that simplified view for as an alchemist and a deeply religious Christian man, he appreciated that all living things have both a visible and an inner, invisible form. He classified diseases as relating to the basic salt, sulphur, and mercury as explained earlier, and proposed that since sulphur could be broken down by four agents, cold, heat, moisture, and dryness, it caused diseases of all four types. Mercury he observed rises and falls as in distillation and so caused diseases characterised by heat, in the worst cases, high fever. He noted salt gave form to all things and is also subjected to four processes. His writing on the diseases caused by salt is complex but notably related to external ulcers, cancers, etc.[29]

Paracelsus wrote prolifically on many subjects including religion and politics, his great work on surgery published in 1536 is most associated with his fame. Always supporting the down trodden, ever recommending use of talents for the benefit of others, he worked to heal the poor for no reward and died a poor man himself in 1541. Through his notoriety, the enthusiasm of his students in collecting his works and study of his publications his ideas were to live on influencing the course of medicine.

In England the closure of Abbeys and other religious houses between 1536 and 1541 had huge social consequences. Monks and nuns were awarded small pensions, but were not the only ones displaced. Many hospitals originated through links with religious houses or were founded by monarchs. Meanwhile the effect on care of the sick in hospitals at the time varied. At the dissolution many books used by monks and nun apothecaries were destroyed. However, in the case of St Thomas' Southwark it re-opened after the dissolution.[30] Merchant and trade guilds often financed small hospitals for care of their members, as with the Hosier's Hospital in Ludlow near the churchyard.[31]

In 1543 in deference to the necessity of midwives and others in treating the poor, the Act which herbalists think of as the Herbalists Charter—to some it was the "quacks charter"—was passed to legislate for a new class of practitioners. This was entitled "An Act That Persons Being No Common Surgeons May Minister Outward Medicines", and it stated the right of "every person being the King's subject, having knowledge and experience of the nature of herbs, roots and waters, to use and minister, according to their cunning, experience and knowledge."[32] Through this Act we see herbal medicine flourishing and herbalists have been indebted to it over the centuries for their legality.

A book translated from the Latin by a scholar, Richard Jonas, called *Of the Birth of Mankind* was constantly in print between 1540 and 1654. This first English edition had been based on Eucharius Rösslin's *Rose Garden*, which contained much from Galen, Avicenna, and Rhazes and was more directed to trainee midwives. As midwives on the Continent were examined by physicians before being licensed to practice, it was necessary for them to know the relevant classical medicine.

The English version left out numerous references to the Greek and Arabic sources and made some alterations to ideas on humoral influences in women, which were now starting to be seen as outdated. Richard Jonas wrote in a way that gave consideration to a pregnant mother reading the book, with gentler presentation of unpleasant procedures and acknowledging the pain involved. He also added a piece dealing with remedies for the infant and helping a woman to conceive.[33] The book was revised by a physician, Thomas Raynalde in 1545. He included new anatomical knowledge from the work of Vesalius.[34] His ground breaking anatomical study *Fabrica* was published just two years earlier, and many more herbal recipes.

Galen had been the previous authority on anatomy and physiology, but, as already pointed out in the chapter on his influence, this depended on anything he had learned as surgeon to the gladiators and dissection of animals, particularly the Barbary ape which led to some mistaken ideas. Although this fact was evident from his writings, later physicians assumed he had dissected human bodies and Vesalius had a hard task to prove him wrong.[35] The correct anatomy of the womb was essential towards a better understanding of the physiology.

The Birth of Mankind excellently researched and edited by Elaine Hobby contains many more recipes than the Trotula. While both refer to a wide range of female conditions relating to pregnancy and childbirth, there are fewer on conditions of children in Trotula. The two texts are in harmony on some points, such as assisting birth with emollient herbs used in bathing, hollyhock in Jonas[36] and mallows in Trotula[37] and oils for anointing. They also agree on the need to make the patient sneeze to speed the birth and the use of suffumigation, directing smoke from burning herbs into the vagina.

As might be expected in the course of centuries and perhaps with a slightly different readership in mind, there are also changes. These appear for instance in ideas on choosing wet nurses. While both agree on avoiding an anxious nurse, Jonas expands on her necessary good moral character and honest conversation. The Book on the Conditions of Women according to Trotula is more concerned with diet, forbidding spicy and pungent foods especially garlic.[38] Dietary restriction does not appear in the later work where there is more emphasis on testing the colour, taste and thickness of the milk. While The Trotula does not discuss when use of a wet nurse is advisable, Jonas makes it plain the mother's milk is most wholesome, and use of a wet nurse is for when she is unable to feed her child. This statement is followed by a quote from Avicenna on feeding times.[39] The Byrth of Mankynd would be a standard work for women and midwives until Culpeper's Directory for Midwives was published in 1654.

We began this chapter considering the influence of Henry VIII through his great interest in medicine and influence from one of his physicians, Thomas Linacre encouraging regulation of medicine in England to be similar to that in Europe. Meanwhile the closure of the monasteries brought more social changes and the publication of books such as Of the Birth of Mankind put more specialised knowledge into the public domain.

Greater changes were heralded by the work of Paracelsus who seems to have had huge impact through his published and collected texts despite being highly unpopular during his lifetime. His attacks on Galen were re-inforced in their effect by the work of Vesalius, proving that Galen had made serious errors in some of his interpretation of human physiology. The brief exploration of some of the practices and beliefs of Paracelsus referring to medicine prepares us for the final note on regulation in this chapter. In 1553 the College of Physicians had been given further power "to survey and examine the stocks of apothecaries, druggists, distillers and sellers of waters and oils, and preparers of chemical medicines".[40] Only twelve years after the death of Paracelsus this inclusion of the chemical category shows his influence in England. Unlike today, aromatic waters were included in this category as they had what was perceived to be a chemical preparation.

References

1. C.J.S. Thompson, The Mystery and Art of the Apothecary (Philadelphia: Lippincott, 1929), 168.
2. Huling E. Ussery, Chaucer's Physician (New Orleans: Tulane University, 1971), 21.
3. Andrew Wear, Knowledge & Practice in English Medicine, 1550–1680. (Cambridge: University press, 2000), 27.
4. Arthur E. Waite, (trans), The Hermetic and Alchemical Writings of Paracelsus the Great (U.S.A: The Alchemical Press, 1992), XI–XII.

5. Waite, *The Hermetic and Alchemical Writings of Paracelsus*, XI.
6. Nicholas Goodrick-Clarke, trans, *Paracelsus Essential Readings* (Northants: Crucible, 1990), 14, 15.
7. Waite, *The Hermetic and Alchemical Writings of Paracelsus*, XII.
8. Ibid, XI.
9. Ibid, 298.
10. Ibid, 259.
11. Ibid, 260.
12. Ibid, 268.
13. Ibid, 270.
14. Ibid, 272.
15. Ibid, Part Two, 172.
16. Ibid, Part Two 174.
17. Ibid, Part Two, 174–175.
18. Ibid, Part Two 184.
19. Ibid, Part Two 176.
20. Ibid, Part Two 174.
21. Ibid, Part two 184.
22. Goodrick-Clarke, *Paracelsus Essential Readings*, 19.
23. Waite, *The Hermetic and Alchemical Writings of Paracelsus*, Part Two, 289.
24. Ibid, Part Two, 292.
25. Carole Rawcliffe, *Medicine and Society in Later Medieval England* (Stroud: Sutton Publishing, 1997), Plate 9.
26. Waite, *The Hermetic and Alchemical Writings of Paracelsus*, Part Two, 62.
27. Ibid, Part Two, 160.
28. Goodrick-Clarke, *Paracelsus Essential Readings*, 106.
29. Ibid, 86.
30. Nicholas Orme and Margaret Webster, *The English Hospital 1070–1570* (London: Yale University Press, 1995), 111.
31. Orme & Webster, *The English Hospital 1070–1570*, 44.
32. Barbara Griggs, *Green Pharmacy* (London: Jill Norman & Hobhouse Ltd., 1981), 62.
33. Elaine Hobby, (ed), *The Birth of Mankind* (Farnham: Ashgate Publishing Ltd., 2009), Appendices 5, 6, 7.
34. Hobby, *The Birth of Mankind*, Introduction XXVII.
35. C.D. O'Malley, *Andreas Vesalius of Brussels 1514–1564* (Berkeley: University of California Press, 1964), 1–17.
36. Hobby, *The Birth of Mankind*, 118.
37. Monica Green, *The Trotula* (Philadelphia: University of Pennsylvania Press, 2002), 79.
38. Green, *The Trotula*, 85.
39. Hobby, *The Birth of Mankind*, 157.
40. G. Urdang, (historical intro), *Pharmacopoeia Londinensis of 1618* (Madison State: Historical Society of Wisconsin, 1944), 6.

CHAPTER 15

The Stillroom—Finding Instruction | 1525–1760

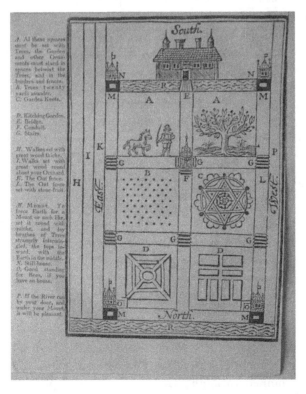

Stillroom Shown (N) on Garden Plan. *New Orchard and Garden*. Lawson.

Use of the stillroom of the lady of the manor as we visualise it today—
emerged in part from the closure of the monasteries. This was also an age
when a strong sense of Christian duty and responsibility for the welfare of
those around her was instilled into such women. A lady of quality might treat not
only her family, but also servants, and, at times, tenants and others who came to
the door for help. In smaller establishments, there might not be a dedicated room
for making medicines and other necessary herbal recipes beyond the kitchen. In the
manor houses and those of the upper classes, there would either have been a room
in the house, or a still-house in one corner of the garden.

We see an example of the second shown in an illustration in William Lawson's
New Orchard and Garden.[1] Distilling could be hazardous, involving fire and steam
at pressure. In earlier times kitchens too were in a separate building due to fire
hazard. So what was a stillroom like? An illustration from the title page of *The
Accomplished Lady's Delight in Preserving, Physick, Beautifying and Cookery* shows a
background of shelving along the walls for the jars, jugs, and bottles either of ingredients or finished preparations, and all the necessary pots and crockery. There is the
lady working at a table, a wooden chest to hold ingredients, and a servant close to
the fire which is heating a still.[2] No doubt there would also be hooks from beams
for hanging bunches of herbs, perhaps a barrel containing liquor and large earthenware crocks containing more ingredients.

In the stillroom, the housewife herself would either make or supervise the making of all manner of necessary supplies for the household, as the title of the book
just quoted tells us. Preserves of fruits and vegetables, including pickles and candied fruits, medicinal conserves, syrups, or honey robs, salves, and what were to
become a stand-by medicine, distilled aromatic waters. Combinations of herbs
in cosmetics and for fragrance, or to use as pest repellents against moths, fleas,
flies, rats and mice, would be essential. From spring through the summer and into
autumn it would be a busy place with the current harvest from the garden being
brought in to make recipes or be dried, pickled, or candied for use at a further time.
Household recipes had already been handed down over many generations but the
newly widened practice of distilling required an extra skill.

The access for the busy housewife to a range of medical and practical knowledge
was transformed by the advent of printing, and particularly the publication of the
Virtuous Book of Distillation. One hundred and fifty-three medical works were published in England between 1486 and 1604.[3] It is to this enormous revolution in book
production that we owe the stream of herbals and books on medicine, surgery, and
botany which we now begin to consider.

The first printed book to be dedicated to herbs was *An Herbal* [1525],[4] known
generally by the name of the printer Banckes, this work is virtually word for word
the fourteenth century manuscript *Agnus Castus*.[5] The language has been updated
slightly, but with limited variation. The order is again alphabetical, sometimes a

herb from the *Agnus Castus* manuscript is left out, or an extra herb added. Otherwise they match through as far as the letter S.

The manuscripts we have available of the *Agnus Castus* stop there, but it is not reasonable to suppose that they always did. Banckes continues with another eight herbs, ending with wormwood. Herbs added include laxatives from Arabic influence, such as senna and scammony. Both Dioscorides and Constantine are quoted as to the source of pepper being India, and further on it is noted "The Saracens dry it in an oven".[6] With many herbs there is little botany and no illustrations to guide the reader. It is a first step in making knowledge previously known to a few people open to a larger public.

The reader would, however, have needed extra knowledge to apply the recipes, as quantities of ingredients are frequently missing, along with dosages. Entries for herbs with several recipes are given to betony, mint, pennyroyal, and rose. The predominant philosophy of the humours is re-inforced as the temperatures of the herbs are given in degrees, so that pennyroyal is recorded as hot and dry in the third degree. Recipes for using this herb are for treating phlegm in the head, with the herb in vinegar, black choler with the juice, and aching legs or arms with a plaster of the herb.[7]

Some years earlier before 1517 possibly the last herbal to be compiled in a monastery was being written at Syon Abbey in London.[8] Syon was the only Brigettine Abbey in England, the nuns following the teachings of St Bridget of Sweden, canonised in 1391. It was founded by Henry V in 1415 and thanks to his generosity became one of the wealthiest nunneries in England.[9] There were many pilgrims to the Abbey who received relief from purgatory in return for their visits and offerings. Scholars also visited to use the growing library. With the advent of printing, manuscripts from Syon were used as copy text by William Caxton's successor, Wynkyn de Worde. He printed a devotional treatise by Thomas Betson, librarian at Syon in 1500.[10] Unfortunately, there is no list of books in the library of the nuns, but volumes in the library catalogued by Thomas Betson grew to over 1300 in number.

Even though there is no evidence that the nuns had more than an infirmary for themselves, they were sixty in number and some literary sources on medicine are likely to have been available to them. The Abbess ruled, as had Hilda at Whitby, over both nuns and the twenty monks who took services and performed various duties. Another parallel with Whitby and Abbess Hilda was that Syon attracted many important visitors. These included Katherine of Aragon and her daughter, Princess Mary.

The herbal we have is written partly in Latin and partly in English, it contains five hundred remedies with some seven hundred ingredients, including native plants and those items necessarily sourced from the apothecary. Such exotics as flowers of pomegranate, cloves, tamarind, shavings of harts horn, burnt ivory, and cantarides

(*Cantharis vesicatoria*) beetles appear. This book is of value as the detail of what was made in the dispensaries of religious houses was largely lost at the dissolution. It is of particular interest that there are over twenty recipes for distilled waters.

The famed Aqua Mirabilis which appears again and again in stillroom books, herbals, and in the Pharmacopoeias through into the eighteenth century, is recorded here. The reputation of this aromatic water, rich in the spices of cloves, galangal, cubebs, mace, cardamoms, nutmeg, and ginger, with a variable selection of herbs, was such that in recent years it provoked commercial interest for sale to herbalists today. There is also a complex water for the eyes, "Pro omni vitio oculorum & experta",[11] containing many of the same herbs in the precious water for eyes we have already reviewed.

Within the day-to-day recipes are others already familiar from the fifteenth century Leechbook. "For the parlous cough"[12] also appears in the fourteenth century, quoting the Harleian manuscript 2378 (MS B), as, "who-so have the perlus cohw"[13] with the same herbs and slightly different instructions, examined in the last chapter. For "man or wommane that hath the perliouse coughe",[14] which is a duplication. In this version there was extra guidance as the herbs are all to be of the same amount. In the Syon Abbey herbal the same recipe reads, "For the perilose kogh: Take Rue and Sauge, Comyn & powdur of Peper and seth them to gidre in hony and make a letuary, and use *therof* a sponfull at eveyn and another at morn".[15]

From the books of recipes already explored we know that distilling had been carried out in England certainly since the fourteenth century. Whether the source of knowledge on the practice was made more widespread by returning crusaders through Salerno or from Spain is conjectural. Social changes laid extra responsibility on the better off ladies to help those around them. That evidently included the wives of yeoman farmers, as well as those of the new middle class which had grown up from increasing foreign trade bringing new wealth, and ladies of the manor distilling herbs for medicine. We see this in the list of seventeen herbs for distilling in summer in Thomas Tusser's *500 Points of Good Husbandry*.[16] In addition to his recommended already well-stocked herb garden for cookery and strewing, many herbs included were medicinal.

The publication of the English translation of the *Virtuous Book of Distillation* in 1527 had given further opportunity for the literate housewife to learn exactly what might be involved. Stressing the Christian acceptability of the work in the preface, the author then gives every direction anyone could possibly need about the equipment and process of the art necessary to produce fine quality aromatic waters.

Distillation is defined as separating the pure from the gross, a main feature of alchemy. Stills might be simple affairs of white clay or made of copper or glass, pewter and lead are mentioned at times. Their shapes also varied, the double flask pelican was for rectifying waters which passed back and forth, up and down between them. The stillatory could refer to different arrangements to supply heat, for instance a furnace or a bain Marie or water bath.

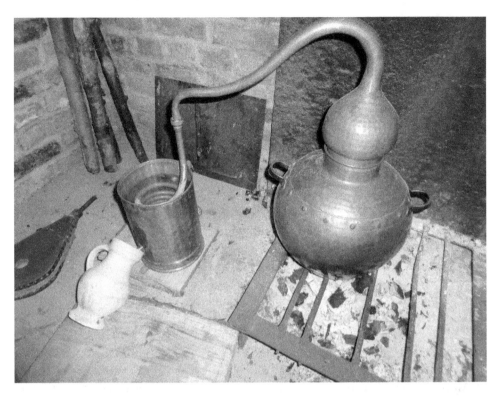

Still in Walderton, Courtesy Weald and Downland Living Museum.

For aromatic waters, I fill my still to one third full with fresh or dried herb and then add water, spring water is ideal, to two thirds, before attaching the helm to cover and seal it. This has a shaped pipe which fits tightly to what is called the worm, a coiled pipe inside the condenser or container for cold water. When the water in the body of the still boils the steam rises, carrying with it the lighter constituents of the herbs and their volatile oils up into the helm and this is then funnelled down through the worm being cooled by the cold water. The resulting aromatic water emerges from a small tap near the bottom of the condenser where it drips or runs into the receiving vessel. The wonderful preceding whiff of the scent of the water which heralds the water itself is a delight I never tire of. Different volatiles come over at different temperatures and so the still will run a little and then appear to stop, and then run again. We find some instructions on keeping the first, second and third runs separate as they may be of different strengths.

How the still is to be heated is the first consideration. I have always used a fire to heat my still but that is not the only way. The Virtuous book gives five ingenious ways to distil without cost, using everything from the sun, to your oven when baking bread, or even the heat from dung or ant hills. Baptista della Porta in his book of *Natural Magic*, written in sixteenth century Italy, comments that the downside of using dung is that it gives the finished water a scurvy scent. He recommends using the sun for best results and describes a form or bench to support the upper glass vessels as their necks pass through custom made holes to fit into the receiving vessels below. The receivers are set in dishes of cold water. Herbs are gathered and placed in the upper vessels with cittern strings in the neck to stop them from falling through. A board is fitted along the side of the bench towards the sun to shade the receivers. The sun then dissolves the herbs into vapours which condense in the cooler receiver below. The herbs are repeatedly replaced each night.[18]

Despite della Porta's comment on dung, in England where the sun is less dependable it could be very effective. If you have ever watched the steam coming from a fresh dung-heap on a farm or used it to heat a cold frame in winter, you will understand the benefit. Ant hills seem more of a challenge. This is followed by five ways of varying ferocity using fire. Distilling in glass was considered to be the best method and required protection for the glass vessel using thick dough in order to be able to bake it in the oven. It might also be set in water for a gentler heat.

To set up a large stillroom might be a requirement of a large house or apothecary and this is catered for as well as a smaller installation. There are full instructions for building a brick furnace heating four stillatories at once. The term stillatory can be applied to the upper helm of the still or might include the whole furnace. Illustrations make clear how the bases containing the herb and liquor to be distilled are contained within the brickwork, and heated by the fire below while the helms sit above.

All of the vessels needed are also illustrated in the *Virtuous Book of Distillation* and include cupels, pans, and helms, pelicans with two arms and alembics. There are wonderfully complex instructions for using clay to anoint the glasses for protection over fire heat, involving horse turds, wine, and flax. Luting might be done in several ways, the term is also used for sealing the joint between the base or body of the still and the helm to ensure no steam escapes. Another precautionary measure was to make linen cloth less flammable by dipping it in salt water, then beaten egg white and leaving it to dry.[19] Regarding gathering of herbs, roots were to be gathered from July to September with the leaves beginning to fall. They were washed, dried and chopped. All herbs were to be gathered in good weather, in an increasing moon. Green herbs were considered better than dried and the very best water to use was dew, gathered by dragging a cloth over the wet grass before sunrise and wringing it out. Distilling might be carried out three times and there were ways of rectifying waters to reduce their fiery nature and help them to keep longer.

The distilled aromatic waters were kept in labelled and dated stone pots with small necks and wooden or carefully made stoppers, and set in a cellar for ambient temperature. Interestingly their expected life was related to the temperatures of the herbs themselves. Waters distilled of hot and dry herbs were regarded as keeping longer than moist herbs.[20] This is something I have found to be true. Lavender, rosemary, dill flowers, and red rose water keep until the end of the third year, especially if they had been rectified in the sun during the second year. I have kept aromatic waters I have distilled from lavender, rosemary, or peppermint in blue bottles in a dark cupboard for at least five years before they have lost their distinctive perfume. It will have changed slightly meanwhile, but they are still good for adding perfume to a room if not for medicine. In my experience it does make a difference that the glass is blue, waters will not keep the same when stored in brown glass.

Very cold waters of mandrake, houseleek, and hemlock were only to be used externally in the first or second year after distilling. During this time they were considered to have maintained strength enough to numb feeling. The very cold herbs kept the waters longest. There are many more categories including tree leaves, fruits, and animal parts. It was clearly important to know when waters should be discarded. This relied on changes in scent, pouring drops on your thumbnail to see whether it ran straight off, or was of a more slimy nature, and looking for a "mother", shown by cloudiness or a reddish colour.[21]

The uses of simple waters, those waters distilled with one herb only, are predictably similar to those of that herb. For instance water of hyssop was listed in the Leechbook of the fifteenth century as "good for the cough and for the lungs".[22] Bancke's Herbal contains a lengthy entry on the red rose and had offered an insight into the usefulness and popularity of, among other preparations, rose water, which is recommended to drink, sprinkle over the face, use for the eyes, and in ointments for the complexion.[23] From the beginning it seems various ways of administering waters were explored. Adding them to hand-baths or areas where the pulse could readily be felt, such as the temples, or at the "pulse box" on the wrist became usual.

For the apothecaries, compendiums of recipes contained lists of waters they should keep in their shops, such as that of Saladini, from 1488, who qualified at Salerno. This contains forty-six herbs as Simple Waters.[24] Ladies were catered for by numerous publications. With exploration of the New World, interest in gardens increased and novel, possibly medicinal plants became available and were eagerly grown. This burst of enthusiasm was fed by the first English gardening book, *The Profitable Art of Gardening* by Thomas Hill in 1568. Just as medicine had taken its lead from Greek and Roman sources, so this author constantly quotes Roman authors, such as Columella, Varro, and Pliny.

Hill gives importance to his astronomical knowledge in growing the herbs, which is not surprising as he also practised as an astrologer. The importance of medicinal herbs in the garden is shown by the index at the end of the book entitled *"A Necessarie Table to the Second Part of this Book, briefly shewing the Physical operations of every hearb and plant therein contained, with the vertues of their distilled waters".*[25] When it comes to the Waters, over forty are given, with the leaves and the root of elecampane distilled separately. The herb and root of valerian are also distilled separately as are strawberry leaves and fruits. His list differs from that of Tusser, featuring more plants that we would now regard as vegetables such as leeks, onions, parsnips, and white beet alongside the familiar thyme, marigolds, lovage, borage, betony, and chervil.

Strawberry leaves may seem surprising and I distilled them myself confirming the water had detectable strength. Historically the water of strawberry leaves has actions including healing wounds and ulcers, cleansing the kidneys, and acting on the liver.[26] Richard Mabey, who edited the modern publication wrote in the introduction that the book seems to have been an instant success, with a new edition the following year and then more. It clearly served a need at the right moment in history.

Gerard, barber surgeon and Superintendant to the gardens of Lord Burghley in London and Hertfordshire for twenty years, was an avid collector of plants. He had an extensive garden of his own in Holborn, London and published a catalogue of his garden trees and plants in 1596, naming over 1,000.[27] He included the benefits of herbal aromatic waters in his copious herbal, largely based on the translation by Dr Priest of Dodoen's Latin herbal of 1583.[28] By the time his herbal is extended in the following century by Johnson, there are some fifty references to waters. His sources of information on the subject included the herbal of Apuleius, Camerarius, who was a practitioner in London and great distillers, such as Arnoldus Villanovus and Conrad Gesner.

There are some imaginative applications, such as gum mastic in rose water to fasten loose teeth firmly, spiced rosemary water for stinking breath, and *Zizyphus* for killing nits and lice. Eye waters and cosmetic waters to clear away spots and blemishes are the most common, but there are also Waters for palsy, migraine, easing the pain from stones in the kidneys and bladder, eating too much (surfet waters) and treating plague sores.

Identifying plants correctly was important for the stillroom products, medicinal and otherwise. Before Gerard's publication, William Turner was greatly concerned with botany and correct identification of plants. In fact he had already written a book on the subject. His *"Libellus de Re Herbaria Novus"* of 1538 was republished in an extended English version *"The Names of Herbes"* in 1548.[29] Later botanists used this in furtherance of their own works. Turner published *A New Herbal* in three parts beginning in 1551 when he was protestant Dean of Wells. After travelling on the Continent in exile during the reign of the Catholic Queen Mary, he published the final part of his herbal in 1568, having returned to England a decade earlier with Queen Elizabeth's reign.[30] His herbal, enriched by his travels and studies of medical botany under Luca Ghini at Pisa, is the first known to have been written for the market provided by the upper-class ladies, however, Turner makes only passing reference to the Waters.

Looking at the many changes for the housewife in the way she can now access information on herbs, we should ask the question as to whether that information on our chosen herbs is also changing by comparing entries in the herbals and some other sources quoted in this chapter. In general, we would expect Banckes to repeat old recipes since it is almost identical with an earlier source and our representative Abbey herbal from Syon is also likely to follow the same pattern as before. It may be that Turner, Gerard, or Markham will indicate signs of a change in approach.

Our Chosen Herbs in Herbals

With betony, popular in the older sources, the familiar emphasis on eye, head, and stomach treatments remains. At Syon four waters for eyes are used, of these, the waters of Peter of Spain and *Pro omni vitio oculorum* are repeated from the previous century. Uses against drunkenness and for vomiting blood continue. Turner writes more on treating venomous bites and using the herb for the bladder and kidneys. He reports that betony scours the liver and helps those who spit out corruption from their lungs.[31] Gerard agrees and gives yellow jaundice and aiding the spleen, as well as sciatica and epilepsy. He describes three ways of internal administration, the flowers beaten with sugar especially for headache, dried leaf in wine for internal bleeding and the root in mead as an emetic.[32] Markham gives a recipe for a beef and herb broth, to strengthen the kidneys and back.[33]

A considerable range of treatments is still given for plantain, classed as cold and dry in the second degree. Ribwort remains recommended for a quartan fever, and ribwort and greater plantain are distilled together. Our oldest sources give almost the same recipe for treating painful gums with plantain juice, honey, and vinegar, variously adding alum or powdered aloes. Gerard notes that although a cold herb the different parts of the plant, leaf, root, and seed vary in temperature and moisture. The root is classed as driest, and not as cold. Plantain oil is made using the heat of sunbeams and dripped into aching ears. This is a use noted in the post-Roman period. Putting this into a syringe and injecting it into the inflamed fundament or anus appears to be a new idea.[34] Instructions for ladies from Markham are to add plantain to other herbs in a compound eye water and generally take advantage of its anti-inflammatory and astringent nature in ointments for burns and scalds, salves for sores and wounds and in a compound bath recipe.[35]

A recipe commented on in Macer in the post-Norman period of using the stimulation of nettle leaves externally to affect the womb appears in the Syon recipes, together with another for foot pain. The most impressive remedy here however gives nettle a new role in a compound recipe for a bath to clear the skin. Together with rosemary, fennel, pellitory of the wall, mallows, violet leaves and more, nettles are first made into a decoction and milk is added to make a luxurious bath which will be sat in with the liquid to the level of the stomach. This is followed by going to bed to sweat.[36] Later in the century, Gerard describes three types of nettles. Cleansing roles regarding the lungs and urinary system have appeared through history and again predominate, and Gerard quotes Apollodorus on nettle as a counter-poison which links us back into the second section of this book. It appears that any nettle is regarded as capable of producing like effects, although the Roman is stipulated as the best.

Elecampane root is eaten to fasten loose teeth, included in a diuretic drink and given as an abortive for a dead child, reminding us of much earlier use. In Gerard the herb is well recommended especially when dried. He feels the moisture of the fresh herb diminishes the hot and dry aspect of treatment and recommends an elecampane lohoch, which is a thick syrupy medicine you lick rather than pour from a spoon. This is for expectorating thick humours and phlegm in the chest, being particularly good for asthmatic patients. He adds the thicker still electuary for coughs and to comfort the stomach, and candying the root. Mixing the boiled root with butter and ginger powder to make an ointment is a new treatment for itchy skin and scabs. Alternatively, the decoction and powdered root were mixed into honey to apply for sores. As ever, Gerard quotes previous authorities including on treating sciatica, and loose joints.[37]

In the older sources for this period, henbane is given generally for pain. Toothache is a main use with the candle remedy repeated as before. A sliver of the root is laid on the tooth which may be loose as well as painful, for three nights in a row. A different recipe in the Syon Herbal is for a compound emetic ointment.[38] Turner gives an interesting instruction to place the dried, bruised seed in warm water and then press out the juice. He comments that this gives a faster acting analgesic than using juice from the fresh plant which is made into little cakes with wheat to preserve it.[39]

Gerard warns that the leaves, seed, and juice as internal medicines can cause a long sleep resembling that from an excess of alcohol, and can be deadly. He denounces charlatans who travelled the country using the painkilling effects of burning henbane seed to persuade the vulnerable who had sat eyes closed over the smoke, that fake worms thrown into water in front of them had been smoked out of their teeth, so that they were cured.[40]

The sweet nature of liquorice and the properties of cooling and moistening found application for the throat and lungs in cough recipes. Gerard tells us he is growing the herb in his garden, although it is not found wild here as it may be on the Continent. From him we learn that the juice of the inner root is solidified and pieces held under the tongue for the cough, to bring up phlegm. Liquorice and ginger are partnered with more spices in gingerbread which, unlike today actually was made with bread, and was seen as medicinal as well as tasty. Liquorice juice was drunk with raisin wine for the liver, chest and kidneys. While it is not surprising that liquorice was recommended to treat all conditions originating in sharp, salty humours, another use is given that I would not like to test. This is taking the dried, powdered root and strewing it into the eyes for pin and web, (conjunctivitis or perhaps cataracts).[41]

Ginger was administered at Syon in two recipes to dissolve and remove phlegm. Powdered ginger is an ingredient in a compound recipe for a laxative, and Aqua Vitae with a mix of herbs and spices.[42] Gerard recounts his trials in obtaining a good description of the plant. He classifies it as heating and drying in the third degree and so useful for the digestion, which indeed it is. While comparing it to pepper, he considers that when fresh, candied or preserved, ginger is actually hot and moist.[43] It is interesting that he divides the temperatures of the fresh and dried in this way when they are, in fact chemically different. As far as our ladies are concerned unless they have a copy of Gerard they will be given an entirely different picture of the properties of ginger from *The English Housewife*. There recipes for the womb feature and ginger appears in the much recommended Doctor Steven's Water for health and long life.[44]

There were plenty of sources providing advice and recipes for the stillroom including the notorious Books of Secrets. These contained animal recipes, pastes for scented beads, customised candles, deodorants, and cosmetics. Magical protection is included with squill bulbs tied to your door. Baptista della Porta (1535–1615) wrote one of these. It is a record of scientific experiments by a group of men who met regularly in Italy to share their knowledge, progenitor of the foundation of the Royal Society in London.[45]

"The Secretes of Alexis of Piedmont" was first published in Italy in four parts between about 1555 and 1569; the English version of part two appeared in 1560, and was reprinted a number of times on through the next century. This contains a recipe for treating deafness using hot eel grease and garlic introduced into the ear which takes us back to much earlier treatments, and a worrying remedy for a red nose which includes borax and ox gall.[46]

There are many other recipes where the herbs are blended with animal parts and chemical powders. I have made a number of the more sensible recipes with groups in workshops and can recommend those involving burning perfumes and aromatic beads. Needless to say the medicinal recipes are highly variable in their safety or probable efficacy and should not be explored by amateurs.

We should also consider that many waters are compound, containing up to thirty-six ingredients. The most famous were often regarded as panaceas for treating infectious disease and serious conditions. One which appears first in

Herbs in Cephalic Waters

References	Q381	Q375	BKS70	QS376	Q373	P145	C286	A99
Lilies of the Valley	2H	1lb	1H	6oz	1H	1lb	1lb	1H
Sage	1H		¼H	1dr (lesser)	1H			1H
Betony	1H		½H		1H	8pugil	8pugil	1H
Rosemary	1H		½H	6oz	1H	6pugil	6pugil	1H
Male Piony								
Rad		6dr			4oz	2½oz	2½	
Seed			6dr	1oz		10dr	10dr	
Flowers					1H	4oz	4oz	
Lavender	1gal	½dr	1gal	1dr	1H	4pugil	4pugil	1gal
Mistletoe-oak		6dr		1oz		2H	2H	
Yellow Sanders	1		1		1			1
Borage	1		1					1
Baum	1		1			1½oz	4pugil	4pugil
Arabian Stoechas	1oz				1	1		
Marjoram	1					1	1	
Squills						1	1	
July Flowers						1	1	
White Dittany						1	1	
Long Birthwort					1			
Angelica					1			
Valerian					1			
Marigolds					1	1		
Lime	1		1oz	1r water	1	1	1	1
Red Rose	1					1		
Cowslip					1			
Violets					1			1
Spikenard	1		1					

Comparison of Ingredients in Cephalic Waters.

Commodious Conceits and Hidden Secrets—Goodhuswives closet of provision for the health of her household (London, 1584), a copy of which is in the Bodleian Library, and is repeated again and again with few alterations over two centuries is Doctor Steven's Water.

I made a comparison of the ingredients and their amounts from seven sources including the Leechbook 1560–1580, Thomas Dawson's *The Good Housewife* 1596, Pechey's *The English Herbal*, 1694, the 1618 London Pharmacopoeia, Quincy's Dispensatory 1736, Eliza Smith's *Complete Housewife* 1739 and *A Book of Simples* dated to between 1700 and 1750. All contained the same amounts of ginger, galingale, cinnamon, aniseed, caraway, rose, thyme, and lavender, one recipe omitted mints, sage, rosemary, and nutmeg, and another household recipe omitted grains of paradise, probably due to cost. Five out of the seven distilled the herbs in Gascoigne wine; Quincy used French brandy, and one household book substituted claret. Considering the range of sources this was very uniform which speaks for the respect for this water. It was said that Doctor Stevens had prolonged his own life by five years beyond the expectation of physicians through taking it. The water subsequently gathered recommendations for treating conditions ranging from palsy to assisting barren women and curing dropsy.

The practice of distilling in wine was common among the ladies and soaking the herbs first was also common to recipes, although the time varied from an hour or more, to two days. The number of spices which must be pounded (brayed) before distilling gives us a first impression of adding heat and perfume to the water, together with any other medicinal properties. If we look in Gervase Markham's compendious guide to every aspect of running a large household, *The English Housewife*, he gives a chapter to distilling and perfuming. Beginning by suggesting stills of tin or sweet earth, he then lists the virtues of several waters. With sage and rosemary, these can be referred directly to the reasoning behind Doctor Steven's Water and the conditions it was believed to treat. Of the herbs, sage had been commonly used to treat palsy for centuries, so it is no surprise to find the water also listed for palsy. Rosemary water is given a long list of virtues, among which are comforting the heart and brain and causing women to be fruitful.[47] As for treating the urinary system, pellitory of the wall was and remains a specific herb for the bladder and kidneys.

To close this chapter, we return to the lady and her need for a stillroom as we catch a glimpse of one sixteenth century charitable lady, Lady Margaret Hoby. who wrote in her diary of her prayers, treating a servant and the poor who came to her door, as well as carrying out her tasks in the house and reading both the Bible and the arball (herbal), all in a few days in 1599.[48] Many of the recipes she was likely to read reflected medicine unchanged, but new ideas were emerging for use of long established herbs and some, such as liquorice and ginger were becoming better known as herbs. Regarding quality of drugs bought from the apothecary, improvements had been made but these still left a lot to be desired.

References

1. William Lawson, *A New Orchard and Garden* (London: Brewster and Sawbridge, 1656), 12.
2. Michael Best, (ed), Gervase Markham, *The English Housewife* (London: McGill-Queen's University Press, 1994), 130.
3. Andrew Wear, *Knowledge & Practice in English Medicine, 1550–1680* (Cambridge: University Press, 2000), 41.
4. Sanford Larkey and Thomas Pyles, (ed), *An Herbal [1525]* (New York: Scholars Facsimiles & Reprints, 1942).
5. Gösta Brodin, (ed), *Agnus Castus* (Cambridge: Harvard University Press, 1950).
6. Larkey and Pyles, (ed), *An Herbal [1525]*, 55.
7. Ibid, 56–58.
8. John Adams and Stuart Forbes, (ed), *The Syon Abbey Herbal. A.D. 1517* (London: AMCD Publishers Ltd., 2015).
9. E. A. Jones, *England's Last Medieval Monastery* (Leominster: Gracewing, 2015), 11–12.
10. Adams & Forbes, *The Syon Abbey Herbal*, 25.
11. Ibid, 257.
12. Warren Dawson, (ed), *A Leechbook of the XVth Century* (London: Macmillan & Co., 1934), (190), 75.
13. G. Henslow, *Medical Works of the Fourteenth Century* (New York: Burt Franklin, 1972), 114.
14. Henslow, *Medical Works of the Fourteenth Century*, 101.
15. Adams & Forbes, *The Syon Abbey Herbal*, 246.
16. Thomas Tusser, *Five Hundred Points of Good Husbandry* (Oxford: Oxford University Press, 1984), 91.
17. Theophrastus von Oberstockstall, (trans), *The Virtuous Book of Distillation* (London: Laurens Andrewes, 1527). (The Restorers of Alchemical Manuscripts Society Digital 2013), Chapters IX–XII.
18. Derek Pryce (ed), John Baptista Porta, *Natural Magick* (New York: Basic Books Inc., 1957), 258.
19. Oberstockstall, *The Virtuous Book of Distillation*, Chapter V.
20. Ibid, Chapter XXIIII.
21. Ibid, Chapter XXIIII.
22. Dawson, *A Leechbook of the XVth Century*, 299.
23. Larkey and Pyles, *An Herbal [1525]*, 68–69.
24. Joannes Mesue, *Opera de Medicamentorum* (Venice: 1581), Supplement, Saladini de Asculo, Simplicibus, 263.
25. Richard Mabey, (ed), *The Gardener's Labyrinth*, Thomas Hill (Oxford: University Press, 1988), 200.
26. Mabey, *The Gardener's Labyrinth*, 213.
27. John Harvey, *Early Gardening Catalogues* (Chichester: Phillimore & Co., 1972), 5.
28. Agnes Arber, *Herbals Their Origin and Evolution* (Cambridge: University Press, 1912), 108.
29. Britten et al., (intro), William Turner. *Libellus de Re Herbaria 1538. The Names of Herbes 1548* (London: The Ray Society, Facsimiles, 1965).

30. George Chapman and Marilyn Tweddle, (ed), *A New Herball*, William Turner 1551 (Manchester: Carcanet Press, 1989), 10–12.
31. Chapman & Tweddle, *A New Herball*, 251–252.
32. Thomas Johnson, *The Herbal*. John Gerard. (New York: Dover Publications Inc., 1975) 714–715.
33. Michael R. Best, (ed), Gervase Markham, *The English Housewife* (London: McGill-Queen's University Press, 1986), 37–38.
34. Johnson, *The Herbal*, 421.
35. Best, *The English Housewife*, 21, 47, 44, 54.
36. Ibid, 54.
37. Johnson, *The Herbal*, 792–3.
38. Adams & Forbes, *The Syon Abbey Herbal*, 282.
39. Chapman & Tweddle, *A New Herball*, 227.
40. Johnson, *The Herbal*, 355.
41. Johnson, *The Herbal*, 1302–1303.
42. Adams & Forbes, *The Syon Abbey Herbal*, 261.
43. Johnson, *The Herbal*, 61–62.
44. Best, *The English Housewife*, 56–57.
45. John Baptista Porta, *Natural Magick* (New York: Basic Books Inc., 1959), V.
46. William Warde and Richard Anglosse, *The Secretes of Maister Alexis* 1558–1569 (Oxford: Atenar, 2000), 70, 101.
47. Best, *The English Housewife*, 131.
48. Joanna Moody, (ed), *The Private Life of an Elizabethan Lady* (Stroud: Sutton Publishing, 2001), 58.

CHAPTER 16

The Physic Garden in Britain | 1536–1648

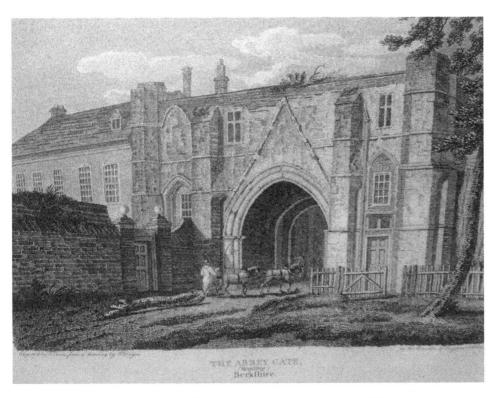

Into The Abbey. *Beauties of England & Wales.* 1808.

The term physic garden is one I am applying firstly to gardens containing plants for medicinal use, which were largely infirmary gardens associated with Abbeys and monasteries until the dissolution in 1536–8. I will then look at the way in which physic gardens planted at Universities and other sites initially for teaching students of medicine and apothecaries became termed botanic gardens, subsequently also serving the allied science of botany. We have little information on the actual monastic gardens in England. The one often quoted plan from St Gall in Switzerland was an ideal for monasteries to aspire to. This shows sixteen beds for the infirmary, containing important herbs such as sage, rue, rosemary, and cumin.[1]

Although the Normans imported many Mediterranean plants and we know that plants as well as books were supplied from mother houses on the Continent of Europe to religious houses here, we do not have a full plant list. There certainly seem to have been areas devoted specifically to plants for physic. For example, Bicester Priory in Oxon had separate gardens for the prior, canon, infirmarian (growing herbs for physic), sacrist, and kitchens, as well as the Great Garden and Orchard.[2]

Some religious orders concentrated on prayers for the sick rather than administering herbs to them. Illness could be regarded as punishment for sin. We saw this idea back in the chapter on Anglo-Saxon medicine. The Benedictine, Augustinian, and Cistercian orders valued treating with herbs alongside prayer. At the Benedictine Abbey at Bury St Edmunds in about 1120 there were extensive gardens. This made it possible for a monk there to paint a number of illustrations for the great Herbal of Apuleius from nature.[3]

I have already included some lines from Walahfrid Strabo's *Hortus* about his own small garden. His plant list is tangible evidence for what was actually grown at his Abbey of Reichenau, not far from St Gall. The garden at Shrewsbury Abbey inspired by the Brother Cadfael books and based on a surviving plan of a monastic garden at Cathedral Priory of Christ Church, Canterbury from about 1165 has sadly closed in the years since my visit. The plan of the Canterbury garden was to record their plumbing system, however, in showing how the water was piped it also reveals a herb garden with a surround of trellis fencing and plants grown in strips close to the infirmary. There was no plant list, however.[5]

A recreation of a monastic garden at Michelham Priory, Sussex may be the best to visit today. I found it inspirational when there as a speaker at a six hundred year celebration in 2003. Their plant list gives a quite comprehensive coverage of useful herbs, medicinal and otherwise and the garden has been recommended to me again recently.

For their horticultural guidance in the medieval period it seems likely that Palladius, the Roman writer on farming was consulted. His fourth century work, under the category *De Re Rustica* (c380–95) was definitely in the religious house libraries of Byland in Yorkshire, Canterbury, Waltham Abbey, and Worcester Cathedral.[6] The main theme is farming but the lay-out in months of the year and detail would have been generally useful across the orchard, vineyard, and other gardens. Palladius took much of his information from the earlier writings of Columella. His common sense preparations are reminiscent of the Aphorisms of Hippocrates. He advises to test the air, soil, and wholesomeness of available water when choosing the site, sowing seeds on warm days with a waxing moon, and the ideal of a garden in a gentle climate with spring water running through it. It is impossible not to smile at some of his remarks, such as, "Three troubles are equally harmful: sterility, disease, neighbours".[7]

Palladius gives specific advice on shape and size of garden beds and a long list of protections from caterpillars, including steeping seeds in houseleek juice and drying all the seeds to be sown in a tortoise shell. He quotes Apuleis on steeping seeds in ox gall against being eaten by mice.[8] Cultivation of herbs is included in his year plan. In March, there are instructions for sowing rue, coriander, creeping thyme, anise, and cumin for instance.[9] When writing on keeping bees he gives us a list of herbs to keep them happy, he writes that thyme gives the best honey, with oregano and creeping thyme next, rosemary and savory as third choice.[10] There is a long list of herbs in the section on veterinary medicine and occasional recipes for herb wines, oils, and other medicines.

At the Reformation dissolution of the monasteries provided opportunities for eager investors who were often courtiers, to buy land with the buildings, and swift redevelopment followed in many places. In 1534 there were 848 religious houses and the smaller houses were closed first. Friaries survived until 1538 and the last monastery to be surrendered was Waltham Abbey in 1540. The majority became secular mansions which meant plants in monastic gardens suffered varied fates.[11] Some were kept by the new owners of the buildings in their gardens, most were removed. Occasionally medicinal plants are found today growing wild in the vicinity of a religious site of the past. Monastic infirmaries were not the only hospitals, where the word appears in documents it may mean a religious house, but also an almshouse, or a house for lepers. A gloss from the fourteenth century on papal canon law made it clear anyone could assign their house for hospitality for the benefit of the poor. In some of the larger towns, there were several leper houses and almshouses.[12]

Later, as already mentioned, Guilds would set up hospitals for their members and there would be many charity hospitals in centuries to come, the eighteenth century was designated as "the Age of Hospitals".[13] The apothecary lived in and supplied medicines from his salary.[14] I have found little mention of hospital gardens, and in many places since the concentration of them was near town centres, they may not have had gardens of any consequence. However, we have a wonderful piece of evidence at the Royal Chelsea Hospital in London where the earliest plan of the gardens from 1690 shows a physic garden over fifty feet wide with a two-storey building marked as the apothecary's laboratory. A short history and photograph of the illustration with more details of the original can be viewed online.[15]

One hospital garden we know a good deal about was at the Smallpox Hospital at St Pancras, this was funded by William Woodville who enters our history in a future chapter. In two of the four acres of ground around the hospital he maintained a botanical garden at his own expense, so that the plants could be provided for the artist to use when etching their forms for the illustrations of his *Medical Botany*, published in 1690.[16]

Returning to considering the sixteenth century there were already plant and mostly tree nurseries in London and a few beyond. The importation of plants from around the world that took place at that period and accelerated from then on caused a rush of excitement and interest in gardening. In a previous chapter on the stillroom, Thomas Hill's book on gardening, which frequently refers to the Roman writers, was mentioned as a guide for gardens being planted to supply the stately houses of the period. Many of which may have given employment to gardeners whose knowledge had been passed down by those formerly cultivating monastic gardens. There was, however, another kind of garden just beginning, one also to be stimulated by introduction of new plants, the botanic garden. In Continental Europe, no doubt encouraged by the more clement weather as well as other factors, these had been planted earlier than in Britain.

The first was planted in Padua where from 1533 students were led on tours of the University garden there.[17] Luca Ghini, a professor in the medical faculty in Bologna became impatient at delays in establishing a garden there and moved to Pisa. As director of the Pisa botanic garden, he improved it by travelling the Apennines gathering plants to display to students. He was as interested in showing plants native to Italy as those from elsewhere in the world. In 1548, the list of plants in the Pisa garden had reached 620.[18]

Identification was crucial to his work and he began pressing samples of plants to have them available for scholars at all times of year. With this he pioneered the hortus siccus (herbarium) collections being careful to show key plant parts, such as both sides of the leaf, flowers, seeds, and roots. To record colours that would fade in time he painted the plants in flower. For this invaluable work he should rightly be more famous but through his generosity in giving samples to others for their work which has remained well known, much of his contribution was lost and he has been left in the background.

In 1551, Ghini sent *hortus siccus* samples to Andrea Mattioli, while Lobelius admired his paintings, some of which he sent to Fuchs as well as fresh herbs for his use.[19] As mentioned in chapter fifteen, William Turner was one of his pupils at the University and must, as with others, surely have been inspired by Ghini's work on identification. The earliest Botanic garden in England was founded by Henry Danvers at Oxford in 1621 with a generous donation of £5,250.[20] John Tradescant the Elder (1570–1638) was chosen as gardener but he does not seem to have taken an active part. It was not until 1642 that Jacob Bobart was appointed and supervised planting.[21] The University has a wonderful treasure in the form of Bobart's bound Hortus Siccus, (herbarium) specimens, with page after page each showing a selection of the plants being grown in the botanic garden and some from the surrounding country in the mid-seventeenth century. The specimens are in alphabetical order, beginning with *Absinthium* and still show the colours of many of the flowers and leaves after almost four hundred years. The record can be checked against the catalogues of the garden contents published in 1648, when some 600 native plants were listed with over 1,000 from overseas.[22]

Originally, these records were kept at the garden, and Jacob Bobart the younger who succeeded his father in 1679 of specimens but at some later date these were cut up into single sheets of paper and are now kept in box volumes. Now they are in the main Oxford University Herbaria along with another bound herbarium of even greater age made in Italy (dated 1606) by an Italian monk, Brother Gregory. Again, this is a very special treasure with Brother Gregory's notes below each plant specimen, written in a neat hand. It is truly inspirational to see the herbs still recognisable after 400 years. Herbal medicine students and I have found visits there really valuable, especially as making herbarium specimens is part of our curriculum.

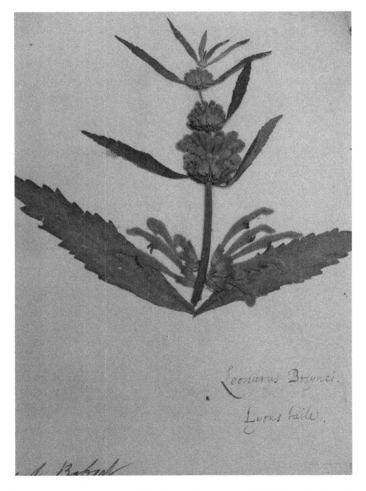

Leonurus Breynei, Jacob Bobart. Courtesy of Oxford Herbaria.

After centuries of additions from expeditions both at home and abroad, the Oxford herbarium now houses some 800,000 specimens. There was a long gap between the botanic garden in Oxford and others. In Scotland, Sir James Balfour 1630–1694 had been largely responsible for founding the College of Physicians in 1681. He and his friend Dr. Robert Sibbald (1641–1715) had much in common.[23] Both had been abroad, undertaking further medical study. Balfour had spent fifteen years in Europe during which time he collected books and surgical instruments among other things. Sibbald had spent time in Leiden and Paris. Despairing of the state of medical knowledge in Scotland, Sibbald began studying indigenous Scottish plants and established a garden of medicinal herbs.[24]

The two physicians planned a physic garden and leased an enclosure of land at St Anne's Yards, Holyrood House, establishing the garden in 1670. Between them contributing plants from their own gardens and more coming from an extraordinary garden owned by Patrick Murray, Laird of Livingston in West Lothian, the Physic Garden, sometimes also referred to as the Botanic Garden, flourished. So much so that it was later moved to a larger site at Trinity Hospital and received a Royal warrant in 1699.[25] Doctor Preston who taught botany at the Edinburgh Physic Garden had begun corresponding with Sir Hans Sloane two years earlier.[26] Sir Hans was to have an important role in supporting another Physic Garden at Chelsea.

The Chelsea Physic Garden was next to be planted for teaching apothecaries who had formerly only gone on simpling days in the countryside during training. The Society of Apothecaries initially rented the three-and-a-half-acre plot from Charles Cheyne in 1673. In 1680, a greenhouse was built and two years later Dr Hermann, professor of botany from Leiden agreed an exchange of plants, so beginning a new chapter for the garden.[27] As the needs of more exotic plants and tending them grew, so did the expenses of running the greenhouse, new plantings of trees and plants and general necessary care and repair.

Sir Hans Sloane, an accomplished physician and botanist was very familiar with the garden when he bought the Manor of Chelsea, including the land of the Apothecaries Garden in 1712. For a small annual charge, he conveyed the relevant land to the Apothecaries Company, providing that each year fifty dried specimens of plants grown in the garden were supplied to the Royal Society of London, of which he was a member. He also inserted a clause stopping the land being sold for building and ensuring its continued role for the centuries to come, additionally giving extra financial support in the following years.[28]

More Botanic Gardens followed with Cambridge in 1762, and after the middle of the century one at Kew House, home of the Dowager Princess of Wales, to become internationally famous in just a couple of decades.[29] It was not until 1790 that the Irish Parliament granted funds to the Royal Dublin Society to establish a public Botanic Garden at Glasnevin. In 1796 Walter Wade was asked to arrange the plants in the new garden at Glasnevin and lecture on botany with regard to medicinal and other uses.[30] Two years earlier he had published a catalogue of approximately

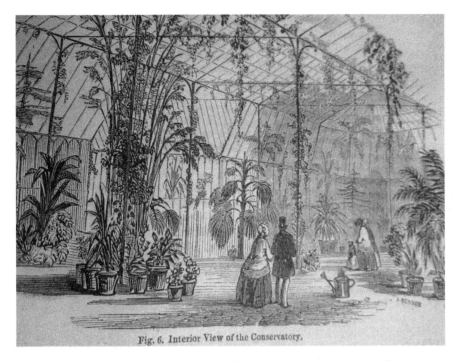

Fig. 6. Interior View of the Conservatory.

Inside the Conservatory, Kew. *The Ladies Companion*. Loudon.

422 County Dublin species, with 132 newly recorded, in which the Linnean system and nomenclature were used for the first time in Irish botany.[31] It had only been half a century since a book written by the physician Caleb Threlkeld described on the title page as the first of its kind, had given botanical details and medicinal uses of the native plants of Ireland with their Irish names. To research the correct names this Englishman who had moved to Ireland had consulted both oral tradition and a pre-1641 manuscript, possibly by the Rev. Heaton.[32]

Ten years after his herbal, an Irishman John Ke'ogh in County Cork, wrote *The Botanologia Universalis Hibernica*, a concise guide to his native herbs, with the Latin and then Irish names written as they were pronounced. He felt this necessary as some letters in the language are silent. Unfortunately, only the translation of these into English is given in the modern reproduction, which contains some interesting local references.[33]

It is disappointing to have to record that Wales, having been ruled by England for so long, waited until 2000 before the National Botanic Garden of Wales was opened at Llanarthney in Carmarthenshire by the Prince of Wales.

References

1. John Harvey, *Mediaeval Gardens* (London: Batsford, 1981), 32.
2. Harvey, *Mediaeval Gardens*, 92.

3. Ibid, 58.
4. R. Whiteman, *Brother Cadfael's Herb Garden* (London: Little, Brown and Co., 1996), 198.
5. Elizabeth and Reginald Peplow, *In A Monastery Garden* (Devon: David and Charles, 1988), 141.
6. Harvey, *Mediæval Gardens*, 21.
7. John Fitch, (trans), *Palladius The Work of Farming* (Devon: Prospect Books, 2013), 40.
8. Fitch, *Palladius The Work of Farming*, 63.
9. Ibid, 126–7.
10. Ibid, 65–66.
11. Mick Aston, *Monasteries in the Landscape* (Stroud, Glos: Tempus, 2000), 160–161.
12. Nicholas Orme and Margaret Webster, *The English Hospital 1070–1570* (London: Yale University Press, 1995), 37.
13. G. Barry and Lesley A. Carruthers, *A History of Britain's Hospitals* (Sussex: Book Guild Publishing, 2005), 57.
14. Barry and Carruthers, *A History of Britain's Hospitals*, 87.
15. "Apothecaries and Physic Gardens: An Early History of the Royal Hospital's Grounds." Royal Hospital Chelsea, October 23, 2020. https://www.chelsea-pensioners.co.uk/news/apothecaries-and-physic-gardens-early-history-royal-hospital%E2%80%99s-grounds.
16. Blanche Henrey, *British Botanical and Horticultural Literature before 1800*. (London: Oxford University Press, 1975), 32.
17. Anna Pavord, *Searching for Order* (London: Bloomsbury, 2009), 169.
18. Pavord, *Searching for Order*, 173–174.
19. Ibid, 178.
20. Stephen A. Harris, Oxford Plant Systematics, *What's in a date?* (Oxford: Department of Plant Sciences, University of Oxford, 2021), 9.
21. Ibid, 9.
22. *A Catalogue of the Plants growing in the Oxford University Botanic Garden and the Harcourt Arboretum* (Oxford: University of Oxford Botanic Garden, 1999).
23. Harold Fletcher and William Brown, *The Royal Botanic Garden Edinburgh* 1670–1970 (Edinburgh: Her Majesty's Stationery Office, 1970), 5–6.
24. Fletcher and Brown, *The Royal Botanic Garden Edinburgh*, 6–14.
25. Ibid, 30.
26. Hazel Le Rougetel, *The Chelsea Gardener* (London: Natural History Museum Publications, 1990), 15.
27. Rougetel, *The Chelsea Gardener*, 22–23.
28. Henrey, *British Botanical and Horticultural Literature before 1800*, 197.
29. Ibid, 156.
30. Ibid, 155.
31. W. Wade, *Catalogus systematicus plantarum indigenarum in comitatu dubliniensi inventarum* (Dublin: 1794).
32. Henrey, *British Botanical and Horticultural Literature before 1800*, 154–55.
33. Michael Scott, (ed), *An Irish Herbal: The Botanalogia Universalis Hibernica* (Northants: The Aquarian Press, 1986).

SECTION VII

REGULATION, REBELLION, AND EMIGRATION | 1581–1812

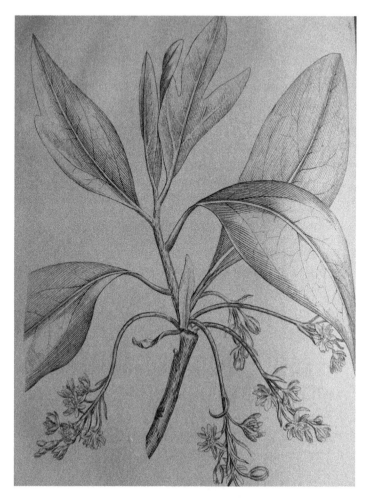

Sassafras. *Medical Botany*, Woodville.

Key Figures

Elizabeth I (reigned 1548–1603), James I (reigned 1603–1625), Thèodore Mayerne, (1573–1655), Thomas Muffet (1553–1604), Charles 1 (reigned 1625–1649), Nicholas Culpeper (1616–1653), William Bradford (1590–1657), John Josselyn (active 1630–1675), John Winthrop Jnr. (1608–1676), Martha Ballard (1735–1812).

Key Texts

Opera de Medicamentorum, 1581, Mesue.
Pharmacopoeia Londinensis, 1618.
Of Plymouth Plantation 1620–1647, Bradford.

Astrological Judgements of Diseases from the Decumbiture of the Sick, 1655, Culpeper.
A Directory for Midwives, 1654, Culpeper.
Culpeper's Complete Herbal and English Physician enlarged, 1652, Culpeper.
New-Englands RARITIES Discovered, 1672, Josselyn.
Pharmacopœia Bateana, 1694, Salmon.
Pharmacopoeia Edinburgensis, 1756.

Roles of Women in Medicine

Nurse, midwife, herb gatherer, herbalist, or cunning woman.

Quality Control

The Pharmacopoeias were intended to set a standard in restricting apothecaries to making only the approved remedies.

Herb Energetics

In the Opera of 1581, the energetics of the herbs are given with details of the individual herbs. The London Pharmacopoeia simply lists recipes without this information. The Edinburgh Pharmacopoeia gives only the part of the plant used in the list of Simplicia or Simples, which lists individual herbs. William Salmon in his translation of Bates Dispensatory does not list energetics with the herbs either. Culpeper gives both the energetics and which planet rules the herb.

Travel and Trade

There would be an ever increasing amount of travel between England and America during this period as settlers set out on perilous voyages to their new lives. New trade opportunities opened up and more plant discoveries and introductions are made. Exploitation of indigenous peoples continues.

Introduction

In the sixteenth century the Act of Uniformity established the authorised *Book of Common Prayer* as the only guide to worship.[1] This was reinforced in 1593. Rising numbers of Puritans who strongly objected were fined and imprisoned if they did not attend church. On Elizabeth's death in 1603, James I, son of catholic Mary Queen of Scots, but brought up with Calvinist doctrine, succeeded her. Both Catholics and Puritans had reason to believe he would lift the fines laid upon them.

After an early promise to do so, he banned Catholic priests and sought to rid England of Puritans altogether.[2] Following many difficulties finding suitable ships and crew, the group later known as the Pilgrim Fathers set sail for America on the Mayflower, and reached New England in 1620. Meanwhile in England the Royal College of Physicians sought to set a standard for medicines by deciding which were acceptable and publishing these in the first Pharmacopoeia. For apothecaries in particular this new regulation of their activities was resented by some. Among these was Nicholas Culpeper who had served as an apprentice apothecary. He believed in the cause of the common person to have access to knowledge of herbs. Since the Pharmacopoeia, written in Latin, contained lists of various medicinal preparations totally without explanation of their contents or the properties of the herbs, he objected to this discriminatory form of information. Culpeper decided to translate it, adding many notes of explanation.[3]

He was not the only rebellious person and other grievances with Charles I who had followed James, led to revolt and the Civil War (1742–45). Both religious and political differences encouraged emigration. Then came the plague in 1665, immediately followed by the great fire of London in September 1666. Both are described in famous diaries of the period.[4,5]

This section ends by following the progress of the Pilgrim Fathers and their descendants in America where trained physicians were scarce and ministers, their wives, midwives, and even the governor of the State, at times, gave medical help.

References

1. Vernon Heaton, *The Mayflower* (Exeter: Webb and Bower, 1980), 13.
2. Heaton, *The Mayflower*, 32.
3. Nicholas Culpeper, *A Physical Directory* (London: P. Cole, 1651).
4. Robert Latham, (ed.) *The Shorter Pepys* (London: Penguin Books, 1985), 500.
5. Austin Dobson (intro), *The Diary of John Evelyn* (London: Cassell and Co., 1909), 70–76.

CHAPTER 17

The Pharmacy Regulated | 1585–1756

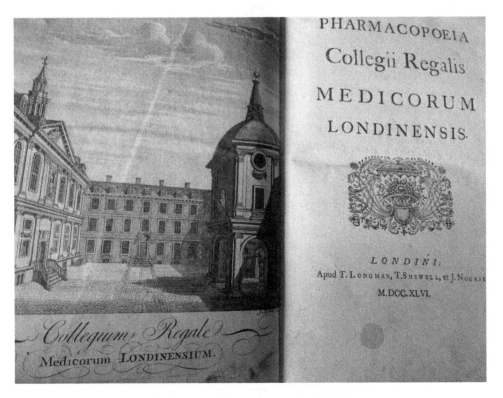

The London Pharmacopoeia. 1746.

Reference has already been made to how far behind England was with setting standards for medical qualifications and quality control in prescribing. An initial plan for a Pharmacopoeia, a collection of those currently acceptable remedies of all kinds supported by the Royal College of Physicians, following the pattern of other countries, was submitted in 1585.[1] The Continental Pharmacopoeia Augustana of 1564 had acknowledged the iatrochemical movement, mentioning Aqua cum Mercurio but without instruction for making it. The London Pharmacopoeia was eventually to take a bolder approach.

Sub-committees met to review prescriptions under specific headings such as syrups, decoctions, and chemical extracts and decide upon acceptable remedies. The physicians responsible for the 1618 London Pharmacopoeia included several past and the current President of the Royal Society and several physicians to the Royal Household, both past and present.[2] The Royal Society sought to dictate which standard recipes apothecaries were to make. Deciding on those acceptable in the twenty-six categories of preparations was not an easy task. After an initial report taking four years, this was submitted to a new committee of examiners. Twenty years later the subject appears again.

Chemicals had been considered for inclusion from the start, although we do not know which. One of the committee of twenty-one physicians was Thomas Muffet, an enthusiastic follower of Paracelsus, since his medical training in Basle and travels in Germany. It seems likely he was responsible for the initial inclusion of "*Extracta, Sales, Chemica, Metallica*".[3] At the time iatrochemistry versus taking a Galenical approach remained controversial and there was still care in inserting preparations that could be classified as in use for some time. Thomas Muffet had written a book on the Hippocratic approach to medicine. He was equally supportive of the chemico-therapeutic movement, which had begun in Arabic pharmacy and progressed in Europe through the work of Arnald de Villanova in Montpellier and then been galvanised by Paracelsus.[4] This was tied to the move away from polypharmacy and will become more obvious as time goes on, finding mention in the next chapter. A Royal physician Thèodore de Mayerne was likely to have been responsible for the introduction of a medicine to become the famous, *Mercurius dulcis*.[5] Still given in the Victorian period as part of the heroic medicine approach, mercuric chloride, later better known as calomel is corrosive to the mucous membranes.

Of the prescriptions themselves, we see in the headings familiar names from earlier collections with no fewer than one hundred and sixty six from Mesue in the second edition,[6] the main authority in the Opera de Medicamentorum. There are forty-six preparations authorised by Nicolai of Salerno and a large representation of Arabic formulas with those of Haly Abbas, Rhazes, and Avicenna. Others are from early in the first Millennium with twenty-seven bearing Galen's name and a pill with Scribonius Largus in the title, the army surgeon with the legions in Britain. This contains sagapeni, myrrh, opium, cardamom, castorei, pepper, and a sufficient quantity of wine to mix.[7] A plaster is attributed to Paracelsus and the compound distilled water of Dr. Stephani (Stevens) is also included.

James I was a man with an apparent phobia about witches and the harm they could do. Witchcraft had been a capital offence since 1484, the year Pope Innocent VIII issued his *Summis desiderantes* against it and there had been executions in the sixteenth century. An Act against witchcraft was passed by Parliament in 1542, making it punishable by death, then repealed five years later, only to be re-instated in 1562. When James I came to the throne he actively encouraged persecution.[8] The Act of 1604 reinforced the 1562 Act making witchcraft a civil offence to be tried in an ordinary, rather than ecclesiastical court. The famous trial of the Pendle witches when three generations of the same family were hanged was not until 1612. Women with knowledge of herbs, some of them midwives, were in danger of finding themselves accused through their clear opportunities to destroy life as well as save it. Men could be equally endangered by such interests as astrology. It would be 1736 before the witchcraft act was repealed finally and replaced by a fine for anyone claiming magical powers.[9]

The king was also deeply interested in regulating professions, particularly when it came to medicine. By 1618 the time was right for the Pharmacopoeia to come to fruition. In 1617, James, encouraged by lobbying from Mayerne, had enforced the separation of the grocers from the apothecaries, granting the Charter of the Royal Society of Apothecaries.[10] With apothecaries now grouped together it made enforcing use of the new Pharmacopoeia easier.

This Pharmacopoeia is concise to say the least when compared to the old collections of recipes with their commentaries from earlier authorities. These were men such as Mesue junior, Christopherus, Avicenna, Rhazes, Serapion junior, Nicolai of Salerno, and Dioscorides whom apothecaries had previously been obliged to depend on. Saladini, whose work is also included in the *Opera de Medicamentorum*, mentions those works he thinks an apothecary should have at his disposal. Along with the Arabic sources already mentioned, he added Nicolai of Salerno, Dioscorides, the *Circa Instans of Platearius*, and the popular *Macer Floridus*.[11]

One work which brought many of these required texts together in a single binding is the *Opera de Medicamentorum*. It was printed in Venice in 1581[12] just as the Pharmacopoeia was perhaps beginning to develop as an idea in England. The first mention of a London Pharmacopoeia appeared in the records of the Royal College of Physicians four years later. The Opera contains not only many prescriptions, with ingredients, amounts, and instructions, but information on individual herbs and other substances, physiology, and medicine. A number of works are bound in one so that the opinions of Mesue can be compared with others. The illustrations are finely etched and realistic, showing roots, stems, and leaves and occasionally flowers if they are pertinent. The plants are accompanied by insects in the manner we see in the embroidery of that period. Capital letters are also decorated with figures and foliage and in the case of Christopherus on pills, a fierce dragon.[13]

In a supplement to the Opera of Mesue, there is a compendium of the work of Francisci de Pedemontium, much recommended in an introduction by the physician, Vincentius Cogogollus. This details diseases of the organs, with sections also on fevers and the temperaments.[14] It is one of a dozen important additional works, including the Antidotarium of Nicolai, Apuleius de Ponderibus & Mensuris, Liber Servitoris of Albuchasis, and another large work from Joannis de Sancto Amando, *Expositio, & dubitationes earum quæ solutiones.*

When it comes to the Pharmacopoeia, there are still portrayals of fantastical beasts at the headings of different sections, but no illustrations of individual herbs. The preparations have brief instructions since no-one who is unfamiliar with pharmacy would be expected to be using the book. Both works are entirely in Latin, the language of educated medical practitioners. In the preface to the Pharmacopoeia, the authors state their intention to replace a "confusing abundance"[15] of older formularies. If even the possible model of the earlier Pharmacopoeia Augustana (first edition 1564) is compared, there is only one half the number of pages with nearly 600 less composita. It is also stated that the emphasis of the recipes is on the older medicine rather than the new chemistry.[16]

Surprisingly, considering how long the preparation of the Pharmacopoeia had taken, a second edition followed in the same year. It was announced that this was because of typographical errors but fundamental changes had been made. A much greater emphasis on a larger number of simples with these as a separate category, rather than lists of ingredients in compound mixtures, is the first to be noticed.[17] There is substantial increase in the numbers of metals and minerals and the multiplication by three times, of animals and animal substances. Young dogs, swans, otters, badgers, and whelks were now being included (almost all had been mentioned in Dioscorides' Materia Medica). The list of waters was also increased. It seems that rather than remaining a handbook for immediate use the authors wished to show a wider knowledge.

Since it is in Latin, the Pharmacopoeia naturally begins with Aqua with a list of simple waters in which the forty-six of Saladini has almost doubled to eighty-four. The compound waters include some that have appeared in earlier collections. With cinnamon water, there are several versions—the older from Matthioli alongside one bearing the name of Mayerne, physician to Henry VIII. More compound waters were already famous, and in household collections, were Aqua Imperialis, Aqua Mirabilis, and Aqua Doctoris Stephani.[18] Aqua Theriacalis on the other hand, which contained theriac of Andromachi and the other great antidote, mithridatium were among the ingredients that were restricted to apothecaries.[19]

Many of the syrups are from Mesue, with a couple from Nicolai of Salerno, the myrtle and oxysaccharum. Syrup may sound simple, but there is a compound syrup of betony which must surely be wonderfully fragrant as it also contains marjoram, thyme, rose, violets, lavender spike, and sage, together with seeds of fennel, anise, and ameos and the roots of peony, polypody, and fennel with betony juice and sugar.[20] We first saw medicinal earths mentioned in Dioscorides, then it was only earth from the island of Lemnos. Now a number of earths from Samos and Silesia among others were in use. The class, *Solis Auxungia* means fat of the earth[21] and they do have a slightly greasy feel. I saw a number of samples from different sources as large round tablets bearing the identifying stamp of where they came from on the upper surface in the Museum of Pharmacy in Basel.

The Arabic Species or mixes of powders are perhaps the recipes I have found of most interest, especially the Dianthos of Nicolai, which is hugely aromatic and can readily be recreated today with an ounce each of rosemary flowers, red roses, violets, and then six drachma of liquorice and clove pinks with a range of spices, aniseed, and ligni Aloes.[22] I included making species in the Stillroom to Dispensary workshop I tutored as a postgraduate course for NIMH in 2010. Powders can be taken in a number of ways and cost less for the patient.

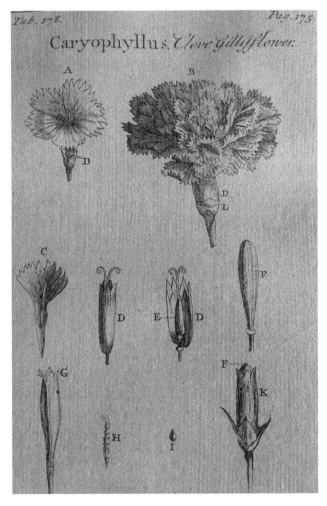

Clove Pink. *The Compleat Herbal*, Tournefort.

Other classifications in the Pharmacopoeia were decoctions, honeys, oxymels of herbs in honey, vinegar, and purified water, and lohochs sweetened with sugar. Under conserves and sugars, we find penidia, which readers may recall from the chapter on medieval pharmacy from the commonplace book. There is a large section on the popular electuaries, followed by purges and pills, then troches mixed with juices such as liquorice, rose water, or wine. Expressed oils are followed by those containing a number of herbs and spices in the composita, then unguents, emplasters, and cerata before distilled chemical oils. This section includes oils of antimony, sulphur, and tartar, flowers of sulphur and mercurius dulcis mentioned earlier. There are no tinctures. A few more preparations bring the reader to the lists of simples, divided into roots, cortex, (bark), woods, flowers, seeds, juices, etc. Finally, there are lists of salts, metals, animal, and marine life.

The Pharmacopoeia did not stay the same for long and has, of course, been regularly updated over the centuries. In 1699 the Royal College of Physicians of Edinburgh issued the first Edinburgh Pharmacopoeia and were, like their counterparts in London, given a charter with the rights to inspect apothecary shops to maintain quality control.[23] This Pharmacopoeia contained approximately 900 drugs and preparations. The 1756 edition in my possession, which is ordered on the same lines, has a very different appearance to the first London Pharmacopoeia. It is altogether smaller. It fits neatly in the hand or in the pocket and is a pleasure to use. Headings are in neat Italic type and lead you in to consider the appropriate nature of some of the prescriptions, such as a cephalic tincture for the head containing valerian, virginia serpentary, and rosemary, digested in white wine, then filtered.[24] Syrups are made with white sugar, the main herb or herbs and fountain water, with violets or ginger being macerated overnight, as I would make them today.[25]

After the familiarity of elderflower unguent and a balsam containing benzoin, balsam of Peru, and aloes in spirit of wine[26] the fifty pages of the chemica section with the fruits of the labours of Geber and Paracelsus in Aqua regia containing sal ammoniac, and corrosive mercury sublimate in other recipes are striking in their contrast. It is a relief to turn back to a sugar conserve containing rosemary and red rose flowers with bitter orange peel and cynosbati fruits, which are like a prickly gooseberry from America, but there my enthusiasm wanes as I take in the first ingredient, a beetle, *cochleariæ hortensis*.[27]

It would be 1794 before a Specimen Pharmacopoeia was circulated among members of the College of Physicians in Ireland and the Dublin Pharmacopoeia followed in 1807.[28] Meanwhile in 1653, the Royal College of Physicians in London had been outraged by an impertinent Culpeper, who had not even finished his training as an apothecary to become sworn in to the Society, setting himself up as if he were a physician translating the London Pharmacopoeia for anyone to read! Others, who were qualified physicians, wrote Dispensatories—collections of formulæ with their commentaries and some of these, such as the *Pharmacopoeia Bateana*, first published

108   *ELECTUARIA.*

Theriaca Edinenſis.

℞ Rad. ſerpentariæ Virgin. uncias decem.

contrayervæ uncias ſex.

Reſinæ guajaci uncias quatuor.

Cardamomi minoris uncias duas.

Croci Anglici,

Myrrhæ,

Opii ana unciam unam.

Rob ſambuci triplum ad pondus

* pulverum.

Vini Canarini q. ſ. *ad ſolvendum opium.*

Miſce, fiat electuarium ſ. a.

Edinburgh Theriac. *Edinburgh Pharmacopoeia.* 1756.

by James Shipton in 1688 were used a great deal by apothecaries. William Salmon brought out his edition with commentary in 1694, which is a mine of information.[29] Those by Quincy and Lewis followed, when studied, the Pharmacopoeia mirror what is happening in the world of the day. They show our native herbs and familiar spices mixed with new exotic imports. In the pages are the animal ingredients of the old world and the chemical minerals and metals of the new.

References

1. G. Urdang, (historical intro) *Pharmacopoeia Londinensis* of 1618, (Facsimile), (Wisconsin: Madison State Historical Society, 1944), 10.
2. *Pharmacopoeia Londinensis*, 11.
3. Ibid, 17.
4. Ibid, 18.
5. Ibid, 62.
6. Ibid, 71.
7. Ibid, 191.
8. John Riddle, *Eve's Herbs* (Cambridge Mass: Harvard University Press, 1997), 126.
9. Witchcraft, Acts of 1562 and 1604. https://www.parliament.uk/about/living-heritage/transformingsociety/private-lives/religion/overview/witchcraft. accessed August 19th 2023.
10. Michael Berlin, *The Worshipful Company of Distillers* (Chichester: Phillimore & Co. Ltd., 1996), 11.
11. C.J.S. Thompson, *The Mystery and Art of the Apothecary* (Philadelphia: Lippincott & Co., 1929), 129.
12. Joannes Mesue, *Opera de Medicamentorum* (Venice: 1581).
13. Mesue, *Opera de Medicamentorum*, 174.
14. Mesue, *Opera de Medicamentorum*, Second Book. 1–158.
15. *Pharmacopoeia Londinensis*, 32.
16. Ibid, 32.
17. Ibid, 34.
18. Ibid, 107.
19. Ibid, 107–8.
20. Ibid, 118.
21. Ibid, 50.
22. Ibid, 154–5.
23. C.J.S. Thompson, *The Mystery and Art of the Apothecary*, 146.
24. *Pharmacopoeia Collegii Regii Medicorum Edinburgensis* (Edinburgh: Hamilton, Balfour, et Neill, 1761), 53.
25. *Pharmacopoeia Collegii Regii Medicorum Edinburgensis*, 87.
26. Ibid, 131.
27. Ibid, 97.
28. Thompson, *The Mystery and Art of the Apothecary*, 150.
29. William Salmon, *Pharmacopœia Bateana* (London: Smith and Walford, 1694).

CHAPTER 18

Culpeper and Astrology | 1619–1654

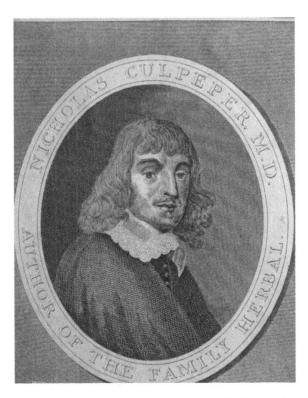

Portrait of Nicholas Culpeper. *Complete Herbal.* Culpeper.

Born in 1619, Nicholas Culpeper grew up in the care of his mother in his grandfather's house as his father died soon after he was born. His grandfather, William Attersoll was a Puritan rector with a keen interest in study and a belief that sickness was good for the soul. He will have encouraged the young Nicholas to read the books in his library. Whether he meant him to choose those on astrology or not, his later mastery of the subject appears to have begun early. His University education was funded by his grandfather in the hope of young Nicholas entering the Church. His grandson had other ideas and after falling in love with a young lady who would not have been approved for him as a match the two planned to elope. Tragically for him his love was struck by lightning and died on her way to meet him.

Such an act of God must have felt like a judgment and after this trauma he abandoned University. William Attersoll again supported him, this time funding his apprenticeship to become an apothecary. His years at Cambridge had given him the ability to meet the first requirement of passing an exam in the rudiments of Latin and, evidently, he could also meet the second requirement. This was being able to decipher the almost illegible writing of physicians which would be a necessary part of his work when making up prescriptions. Simpling days spent identifying herbs would have been part of his eight-year training.[1]

It seemed that ill fortune dogged his steps, as his first master left the country being unable to meet his debts and so Culpeper's payment for the remaining years was lost. The Society of Apothecaries transferred his apprenticeship to a second master, Drake, but, unfortunately, he had two years still to serve when Drake died in 1639. The Society allotted him a third master but Culpeper had other plans. His mother was now dead and he had been left only a small sum by his disappointed grandfather.

His friend Leadbetter had just finished his apprenticeship, taking over Drake's shop in Threadneedle Street and Culpeper decided to set up as an unlicensed apothecary with him, in direct contravention of the rules he had sworn to follow. In that same year of 1640 he married Alice Fields, a wealthy young woman whose dowry funded their new home and his practice which enabled him to treat the poor at no charge. Their home was in Spitalfields, close to the site of St Mary's hospital.[2] The hospital had been gone since the reformation, but there may well have been herbs still growing nearby. In his herbal he links herb descriptions with local habitats.

Culpeper's political beliefs are evident in both his herbal and other writings and his whole career. He stood for the rights of the common people against authority in all things, including, when it came to the Civil War, joining the Parliamentary troops. He preferred to treat the poor without recompense to visiting the wealthy, and he supported using herbs which could be grown nearby rather than the dearer imported drugs. He, therefore, came into direct opposition to the Society of Apothecaries which commonly sold the exotic and more expensive in order to make more profit. He defied the Royal College of Physicians who had the right to examine apprentices, fining those practising as unlicensed practitioners and it is not clear whether his failure to qualify was due to them or his own rebellious opinion of what they stood for.

In their effort to restrict the practice of the Apothecaries the College of Physicians had also laid out in the Pharmacopoeia of 1618 those recipes to be made in their shops. There are no elaborate instructions as has already been discussed and Culpeper evidently saw this as a challenge. Determined to stand up for his principles, Culpeper translated the Pharmacopoeia, entitling it *A Physical Directory* so that all could read it, attracting more trouble. The fury of the College shows in the huge lash-back of fierce criticism which followed.[3] Undeterred he worked on.

He was keeping company with men of dangerous politics and publishing almanacs prophesying the coming of a new order. That alone could have triggered a charge of witchcraft, something which had happened to other astrologers. William Lilly, a contemporary of Culpeper was careful to entitle his book, *Christian Astrology*. However, Culpeper was actually accused of witchcraft by a patient who had wasted away after treatment from him. Whether the Society of Apothecaries or physicians were behind this we will never know, but he was in court in the December and was acquitted of the witchcraft charge. When he returned home from the Battle of Newbury, wounded in the shoulder, it was to find that The Royal Society of Apothecaries had warned Leadbetter to cut ties with him and he finally did so in 1643.[4] Culpeper then practised from his home and continued writing.

The edition of *Culpeper's Complete Herbal* in my possession, printed in 1815, contains his last epistle for readers dated as written at his house in Spitalfields, September 5th 1653, four months before his death. It was later published by his wife and his message to her on publishing his works follows.

This edition is not simply his herbal with details of plants; *The English Physician Enlarged* and *Family Dispensatory* has been added to it, so that the work offers a guide to understanding the use of herbs from the Pharmacopoeia. With the further addition of his Key to Galen's Method of Physic it gives a guide to medicine plus plain instructions for making medicinal preparations. It contains much normally restricted to an official dispensatory but is intended for use by families rather than the apothecary.[5] By then his Herbal had attracted copyists seeking to profit from his work and he gives instructions as to how to tell the forgeries with all their mistakes, from his own work.

He describes his study of the most approved authors on medicine. Within the text he quotes Hippocrates, Galen, Dioscorides, Pliny, Matthiolus, and Camerarius, a physician in London. He criticises Gerard and Parkinson for not understanding why they are repeating earlier writers and goes on to describe his wish to know what causes illness and why the herbs can cure it. Culpeper makes clear the importance of astrology when he writes, "I always found the disease vary according to the various motions of the Stars; and this is enough, one would think, to teach a man by the effect where the cause lies".[6]

Astrology in medicine is not new, instructions to consider the "rising and set-ting of the stars"[7] go back beyond the Hippocratic Corpus to Egypt and possibly Babylon. After initial acceptance the Church had doubts and in the thirteenth century Albertus Magnus made a distinction between the astrology used by sailors in navigation and physicians in treating disease and the sort which made more general predictions, which was soothsaying and not acceptable.[8]

Arabic influence in the *Introductorium in Astronomiam* of Abu Ma'shar who had died in the ninth century, added credibility to astrological medicine when the text became available in twelfth century Europe.[9] This work explained the connections between the twelve signs of the zodiac and the parts of the body, often illustrated by elaborate drawings of the zodiac man. Starting with the ram of Aries at the head, parts of the body are decorated with zodiac symbols and names of the houses until with some it is difficult to make out the main message. With the symbols of the bull of Taurus around the neck, the crab of Cancer over the lungs and the lion of Leo over the heart, it is a good thing the twins of Gemini can be placed alongside the arms, rather than being restricted to the shoulders. Virgo for the stomach and bowels and the scales of Libra relating to the kidneys and bladder must also fit into the lower torso with the scorpion of Scorpio lowest, governing the sexual organs. This slightly simplified list leaves us with the centaur archer of Sagittarius at the hips, Capricorn's goat at the knees, and Aquarius pouring water suitably down over Pisces fishes at the feet.[10]

Culpeper connects this concept together with the plants through their planetary associations. In his epistle to the reader with instructions on use of his complete herbal, the reason he has already recommended his earlier work, *Astrological Judg-ment of Diseases from the Decumbiture of the Sick* quickly becomes apparent. He lists five points to consider, the first three are simple, the planet causing the disease, the part of the body affected and the planet governing that part of the body, and he refers to his Judgement of Diseases for the details. The fourth and fifth points reveal the complexity of this system of medicine.

"Fourthly, You may oppose diseases by Herbs of the planet, opposite to the planet that causes them: as diseases of *Jupiter* by Herbs of *Mercury*, and the con-trary: diseases of the *Luminaries* by Herbs of *Saturn*, and the contrary; diseases of *Mars* by Herbs of *Venus*, and the contrary.

Fifthly, there is a way to cure diseases sometimes by *Sympathy*, and so every planet cures his own disease; as the *Sun* and *Moon* by their Herbs cure the Eyes, *Saturn* the Spleen, *Jupiter* the Liver, *Mars* the Gall and diseases of choler, and *Venus* diseases of the instruments of Generation."[11]

Although the reader of the herbal is directed to his earlier work on the judgement of diseases to make the necessary astrological calculations, Culpeper puts much of the simple instruction into his herbal, accentuating certain necessary steps with par-ticular herbs. If all the herbs under a particular planet are selected and compared, much can be learned. When we add to this his explanations of the links of the herbs and their planetary rulerships to the zodiac signs, the outline of the system and back-ground reasoning emerges and we can also find references to humoral classification.

For instance, the Sun is naturally associated with the element fire, and plants ruled by the Sun include angelica, greater celandine, chamomile, eyebright, juniper, rosemary and rue—hot and dry herbs by the Hippocratic classification. The Sun rules the heart, as does the zodiac sign Leo. Culpeper writes under saffron "It is an herb of the Sun, and under the Lion, and therefore you need not demand a reason why it strengthens the heart so exceedingly … . It quickens the brain, for the Sun is exalted in Aries, as he hath his house in Leo".[12]

The Sun also rules the sight and eyes, the left eye of a woman and the right eye of a man. The list above contains some of the most used eye herbs, under Celandine he writes "all that know anything in astrology, know that the eyes are subject to the luminaries: let it then be gathered when the Sun is in Leo, and the Moon in Aries, applying to this time; let Leo arise, then may you make into an oil or ointment..".[13] With butterbur, another herb of the Sun that is given as a great strengthener of the heart, his feelings for the poor enter the text when he writes, "It were well if gentle-women would keep this root preserved, to help their poor neighbours. *It is fit the rich should help the poor, for the poor cannot help themselves*".[14]

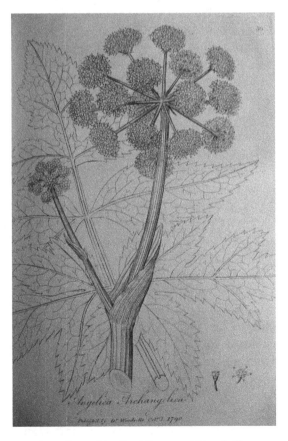

Angelica, *Medical Botany*, Woodville.

There are truly detailed instructions under angelica—"It is an herb of the Sun in Leo; let it be gathered when he is there, the Moon applying to his good aspect; let it be gathered either in his hour, or in the hour of Jupiter, let Sol be angular; observe the like in gathering the herbs, of other planets, and you may happen to do wonders. In all epidemical diseases caused by Saturn, that is as good a preservative as grows: It resists poison, by defending and comforting the heart, blood, and spirits".[15]

In opposition to the Sun is the Moon, identified with the element water. Plants under the Moon include chickweed, cleavers, wild lettuce, opium poppy, water lily, and willow. The Moon rules the brain and eyes, and is linked with cooling and moistening herbs. Culpeper states of lettuce, "The Moon owns them, and that is the reason they cool and moisten what heat and dryness Mars causeth".[16] Cool, watery Moon herbs also oppose the effects of Mars, which, like the Sun is identified with fire.

So far, the relationships given are simple but there is more to them. Martian plants are heating and often of a prickly nature, such as nettle, hawthorn, blessed thistle, and basil. The related signs are Scorpio, governing the sexual organs and lower abdomen, and Aries. We find the greatest guidance under blessed thistle where Culpeper explains that this herb helps vertigo, because it is martian and under Aries, the sign ruling the head. It is effective for diseases related to gall because Mars governs choler. Mars also causes boils, itchy conditions, and plague. These conditions a martian herb cures by sympathy, while blessed thistle cures French pox by antipathy with the opposing planet. At the beginning of guidance under blessed thistle, the reader is advised to apply all that is written there on the astrological influences to using every other herb in medicine.[17] He does not always agree with earlier authorities, writing that although almost all astrologer-physicians set plantain under Mars because it cures diseases of the head and private parts that come under Mars, Aries, and Scorpio, he believes it to be under Venus, curing the head by antipathy to Mars, and the privities by sympathy to Venus.[18]

In opposition to hot Mars is cooling Venus with her herbs for treating the womb, yarrow, motherwort, tansy, vervain, and mugwort. Of mugwort, Culpeper writes that as a herb of Venus it "maintains the parts of the body she rules, remedies the diseases of the parts that are under her signs, Taurus and Libra".[19] Mugwort is recommended for treating the womb and urinary passages (Libra), and throat and neck (under Taurus).

Herbs under Jupiter, a planet that protects the earth from asteroids entering our universe are also protective. The list includes such cooling, cleansing herbs as dandelion, dock, and houseleek. Of hyssop, Culpeper writes it "strengthens all the parts of the body under Cancer and Jupiter".[20] Cancer rules the chest and lungs. Culpeper links betony to Jupiter and the sign, Aries.

Herbs under Mercury relate to the signs Gemini and Virgo, which rule the shoulders and arms, stomach and bowels. They can be heating and carminative, such as caraway, fennel, and elecampane—hot and moist. Some, such as lavender and valerian, can be sedative or alerting in differing dosages and patients, both illustrate the variable effects of Mercury, commented on by Culpeper when writing of the mulberry tree.[21]

Herbs under Saturn are cold and moist, with mullein, comfrey, heartsease, Solomon's seal, henbane, and fumitory as examples. Of Solomon's seal Culpeper comments, "Saturn owns the plant, for he loves his bones well".[22] The reader is advised to keep syrup of fumitory readily available as he writes, "If by my astrological judgment of diseases, from the decumbiture, you find Saturn author of the disease, or if by direction from a nativity you fear a saturnine disease approaching, you may by this herb prevent it in the one, and cure it in the other".[23]

We have already seen the importance of astrology in medicine in the fourteenth and fifteenth centuries illustrated by the charts of the zodiac man in chapter fourteen. This is the kind of detail for the University-trained physician to use—equipped with astrological tables hung from his belt. Self-help manuals with bare essentials of astronomical knowledge were also available for the less well-educated leech.[24] He would make a horoscope for the birth of the patient as well as a decumbiture. A horoscope was cast using information about the birth of a person. A decumbiture was a chart resulting from calculations using similar celestial information for when they became ill or, alternatively, the the time the physician was consulted. Full details of how to calculate them with explanations are given in Culpeper's *Astrological Judgement of Diseases*.[25]

There is not space here to explain the hours of the planets and these exacting rules for gathering and making of medicines; for this, it is recommended to consult either Culpeper's *Astrological Judgment of Diseases* or if not already familiar with astrology, Graeme Tobyn's book, *Culpeper's Medicine*.[26]

Culpeper derided the physicians for casting decumbitures on the positions of the planets when they had only looked at a urine sample and not seen the patient. He makes it clear that whatever the astrology says must agree with the patient's symptoms and observable signs to be valid. Like Paracelsus and Galen before him, Culpeper was forthright in his scathing attacks on others. His keen wit and honesty shine out not only in the herbal with the imaginary characters of Dr Reason and Dr Experience making comments in the text, found frequently in his *Astrological Judgement of Diseases*, but also in his comments below certain College recipes in *The English Physician Enlarged*.

Although favouring simple remedies, Culpeper includes a recipe mentioned several times before but not detailed, *Matthiolus's great antidote against Poison and Pestilence* with, by my reckoning, about one hundred and twenty-nine ingredients including spices, gems, resins, parts of animals, roots, seeds, and herbs. Below he writes, "The title shews you the scope … I believe it is excellent for those uses … . I am very loth to leave out this medicine, which if it were stretched out, and cut in thongs, would reach round the world".[27]

Detailed instructions on pharmacy appear in *The English Physician Enlarged*, and in my copy, these are followed by *A Key to Galen's Method of Physic*. Culpeper describes this as being suitable instruction for the vulgar, by which he means those with no knowledge of astrology. For the astrologer, the only person he sees as fit to practice physic, he gives deeper guidance.

While he refers to Galen's methods in the English Physician, in the *Astrological Judgement of Diseases* Culpeper lists presages on various signs, which are based on those of Hippocrates. He writes of Hippocrates as a brave physician and compares the way in which Galen improved on his work with the way in which Aristotle improved on Plato's philosophy.[28] The temperament characteristics we last saw in the *Regimen of Health*[29] are repeated and enlarged upon in his works. He explains humoral causes for stature and nature with each and includes compound temperaments and the temperaments of the organs in agreement with Avicenna's interpretations of Galen.

In recommending treating by sympathy in order to add strength to those organs for the body to be enabled to fight the disease naturally, he was also following Hippocrates. Treatments by antipathy were to be reserved for acute situations, as they could often be damaging. He also supported aspects of Paracelsian chemical medicine and may have dabbled in alchemy.

Bearing in mind that his wife Alice appears to have lost four of their six children either as stillbirths or soon after birth, it is perhaps not surprising that he was keen to find out and pass on as much information on pregnancy, birth, and care of small children as possible. In his *Directory for Midwives*, he approaches that well-worn subject of the character and diet of the woman who feeds the baby, whether mother or wet nurse. After stating that all authors give a description and favour the mother, he makes a touching statement, "Myself having buried many of my Children young, caused me to fix my Thoughts, intently upon this Business".[30] Culpeper goes on to remind readers of the multitude of children who have died while suckling and ponders on one possible cause being from the milk. After researching as best he can he sets out as much information as possible in the following pages. His beliefs and current knowledge about conception, the formation of the foetus and natural and complicated births and how to deal with them, gives much well-ordered information. It is fascinating to read of the ideas of the time, particularly that the prolapsed womb might be attracted back into the body by placing a herb on the top of the patients' head! Knowledge of physiology has come a long way since the seventeenth century.

His Directory is thorough covering everything from desire for copulation and signs of conception to weaning the child and much between. He also includes a great deal of medicine referring to problems with various organs of the mother before and after the birth. It is typical of him to write the book for female midwives telling them to consult his work rather than going to the College of Physicians for teaching. His book is indeed full of practical information as a manual should be. Nicholas Culpeper died in January 1654. Sadly he was survived by only one daughter.

The compassion he expresses in his directory and support for midwives in general against the hostile views of their competence from medical authority is typical of his persistence in standing up for the oppressed. In his introduction he writes that if his rules are followed the work of delivery will be easy, followed by the telling statement, "… and you need not call for the help of a Man-Midwife, which is a Disparagement, not only to yourselves, but also to your Profession …".[31] He ends by asking that if any midwife finds failings in his book, she should judge him charitably as he is only a man, and acquaint him with his mistake.

Paracelsus and Culpeper both championed the cause of the poor and attracted the wrath of authorities. Both men held a respectful attitude to creation and the creator. Although Culpeper is undeniably most remembered for his emphasis on medical astrology, he opened a wider view of medicine and humoral teachings to the lay reader. His herbal has never lost popularity, out-living consultation of his other books by the majority. It seems ironic that although astrology in medicine meant everything to him it is not the reason for his fame and has been decried many times. Few readers of his herbal today understand his main message, or read it at the deeper level alongside his *Astrological Judgment of Diseases* as instructed in order to use the remedies as he intended. Even so if anyone is stopped in the street and asked to name a herbalist of the past, Culpeper is often the only one they know.

References

1. C.J.S. Thompson, *The Mystery and Art of the Apothecary* (Philadelphia: Lippincott, 1929), 182–184.
2. Benjamin Woolley, *The Herbalist* (London: Harper Collins, 2004), 158–9.
3. Graeme Tobyn, *Culpeper's Medicine* (Dorset: Element, 1977), 15.
4. Woolley, *The Herbalist*, 233.
5. Nicholas Culpeper, *Culpeper's Complete Herbal* (London: Richard Evans, 1815 edition). Title page.
6. Culpeper, *Culpeper's Complete Herbal*, IV.
7. W.H.S. Jones, (trans), Hippocrates, Vol. IV (London: Harvard University Press, 1931), 229.
8. Carole Rawcliffe, *Medicine and Society in Later Medieval England* (Stroud: Sutton Publishing, 1997), 85.
9. Rawcliffe, *Medicine and Society in Later Medieval England*, 86.
10. Ibid, Plate 9.
11. Culpeper, *Culpeper's Complete Herbal*, V–VI.
12. Ibid, 161.
13. Culpeper, *Culpeper's Complete Herbal*, 42.
14. Ibid, 36.
15. Ibid, 8.
16. Ibid, 104.

17. Ibid, 41.
18. Ibid, 141.
19. Ibid, 123.
20. Ibid, 95.
21. Ibid, 123.
22. Ibid, 163.
23. Ibid, 81.
24. Rawcliffe, *Medicine and Society in Later Medieval England*, 89.
25. Nicholas Culpeper, *Astrological Judgement of Diseases from the Decumbiture of the Sick* (Bel Air: Astrology Classics, 2003), 1–133.
26. Tobyn, *Culpeper's Medicine*, Part Three, 130–173.
27. Culpeper, *Culpeper's Complete Herbal*, 338.
28. Nicholas Culpeper, *Astrological Judgement of Diseases from the Decumbiture of the Sick*, 147.
29. Sir John Harington, *The School of Salernum. Regimen Sanitatis Salerni* (Salerno, Rome: Ente Provinciale per Il Turismo,1957), 71–82.
30. Nicholas Culpeper, *A Directory for Midwives*, 1762 (Gale ECCO Print Editions, 2022), 127.
31. Culpeper, *A Directory for Midwives*, V.

CHAPTER 19

The New World | 1606–1812

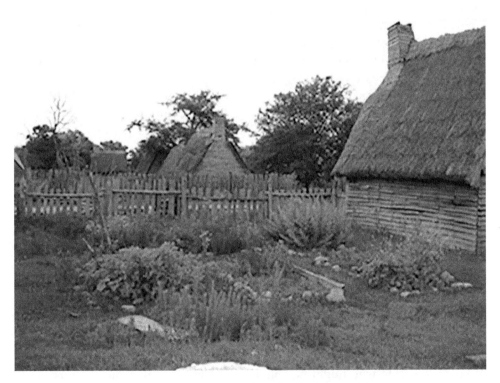

Pilgrim Cabins. Courtesy Plimoth Plantation Museum.

Between the time of the publication of the first London Pharmacopoeia in 1618 and the mid-century, increasing numbers of people decided, either due to religious or political considerations, to try to make a new life in America. Of the 102 pilgrims who set out to found the Colony of New Plymouth in 1620, fifty had died by the following summer.[1] The Plymouth settlers had planned to take everything they thought they would need for their first year, including tools, rope, arms, utensils, trees to be planted for fruits, and seeds for vegetables and herbs. However, due to the loss of one of the two ships at the outset of their journey, the Mayflower was overloaded with passengers and could not take all their provisions. Going on board the replica of The Mayflower anchored offshore is an experience that left me in no doubt of the horrendous overcrowding and how difficult the voyage would have been coping with sea sickness, lack of privacy, limited food, and sheer anxiety.

With two months as the shortest time at sea if all went well, thought went into provisions for health on the journey. In 1638, John Josselyn on his first visit to New England wrote in his journal a list of provisions to take on board. Among these were conserves of roses and clove gillyflowers, pepper, green ginger, nutmeg, dried fruits, wormwood, cinnamon, mace, and juice of lemons to cure or prevent scurvy.[2] On a second visit, this time for eight years he wrote the first full account of the animals, birds, fishes, insects, and plants he saw there, with details of their medicinal uses by Native Americans and the settlers.[3]

Had it not been for the friendliness of the Native Americans despite finding on their first discovery of the settlers that these strangers had already helped themselves to a buried store of their food; it is unlikely any of the early pilgrims would have survived. They were soon joined by others, but in England there remained great confusion about the climate and what would or would not grow in the new land. Much expectation of a semi-tropical climate led to seeds or grafts being taken for the pomegranate, mulberry for silkworms, and grape vines to provide wine for England. There were numerous disappointments. Fortunately, wild strawberries and raspberries, cranberries and blueberries abounded.

Settlements in Virginia, the first founded in 1606, were already sending cargoes of sassafras and tobacco back to England before the pilgrims arrived, and many voyages were funded by underwriters who, seeing this early commercial success, expected more profitable drugs to be returned to England as repayment.[4] However, New Plymouth did not offer such discoveries. For the health of the settlers underwriters tried to send at least one barber surgeon with each ship. A few physicians elected to go, but either did not stay or changed their profession as there were not enough rich patients for them to treat.

It was considered desirable for clergymen to marry women with knowledge of home medicine who might be able to treat the ills of their neighbours in the way the lady of the manor traditionally functioned in society in England. This is emphasised later in George Herbert's *Country Parson*, published in 1652, a guide on behaviour including expectations of their wives. The second requirement is for his wife to cure and heal, using her knowledge already gained. If she does not have such knowledge, he is to ensure she gains it from "some religious neighbour".[5] It is also related that the parson in his role as physician to the sick, required only three books in his library to help him, one on anatomy, another on physic, and the third a herbal to encourage use of home grown medicines rather than drugs from the apothecary. On finding sick persons in houses he visits he should use his access to books presumably, to provide them with receipts, (recipes). Two examples of suitable receipts are quoted, a poultice of "Elder, camomill, mallowes, comphrey and smallage" and a salve of "hyssop, valerian, mercury, adders tongue, yarrow, melilot, and *Saint Johns* wort".[6]

In workshops at the Weald and Downland Living Museum, we made both the poultice and a slightly adapted form of the suggested salve, containing hyssop, valerian flowers, yarrow, melilot, St John's wort, and wild marjoram. This has remained a very popular ointment for those taking a jar home after workshops and I am still asked at intervals for another jar, years later, as it is so useful.

As the new social order was set up and wilderness tamed, it appears, that at first magistrates and even the Governor of Connecticut himself, could also be asked for medicinal advice in serious cases. However, with parsons and ministers it was usually their wives who ministered to the sick. From William Bradford writing of the Plymouth Colony, we find both Mrs John Cotton and Mrs John Eliot, whose husband gained fame for giving the indigenous people a written language and then translating the Bible into it, have been singled out for praise. Cotton Mather wrote of Mrs. Eliot's considerable skill in both physic and chirurgy.[7]

One Governor who might have been equipped to offer medical advice, although he was not a physician, was John Winthrop Junior. He crossed the Atlantic to join his father and brothers in the New World in 1631. He took foodstuffs, seeds, and necessities and his list of seeds bought from the grocer Robert Hill is our best guide for those taken to Boston at this time. We find some of the same herbs Tusser considered necessary for stilling, dill, endive, sorrel, fennel, and hyssop, together with blessed thistle. Purslane, parsley, marigold, rosemary, savory, thyme are also there, with lovage, borage, and more.[8] Young John Winthrop had a deep interest in books and even with the restrictions on what he was able to take on board managed to include many of his precious volumes, packed in a barrel for safety. They were recorded as mainly on chemistry.[9] He also took distilling apparatus.

John Winthrop was chosen governor twelve times between 1631 and 1648, several times, it has to be said, in his absence. He travelled widely, not only in the service of the Massachusetts Bay Company but also on establishing new schemes of his own. Amid a great deal of business back in England in 1635, he accepted provisional governorship of the River Connecticut and adjoining harbours and places. In addition to marrying his second wife on the previous day (the first had died in childbirth), he spent time with two German physicians on that trip, one of whom gave him a book on alchemy in which he later made notes.[10] He was to remain governor of Connecticut for the rest of his life in spite of several tries at resignation which were not accepted after many years of valued service.

As the medicinal needs of the community grew he searched unsuccessfully for a regular physician and having already given medical help he found himself filling the role. Not surprisingly with his alchemical interests, he favoured Paracelsian medicine. He prescribed compounds containing the poisonous antimony, mercury, and white vitriol, also rosin, red coral, and balsam. Sometimes he used herbs such as saffron, sassafras, wormwood, and anise. Experimenting, he invented an all-purpose treatment with his purgative rubila powder.[11] Rubila powder became famous but sounds particularly unattractive from the noted difficulty of keeping it down and the powerful side effects.

John Winthrop was not trained as a physician but his approach was in keeping with the times and he certainly had the confidence of his patients. Despite his very active political life his regular records of prescribing between 1656–7 and 1669, show that he treated at least seven hundred individual patients.[12]

In 2011 I spent a week tutoring workshops at Plimoth Plantation Museum where the new Colony of Plymouth is brought to life for visitors. A dusty road leads between lines of thatched, wooden cabins, with neat, fenced gardens of vegetables and herbs. The settlement is on a hillside looking out to sea and daily life is portrayed by staff and volunteers in costume, who tend their gardens, cook their meals and keep house, talking to visitors strictly "in period". Their diet they tell visitors is ordered according to their humoral needs and a humoral garden shows the herbs in their categories to explain this to the public.

It was summer and the temperature was thirty-four degrees centigrade that week. With linen clothing worn, this ensured better comfort than modern dress. Inside the cabin the windows could be shut as needed by sliding wooden shutters, but were of course open, along with the door, for light. The thatch gave insulation and although the fire was needed for cooking, the heat did not feel too oppressive. The furniture was limited to a bed with curtains, table, benches, chest, and cupboard with shelving. All were simply made and little different to furnishings in a cottage of the period in England. The pottery made on site served admirably for plates, drinking vessels, and pots for cooking and I was delighted to demonstrate using it. Equipped with gathering baskets and plentiful herbs growing nearby, I felt I would have been happy to move in—until winter, with all the hardships that would entail.

In workshops we looked first at life in England at the time and English expectations, herbals, and books on gardening that would have been taken to the new world as guides. *Dodoen's Herbal*, first published in Flemish in 1554, may have been taken on board the Mayflower. The herbal that quotes much from it that we know rather better and was often consulted later was Gerard's *Herbal*, extended by Johnson in 1633. *Culpeper's Herbal* was also popular there. John Parkinson's *Paradisi in Sole*, published in 1629, provided ambitious inspiration for gardens of the wealthy.

We are reminded that this beautiful book was written by the royal apothecary and botanist to James I, by the inclusion of the medicinal virtues of the plants where applicable. He also appears to give more attention and detail to the virtues of herbs new on the scene.

Parkinson takes us first into the flower garden emphasising beauty and variety, including bulbs such as the tulip and crocus. After each group of related plants he then gives the virtues of any medicinal herb in that group. So we have the virtues of saffron under crocus used against smallpox, measles, jaundice and plague.[13] With the violets and pansies he writes their virtues are so well known that he comments only on the purging qualities of violets and use of the distilled water of heartsease for the French disease.[14]

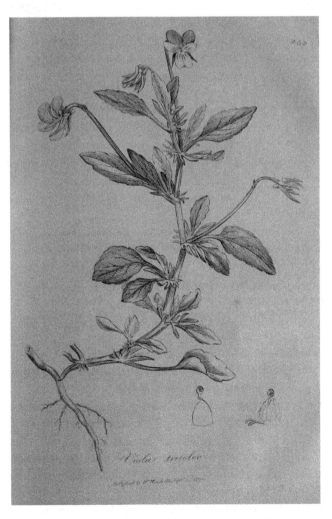

Heartsease, *Medical Botany*, Woodville.

Many pot herbs which are also medicinal can be found in his kitchen garden list. Sage, mints, purslane, angelica, and liquorice, are included. Parkinson has added some specifically for the skill of the gentlewoman who may not live near a physician and who cares for her family and poor neighbours. A much larger physic garden is hinted at for the future, which, in time will be his *Theatrum Botanicum*. Throughout the book, it is the botanist who shines through most powerfully, a botanist with an eye for beauty he wishes to share. *Theatrum Botanicum* was a herbal to rival Gerard's work but never to become as well known.

There were, of course, more books offering advice, with Andrew Boorde's *Breviary of Health* 1587, and William Lawson's *A New Orchard and Garden* 1648. Looking at herbs of the early settlers included the list of suggested provisions for the voyage from England and Sir Hugh Plat's *Delights for Ladies* published in 1609 provided recipes for troches of the sea which we made with cinnamon, ginger, sugar, gum tragacanth, and rose water.[15] Sugar was soon to be plentifully available, more than in England as ships from the West Indies came with supplies of fruits, such as lemons, spices, and sugar. An Ipswich storekeeper's account book supplied the inspiration for a syrup for back pain, although we left out the gunpowder![16]

Many herbs could soon be picked in the gardens for recipes as this was a time when home medicine was encouraged with herbs growing around you. For this John Josselyn's *New England Rarities* offered us a guide. He lists not only what the settlers found to be growing, but also those plants that had appeared since the settlers had arrived and kept cattle there. These included stinging nettles, dandelion, chickweed, mayweed, noted as making a good unguent, and plantain "which the Indians call *English-Man's Foot*".[17]

He also names garden herbs that thrive and those that did not. Marigolds, savory, feverfew, tansy, sage, and spear mint were all given by him as thriving and borage was plentiful. Yarrow and angelica were both already growing there. Borage and angelica, we candied. One herb I felt sure must have been cultivated as an essential was soapwort. On enquiry while the workshops were still at the planning stage, I found to my surprise there was none in the gardens or growing wild. Planning took two years and in the spring before my arrival soapwort sprang up where no-one had seen it before. To my joy I found it at the side of the path. I demonstrated that even in water heated only by the air temperature, it removed the stains of oil and herbs from an ointment straining cloth, leaving perfectly white muslin with all the globules of oil on the surface of the water.

Other herbs did not grow so well. Josselyn recorded that rue would hardly grow and lavender and rosemary were not for that country, which must have caused concern when thinking of times of pestilence. He also lists the most common diseases affecting the settlers, which included, "*The Black pox, the Spotted Feaver, the Griping of the Guts*" and others[18] When writing of native plants he often quotes local tribal use as with powdered white hellebore for wounds following an application of racoon grease, or a strong decoction of tobacco as a wash for burns and scalds, followed by strewing on the dried powder. He also writes birch bark was used by the Native Americans for bruised wounds and cuts and describes how they prepared it.

Thinking of fruits and nuts, haws are described as big as services, which are a slightly smaller fruit than a pear, and he notes the walnuts, presumably from the black walnut, *Juglans nigra*, are very different from those in Europe. Many trees were used medicinally, including oak, alder, birch, sumach, board pine, fir, and spruce. Of the plants, it appears the sarsaparilla was the best hope for export, although I do not know of any evidence it was traded from this area. Gardens at the museum represent the early small kitchen gardens grown.

In the April of 1621 the Mayflower which had remained as a precaution with so many of its former passengers falling sick, departed. Then their new friend Squanto showed them how to set corn and tend it.[19] Help with cultivation would be their saving, as the seeds of wheat and peas they had brought did not grow. Their first harvest of corn was good but in the following years more ships arrived and those who had established homes found they were sharing what they had with others, some of whom had great need of help. William Bradford's account gives a detailed picture of arrivals, trading beaver skins with the help of the Wompanaog and the difficulties this made with other tribes.

As mentioned, John Winthrop Junior lost his first wife, along with their baby in childbirth. I do not know of a record of midwives setting out for the New World and it was clearly usual for neighbours to give support. Previously in England, more than one woman is pictured with the woman in labour. A deposition in Essex County in America in 1657 places a dozen women with the labouring mother to be.[20] Women might gain considerable experience in attending births and giving birth themselves.

In the following century the diary of Martha Ballard who was born in 1735 records her delivering 814 babies from her fiftieth year until her death twenty-seven years later.[21] She had earlier given birth to nine babies herself and was clearly experienced also with growing and preparing herbal remedies for conditions beyond pregnancy and labour. Martha does not mention learning recipes from books, although the herbs in her remedies can be found in Culpeper and books of housekeeping containing physic, such as Eliza Smith's guide to housekeeping from earlier in the century.[22] Culpeper's *Complete Herbal* was re-printed many times in America. Her main herbs are those also grown in England. With an uncle and two brother-in-law physicians she would certainly have had opportunities to become interested in medicine. Her diary records visits, who had called her out, the patient's condition, and when payment was made.

Martha regularly stayed overnight tending to women about to give birth, or occasionally with the grievously sick in epidemics, laying them out if they died, but still had to carry on her daily duties at home, assisted by her daughters. While they sometimes did the washing and are always preparing thread and weaving, Martha was also out picking saffron for infants with jaundice, digging roots for treatments, or attending births. Along with churning butter, brewing and baking she was preparing specific herbal medications. Martha mentions various syrups for treatments, including mullein, currant, or Balson on occasions and a compound of comfrey, plantain, agrimony, and Solomon's seal for her niece on another.[23]

There are also mentions of plasters of comfrey and decoctions. Martha cut hyssop for inclusion in a bath to give ease after complications in childbirth, together with tansy, chamomile, hyssop and mugwort in 1790.[24] People also came to the house for healing herbs that she either grew along with the family supplies of vegetables and fruits, or wild-gathered. Always when she was waiting and watching during a long labour she knits for her growing family, mostly gloves and mitts.

In the diary, her accounts deal with trading cloth and bartering as well as cash transactions. Although she was the one in charge at a delivery, unless a physician was needed, she also called the patient's "women" to be present and support her. Very occasionally she mentions the doctor was also present, and although there may have been tensions when she did not necessarily agree with his treatment, there does not seem to have been real animosity. Martha attended some autopsies and dissections and on one occasion in 1808, records twelve doctors and three midwives being present together at an autopsy.[25] Within twenty years, this situation would begin to change as the scientific aspect of such training was presented as being likely to destroy the compassionate approach of a woman for her patients. There was much turmoil in medicine to come, on both sides of the Atlantic.

We have looked at the herbs introduced into America and noted the early importance of sassafras and tobacco. In 1613 John Rolfe crossed seed from a local plant in Virginia with one from the West Indies to produce his first crop.[26] Many herbs would be brought across the Atlantic, which did not make fortunes for those who transported them but became incorporated into later herbal prescribing.

In the seventeenth century, these included witch hazel introduced into England in 1656 from East North America. The black walnut, already mentioned by Josselyn, came from Eastern America in the same year. In 1658, wild rosemary was introduced and the American mandrake was also introduced in 1664. Milkweed came in 1670, sumach arrived in 1688, and sweet gum in 1690.[27] The introduction of some plants was, in part through the influence of Gerard's herbal updated by Johnson. Excitement at having already received new plants and trees from South America into English gardens had already begun with the nasturtium also known as yellow lark's heels from Peru in 1535, Thuja in the following year and passionflower in 1568.[28] Josselyn's descriptions of the rarities in New England must also have raised interest. Black cohosh and Wintergreen were eighteenth century introductions.[29]

Having followed the fortunes of those brave enough to leave a troubled England for a fresh start and freedom in the unknown New World and appreciated some of their struggles to survive, the reader may understand the value they must have placed on those medicinal remedies and whatever knowledge of physic they took with them. With Boorde, Gerard, and Culpeper as known guides and a growing interchange between native Americans and the settlers on the medicinal uses of native plants new to them, so the foundation of a distinctive American manner of prescribing was laid.

References

1. William Bradford, *Of Plymouth Plantation 1620–1647* (New York: Random House Inc., 1981), 85.
2. Ann Leighton, *Early American Gardens. "For Meate or Medicine"* (Boston Mass: Houghton Mifflin Company, 1970), 49.
3. John Josselyn, *New-Englands RARITIES Discovered* (Bedford: Applewood Books: 1672).
4. Josselyn, *New-Englands RARITIES Discovered*, 105.
5. George Herbert, *The Country Parson* (Norwich: Canterbury Press, 2003), 23.
6. Herbert, *The Country Parson*, 54.
7. Leighton, *Early American Gardens*, 65.
8. Ibid, 190.
9. Robert C. Black III, *The Younger John Winthrop* (New York: Columbia University Press, 1966), 55.
10. Black, *The Younger John Winthrop*, 87–88.
11. Ibid, 169.
12. Ibid, 170.
13. John Parkinson, *Paradisi in Sole, Paradisus Terrestris* (New York: Dover Publications, Inc., 1976), 306.
14. Parkinson, *Paradisi in Sole, Paradisus Terrestris*, 282.
15. Sir Hugh Plat, *Delights for Ladies* (1609) (Crosby Lockwood & Son Ltd., 1955), 35.
16. Leighton, *Early American Gardens*, 131.
17. Josselyn, *New-Englands RARITIES Discovered*, 86.
18. Ibid, 63.
19. Bradford, *Of Plymouth Plantation*, 94.
20. Laurel Thatcher Ulrich, *Good Wives* (New York: Vintage Books, 1991), 126.
21. Laurel Thatcher Ulrich, *A Midwife's Tale* (New York: Vintage Books, 1991), 33
22. Ulrich, *A Midwife's Tale*, 50.
23. Ibid, 354.
24. Ibid, 192.
25. Ibid, 250.
26. Maggie Campbell-Culver, *The Origin of Plants* (London: Headline Book Publishing, 2001), 145.
27. Campbell-Culver, *The Origin of Plants*, 145–146.
28. Ibid, 117–118.
29. Ibid, 180.

SECTION VIII

FAMILY HEALTH AND A STANDARD
FOR HERBS | 1638–1878

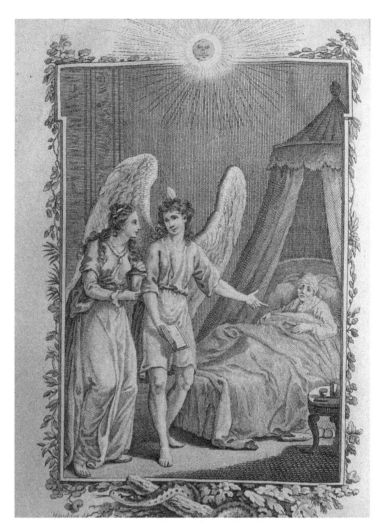

Frontispiece from *The New Family Herbal*, Meyrick.

Key Figures

Sir Francis Bacon (1561–1626), Dr A. F. M. Willich (active 1800), William Withering (1741–1799), William Meyrick (c1770–post 1799), Joseph Miller (died 1748), William Woodville (1752–1805), William Buchan (1729–1805), Elizabeth Blackwell (born c1700), Prof. Phelps Brown (1825–1878).

Key Texts

History Naturall and Experimentall of Life and Death, 1650, Lord Verulam.
Botanicum Officinale, 1722, Miller.

Account of the Foxglove, 1785, Withering.
Gentleman's Magazines, 1753 and 1788, Sylvanus.
Medical Botany, 1790, Woodville.
Domestic Herbal, 1776, Buchan.

Roles of Women in Medicine

Nurse, midwife, herbalist, herb gatherer, botanical artist.

Quality Control

Regular assessment of recipes in the Pharmacopoeia, and conformity of Officinal medicines in apothecary shops to the standard of the College of Physicians. Despite this there was considerable complaint about herb-women who gathered herbs for sale substituting more common herbs when they could not find what the apothecary had ordered.

Herb Energetics

Some are given but without degrees. A herb might be classed as cooling and binding or astringent rather than cold and dry.

Travel and Trade

Spices are increasingly imported from Jamaica and the Caribbean where enslaved people are subjected to harsh conditions working on plantations. Chocolate, tea, and coffee were introduced and were initially very expensive. Plant hunters are travelling the world searching for new exotics, some of which will be adopted as medicines.

Introduction

In the late seventeenth and on into the eighteenth-century Britain still had a largely agricultural-based economy and the industrial revolution with all the evils it brings, is not greatly in evidence until the last quarter of the eighteenth century. The British Empire was growing and men in business were thriving, yet the situation for the workers was often one of dangers from machinery and polluted air at work with long hours and little to eat. Child labour was common and living conditions poor. Child mortality was high and a large figure for deaths aged between twenty and thirty due more to endemic tuberculosis and epidemics, particularly plague in 1666, kept the average lifespan at forty, although many lived to a ripe old age. The late 1700s saw many centenarians if the mortality bills in Gentleman's Magazines are anything to go by. Looking carefully, it becomes apparent that many of these long-lived people were poor and living not as the rich on extraordinarily sweet and fatty food, but often mostly on simple bread and what we would term cottage cheese.

The construction of a growing network of canals in the second half of the eighteenth century made transport easier and provided faster supply of raw materials and distribution for the increased output of goods aided by new machinery in manufacturing centres. Cottage industries are beginning to dwindle in importance. Herbs are less used by physicians as the century passes and the increased enthusiasm for powerful drugs will add to the decline in general health during the next century.

CHAPTER 20

A New Regimen for Health
and Longevity | 1638–1878

Mortality Bill for London 1746–1747. *Gentleman's Magazine*. Sylvanus.

In the early chapters we explored the philosophy of Hippocrates on supporting the body in order to maintain health, as well as in assisting the natural processes of overcoming disease. In the first century AD the extension of these theories in the work and writings of Galen ensured their persistence for many centuries. After the Anglo-Saxon period when the light of Greek philosophy was dimmed by other influences, the regimen of health re-appeared from the teaching centre of Salerno. Arabic works, in particular the *Canon of Avicenna*, gave a detailed study of Galen's humoral medicine and how to apply it. For the lay person the *Tacuinem Sanitatis* was the ultimate guide to health, translated into English by Sir John Harington in the reign of Elizabeth I. We explored this set of instructions on identifying humoral temperaments and ways in which to recognise and treat humoral imbalances in daily life in chapter twelve. It includes dietary advice, the effects of weather conditions and those of emotional states on health.

In the last chapter we saw that these instructions were still being followed, having travelled to New England, despite the best efforts of Paracelsus who burned Avicenna's work publicly. Nevertheless, Paracelsus did have a strong influence on the development of pharmacy and specific treatments and we find science and scientists keen to make progress in many fields in the eighteenth century and onwards.

Sir Francis Bacon, known also as Baron Verulam (1561–1626) was a highly intelligent philosopher and scientist. Also a lawyer and politician, he was unsuccessful during Elizabeth's reign and after speaking in Parliament against proposals for a subsidy, was banned from Elizabeth's Court. The reign of James I opened new opportunities for him as he supported the view that the royal prerogative should be more important than the workings of Parliament. He also supported union of England with Scotland, a project dear to James. In 1618 he was appointed Lord Chancellor and lived in style. It was unfortunate that he had never been good at managing his money, to the extent of being briefly imprisoned for debt early in his career. This may have led to his downfall as he was impeached in 1621 for accepting bribes while drafting patents for monopolies.

Fined £40,000, Bacon retired from Court and spent the last five years of his life writing. He had already written his Novum Organum in the previous year setting out a plan to reorganise scientific method.[1] He criticised science as following old learning and he seemed to be particularly offended by the thinking of Aristotle. Bacon proposed that science should both follow nature and be founded on experiment. He therefore looked at the physical properties of all manner of natural phenomena, from that concerning inanimate objects to plants, insects, animals, and man. It was not surprising then that when it came to addressing the subject of longevity, he followed this method using deep questioning on causes and comparisons and experiment to reveal effects.

Francis Bacon's *History Naturall and Experimentall, of Life and Death* first printed in 1638, had reached its sixth edition by 1651 and this is bound together with his fascinating exploration of Natural History and ideas for a college for interpreting nature, *New Atlantis. A Worke unfinished*. This is a favourite volume in my library as it reveals so much of the thought processes of his time. The breadth and depth of Bacon's constant careful questioning and observation is inspirational in our world of microscopic perspectives that ignore the context of the whole.

Interest in long life was high in the seventeenth and eighteenth centuries and Britain became one of the select countries known abroad as fostering longevity. Once the Bible became available in English, more notice was taken of the incredible ages of men listed in the Old Testament. The question was asked why people now lived such a comparatively short time and what might be done to regain this ability. Bacon looked at the subject dispassionately. He was no physician and felt that curing disease was a sordid affair and some physicians should take a nobler stance to concentrate more on prolonging and renewing life.[2]

Bacon suggests that prolonging life can be done safely and conveniently, with the aim of travelling through this world with our bodies little worn or impaired. As a herbal practitioner, I have seen many elderly patients and as a result of helping them, researched and written two courses on ageing successfully. I was, then, particularly interested to read of his three intentions, namely examining how to stop wasting of the body, how it is repaired, and how to renew oldness. Supporting digestion in obtaining nourishment, moisturising hardened tissues, and cleansing the system of old matter are aims I can relate to.

In studying natural history, Bacon had already made many observations on longevity of animals relating to how long they take to reach maturity, including the effects of hibernation.[3] He had also experimented with imaginative preservation of life, immersing clove gillyflowers in quicksilver.[4] His symbolism in observing that trees are long-lived by virtue of their loss of leaves in winter and provision of new leaves each spring speaks vibrantly of renewal. When Bacon turns to considering all manner of the circumstances of human birth and growth, he first references the Biblical ages in the Old Testament in order to engage his readers. He carefully lists observations on long-lived people in history and then reviews ideas on rejuvenation. Some from the alchemical works of Paracelsus such as medicines made of gold, or balsams made from serpents or eagles, he dismisses as fabulous and superstitious vanities.[5]

Of lifestyles, Bacon selects a monastic life as offering leisure for contemplation of heavenly things, austere diet and humbling penances to be helpful to long life. A thorough investigation of every possible factor, from heredity to climate appears in the pages, with the usual regimen for health presented critically. Consideration is given to whether when age has weakened digestion extra nourishment might be given through the skin in baths or into the bowel with nourishing clysters, (fluids injected up into the bowel).[6] All of this is investigated before suggesting medicines. At the time gold, amber-grise and the bezoar stone from a goat were recommended. Bacon supported the last two and then favoured simple cordials. these he divided into hot—saffron, *folium indicum*, *lignum aloes*, citron peel or rind, balm, basil, clove, gillyflowers, orange flowers, rosemary, mint, betony, *Carduus benedictus*—and cold—nitre, roses, violets, strawberry-leaves, strawberries, juice of sweet lemons, juice of sweet oranges, juice of pearmains, borage, bugloss, burnet, sanders, camphor.[7]

The instructions include the caveat that some things helpful to long life are not without peril. He therefore offers sundry remedies for everyone to make their own choice to suit their age and temperament. The intentions of these are to renew vigour of the spirits, and he lists ten operations to this end, including on the blood, juices of the body, bowel action, aliment (nutrition), purging of old juice, and supply of new.

He writes, "in every Consumption, whether it be by Fire, or by Age, the more the *Spirit* of the Body, or the Heat, preyeth upon the Moisture, the lesser is the duration of that Thing. This occurres every where and is manifest".[8] After more discussion on kinds of heat and the objectives with the spirit, we read, "Whatsoever is given with good successe, in the curing of *Pestilentiall* and *Malignant Diseases*; to stop and bridle the *Spirits, ...* may very happily be transferred to prolongation of life: For one thing is effectuall unto both; namely the *condensation* of the *Spirits*: Now there is nothing better for that than *Opiates*".[9] Here he is agreeing with Paracelsus, who also suggested opiates.

Bacon makes an interesting comment on some melancholic humours made in the body being like opiates and sees them as a sign of long life. There follows the recommendation—"Let there be therefore, every year, from Adult years of youth, an *Opiate* diet; let it be taken about the end of *May*; because the Spirits in the Summer, are more loose, and attenuated; and there is lesse danger from cold humours; .... This medicine to be taken onely each other day, and to be continued for a Fortnight: this Designation in our judgement, comes home to the intention".[10]

A "*Suffumigation of Tobacco, Lignum Aloes, Rosemary-leaves* dried, and a little *Myrrhe,* snuffed up in the morning, at the Mouth and Nostrils, would be very good" is one of his prescriptions.[11] Waters are, in his opinion, a better form than Grand Opiates such as Mithridate, and he lists safer medicines, principally saffron, since opiates are to be taken very sparingly, and at certain times, he gives more herbs for daily diet to prolong life.[12] The robust heat of elecampane, garlic, *Carduus benedictus*, young watercresses, germander, angelica, zedoary, vervain, valerian, myrrh, pepper-wort, elderflowers, and garden chervil is to be preferred to spices, wine, and strong drinks, together with savory, wild marjoram, and pennyroyal, for their heat is predatory.[13] Diet should not be too rigorous, but constant and sparing, water to drink, a hard bed and moderate sleep, venery, and exercise. He is of the opinion that either great joy or great fear will shorten life, while envy is the worst passion as it feeds on the spirit which in turn feeds on the body. Hope is seen as the most beneficial of the affections.

A great deal of more detailed advice follows and forms a basic exploration on which others were to build. Two famous allegedly supercentenarians, Thomas Parr, from Shropshire, buried in Westminster Abbey in 1635, in honour of his supposed age of 152 years, and Henry Jenkins who died at the reputed age of 169 in 1670, brought fame to England as news of their stories spread in Europe. In the case of Henry Jenkins, Dr Tancred Robinson in an account sent to the Royal Society recorded that four or five men of Ellerton, all close to 100 years old themselves vouched that he had been elderly ever since they had known him.[14]

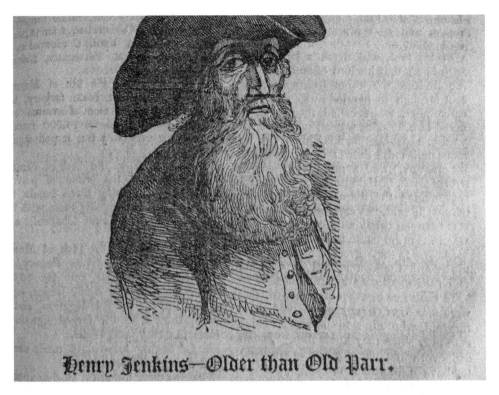

Henry Jenkins, *The Every-Day Book*, Hone.

Francis Bacon gives us a picture of rural England very unlike the common modern understanding of the time; "I suppose there is scarce a *Village*, with us in *England*, if it be any whit populous, but it affords some Man or Woman of fourscore yeares of age: Nay, a few yeares since, there was in the County of *Hereford*, a Maygame, or Morris-Dance, consisting of Eight Men, whose Age computed together, made up eight hundred years; Insomuch, that what some of them wanted of an hundred, others exceeded as much."[15]

In the eighteenth century, Swiss anatomist and botanist, Albrecht von Haller, who was familiar with the story of Henry Jenkins, wrote that England seemed to exceed all other nations in the number of those who lived to an advanced age. To gain a sense of whether that statement was correct, we can find hard data in the copies of The Gentleman's Magazines for the eighteenth century. These contain many interesting obituaries.

On February 24th 1753 widow Coxson died in Derbyshire aged 117, leaving a total of 173 children, grandchildren, and great grandchildren. The two previous entries were aged 113 and 101 respectively and the first in the March list, died in Bordeaux aged 108, having suckled 22 children. Her father had lived to 101 and her mother to 104 years.[16]

In 1788 Daniel Prim of Whitechapel died at the age of 103. The obituary records he was bound apprentice to a weaver in London in the reign of King William and he followed that business till he reached his ninetieth year.[17] There are many more and the regular Bills of Mortality for London, which was not the healthiest place to live, often record someone dying at over 100 years. In 1738 when 9,600 infants died under two years of age, there were 101 deaths aged between 90–100, then two aged 100, four aged 102, two aged 103, one at 105 and one person aged 111.[18]

It can be seen that the life expectancy of that period at forty years, rising to forty-five years by the end of the century, has been greatly reduced by infant mortality and high death rates between the ages of twenty and sixty. . Persistent major killers included convulsions, with the highest figure of 7,524 out of 25,825 deaths in London in 1738.[19] Endemic consumption and outbreaks of smallpox took their toll.

Dr Anthony Willich, born in what is now Poland, was living in London in 1800 when his *Lectures on Diet and Regimen* for the use of families was sufficiently popular to run to a third edition. He appears to have been well known at the time, although little of his life is known today beyond his popularity. He valued the opinions of both German and English physicians, crediting the work of William Cullen M.D. in Scotland and Hahnemann.[20] He was a man who says what he means and is not shy to discuss the attitude of a society in which everyone now claims to be their own personal physician. He comments bluntly that while people distrust physicians, judging them to have self-interest or professional motives, in avoiding them they so frequently prescribe for themselves as to be unable to tell whether they are healthy or diseased.[21]

This state of affairs, so damaging to the health of the patient, he traces to the differing opinions of the various medical schools as to the causes of disease. In the meanwhile, he observes that as luxury increases in a nation so does the number and variety of diseases. His lectures, published for the benefit of the eager public, explore every aspect of preserving health and prolonging life. Dr Willich was an enthusiast when it came to the six Galenical non-naturals and he adds scientific detail where he can and on the effects of air and weather on the patient, which readers will recall from Galen, he gives a concise history of oxygen. Writing of consumption under his topic Air and Weather, he states, "consumption cuts off about 80,000 persons every year, in Great Britain alone, and these generally in the prime of life".[22] He also went to the London Bills of Mortality for his information, quoting the average of deaths from three years, 1796, 1797 and 1799 he writes, "we shall find that this uncontrollable disorder destroys annually 5,853 out of 17,412 individuals, or upwards of ONE THIRD of the inhabitants of London".[23]

He considers the properties of many foods, including coffee and sugar, approving of both when taken sensibly. Of spices he views cubebs, cardamoms, vanilla, and cloves as hot and pungent and so improper for daily use. Ginger he regards as one of the most wholesome spices, but, in his opinion "The indigenous, spicy, and balsamic herbs, such as *parsley, marjoram, thyme, sage,* and the like, cannot be too much recommended for culinary use, especially in broths; ... Among all the native spices, there is none, in my opinion, which excels, in medicinal virtues, the common *Caraway*".[24]

On sleep he agrees with the famed Dr Mead and gives an ideal of six hours in twenty-four. Assessing both active and passive exercise, Willich recommends passive exercise such as swinging or sailing for infants, asthmatic cases, and the old and emaciated. He regards speaking as a most necessary and healthful exercise, especially for females since they are more confined at home, although not to excess.[25] So detail continues regarding the familiar classifications of sleep and wakefulness, evacuations which include semen and forthright statements about sexual activity, and passions of the mind. He has strong views on the dangers from disappointed love, jealousy, fear, and anger. These last taking us back to the *Tacuinem Sanitatis*. The wisdom of the ages is all there.

Willich seeks to bring the humoral system up to date, referring to the doctrine of four temperaments, he adds another four. These are listed as varieties of the sanguine and phlegmatic, being: the sanguine-choleric; the hypochondriacal; the rustic, which combines the sanguine qualities with the phlegmatic; and the gentle temperament, which combines the sanguine, choleric, and phlegmatic.[26] One of his eight conditions required for the attainment of long life is a hereditary disposition to longevity.[27]

Examples of this were seen in reports in the Gentleman's Magazines:

In 1753, the obituary of Margaret Plantinet, at Bourdaux in France, aged 108, she suckled twenty-two children herself, her father lived to 101, and her mother to 104.[28] In August 1761 John Newell Esq; at Michaelstown, Ireland, aged 127, was the grandson of Thomas Parr, reputed to have lived to 152.[29]

Willich refers to the "illustrious Lord Bacon" repeating his assertion that since man takes twenty to twenty-five years to reach maturity, following the pattern observed with animals he should also live to be eight times that number, which is 200 years.[30] They agreed on many points, only differing on the use of opiates.

We find the search for a recipe for longevity reaching similar conclusions in 1878 when Professor O Phelps Brown, arrived in London from America. His personal approach to herbal medicine is revealed as he states, "In our present artificial state of society, it is not probable that one in a thousand persons dies a natural death".[31] Having discussed how numerous the examples of extreme longevity are in history, he also quotes Haller who collected the cases of more than a thousand supercentenarians, aged from one hundred to one hundred and seventy in Europe in the eighteenth century. The Professor recommends a plain, simple diet and to refrain from excesses of all kinds, physical or mental. In order to assist nature, he advertises his "renovating pills" to be taken alongside the diet and hygiene indicated. Hygeine refers to air, light, drink, food, temperature, exercise, clothing, sleep, bathing, exertions, and control of passions. Best of all he says, is a "cheerful, equitable temper of mind".[32]

Jeanne Calment remains the oldest person whose age has been verified. She lived to be 122 years 164 days, dying in 1997. According to the site for the Guinness book of records she gave as her lifestyle, olive oil in her diet as well as rubbed on her skin, a modest taste for wine and love of chocolate. She also smoked cigarettes. Jeanne took up fencing at the age of eighty-five and still cycled at age 100.[33]

Do the supercentenarians have genes that protect them from hazards that would prove fatal to a weaker person? It is an interesting question. Science has come a long way and researchers are now looking into the different rates at which people age at a cellular level. Telomeres, repeating segments of non-coding DNA on the ends of our chromosomes shorten when the cell divides and help to determine how fast we age. The good and formerly unexpected news is that in some circumstances they can also lengthen, slowing degeneration. The way we live, eat, exercise, and think positively or negatively, can cause changes for better or worse.[34] The idea that there might one day be an elixir of life to affect this process safely is surely worthy of Paracelsus, but there are too many other factors for this to be a simple answer.

References

1. C.P. Hill, *Who's Who in History*, Vol. III, 1603–1714 (Oxford: Basil Blackwell, 1965), 23–26.
2. Francis Lord Verulam, Vis-Count Saint Alban. *History Naturall and Experimentall, of Life and Death or Of the Prolongation of Life* (London: William Lee and Humphrey Moseley, 1650), Preface.
3. Verulam, *History Naturall and Experimentall*, Century IX, 194.
4. Ibid, Century VIII, 168.
5. Ibid, The History of life and Death, 26.
6. Ibid, 14.
7. Ibid, 25.
8. Ibid, 28.
9. Ibid, 29.
10. Ibid, 29.
11. Ibid, 30.
12. Ibid, 30.
13. Ibid, 32.
14. D.B. Haycock, *Mortal Coil. A Short History of Living Longer* (London: Yale University Press, 2008), 16.
15. Verulam, *The History of life and Death*, 20.
16. Urban Sylvanus, *The Gentleman's Magazine, and Historical Chronicle* (London: Edward Cave, 1753), 148.
17. Sylvanus, *The Gentleman's Magazine*, 1788, 179.
18. Sylvanus, *The Gentleman's Magazine*, 1738, 662.
19. Ibid, 662.
20. A. F. M. Willich, *Lectures on Diet and Regimen* (London: Longman and Rees, 1800), a2.
21. Willich, *Lectures on Diet and Regimen*, 26–27.

22. Ibid, 219.
23. Ibid, 219.
24. Ibid, 432.
25. Ibid, 459.
26. Ibid, 45–47.
27. Ibid, 161.
28. Sylvanus, *The Gentleman's Magazine*, 1753, 148.
29. Sylvanus, *The Gentleman's Magazine*, 1761, 382.
30. Willich, *Lectures on Diet and Regimen*, 162–163.
31. Prof. O. Phelps Brown, *The Complete Herbalist* (London: Published by the author, 1878), 194.
32. Phelps Brown, *The Complete Herbalist*, 199.
33. "Oldest Woman Ever." Guinness World Records. Accessed July 31, 2023. https://www.guinnessworldrecords.com/world-records/oldest-person.
34. E. Blackburn and London E. Epel, *The Telomere Effect* (London: Orion Spring, 2018), 7.

CHAPTER 21

Home Medicine and Aromatic Waters | 1694–1776

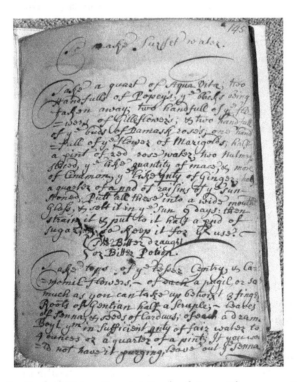

To Make Surfet Water. Receipt Book of Anne Blencowe, 1694.
Courtesy of William Sitwell.

In Chapter eighteen, we looked at the sources of information available to ladies for distilling and making home medicines, beginning in the sixteenth century and ending our review in the first quarter of the seventeenth. Through later works and analysis I have carried out on recipes from the whole period of distilling in the home we can put together a broader view of recipes adopted by lay persons and those in the editions of the Pharmacopoeia. The results may be enlightening regarding differences of opinion on efficacy between the two and we can trace the most successful herbs for this form of administration as far as today.

The seventeenth century sees the waters included as an important part of mainstream medicine where their actions are praised when made well. Culpeper, ever critical, looks upon them as artificial medicines.[1] He recommends distilling in sand, which he believes results in waters twice as strong and gives details of the effects and appropriate uses of many simple waters of individual herbs. The 'compound and sprituous waters' he regards as heating and warns against use in health and youth but writes that they are more beneficial in summer, "because in summer the body is always coldest within, and digestion weakest, and that is the reason why men and women eat less in Summer than in Winter".[2]

As the name suggests, most Aqua in the Pharmacopoeia are of herbs distilled in water. However, it was common practice for the ladies distilling herbs to use white wine or ale as a base liquor. Very occasionally a sherry, sack, or brandy was used. Tinctures are rare in household recipes and are found used for gums and resins, such as myrrh and frankincense or tree balsams.[3] Specific recipes with a milk base are generally to treat the lungs, mostly consumption. They also either contain parts of snails or a mucilaginous herb. Where there is no marshmallow, snails, or houseleek, Carduus appears to be a common factor. Generally, the amount of liquid added was twice the weight of other ingredients.

Herbs and spices were macerated in the liquid for anywhere from a few hours to several days before distillation. The spices of nutmeg and to a lesser extent, cardamom, cloves, ginger, and mace, were popular ingredients. The herbal spice that appears in the most recipes reviewed between 1393 and 1892 is cinnamon appearing in forty-nine of several hundred. Cinnamon water is still made for herbal dispensaries today. While thirty-eight contain nutmeg, these favourites are followed by slightly lower figures in descending order with rosemary, mints, lemon balm, aniseed, then angelica, rose, sage, fennel, betony, rue, and lavender.

It will be noted that the most popular herbs and spices above, with the exception of betony, are rich in volatile oils which are well extracted via distillation. Others, such as plantain and endive, appear to have little to offer; however, plantain water has filled a role of softening the effects of potentially damaging medicines and plantain hydrosols are popular today. A hydrosol is a by-product of steam distillation producing essential oil. An aromatic water is distilled for the water which contains a small amount of the essential oil. We should not imagine the housewife entirely made up her own complex remedies with the waters, as she did with other commonly made medicinal recipes. In the printed recipe books, we find some recipes given authority by having the name of a famous person in the title, as with the Queen of Hungary's Water, and Dr Steven's Water. This last was made with great consistency of the many ingredients, between 1560 and 1736. Others with great popularity in recipe books are Aqua Mirabilis, Aqua Imperialis, Plague and Epidemick waters and Cephalic waters for the head, nerves and to treat palsy. The last was most often applied to the skin where the pulse is close to the surface. Waters were also added to hand-baths as well as taken internally.

The requirement for plague and epidemic waters was high as the Great Plague of 1666 was still in living memory at the beginning of this period. A second scourge was smallpox, which if it did not kill could lead to horrible disfigurement. Recipes entitled for plague, poxe, measles, and fevers are records of the main fears. If we look at a number of household books, it becomes evident that of the herbs we have been following, with the exception of nettle, these are much used in the compound waters. Betony and liquorice appear in the highest number. Betony predictably appears in palsy water which covers conditions involving the head and nerves, also vertigo water, a water to strengthen eyesight, one for convulsions, and cordial waters that generally treat many conditions, including infectious diseases. Liquorice also follows main uses in other types of preparation appearing in surfeit waters for over indulgence, snail water for the chest and lungs, pleurisy water and cordial water.

Elecampane is a strong antibacterial and is found in epidemic and plague waters and cordial waters that also cover treating infectious diseases. It is present in five recipes. Ginger is included in surfeit waters, stitch water, two cordial waters, one version of Aqua Mirabilis, and Dr Steven's water. Plantain appears in milk water for cancer and the King's Evil or scrofula (tubercular abscesses of the cervical lymph glands), snail water which is again made with milk, and a cordial. Plantain water is recommended with rose water for after-pains from childbirth and in a recipe for drying old sores.

The earliest book of recipes in my analysis covering household books from 1694 to 1750 was that of Anne, Lady Blencowe. She was born in 1656, daughter of mathematician and cryptographer John Wallis, who is mentioned in the diaries of both Samuel Pepys and John Evelyn. Professor of geometry at Oxford, Wallis could provide well for his family and the education of his son and daughters. The portrait of Anne as a young attractive woman shows her as a self-assured lady of consequence shortly to be married to John Blencowe who had inherited a large, beautiful house near Banbury, in the previous year. Their first son was born a year later in 1676 followed by six more children, the last born in 1688. John Blencowe was knighted and became a judge and member of parliament.[4] Anne would frequently have entertained guests as her elegant cookery recipes show.

Her father's influence may be evident in her choice of physic remedies in that she clearly favoured the newer chemical medicine. He was a member of the Royal

Society, along with men of science such as the chemist Robert Boyle. As in other household books, she included one or two recipes bearing the names of physicians, Dr Mead and Dr Nintle, and gathered several more from family or visiting guests, adding their names. She is interested in remedies for dropsy and asthma, and more surprisingly for treating scrofula. In this recipe the sieved ashes from burning sponge are given in milk. The patient is also to drink sanicle tea.[5] Sanicle is a wild herb found in shady situations that was popular in Anglo-Saxon and medieval times for healing wounds, often used alongside bugle or yarrow. It is suited to cleansing ulcers. The sponge would have contained iodine, probably not as helpful for scrofula but it is necessary for an active thyroid. There are a number for nervous conditions and several mention suitability for children. With the great plague in her childhood, it is not surprising that she gives the most careful attention to writing out the following recipe—"Cordiall Water: good against any infections as ye Plague, Poxe, Measles, burning feaver, & to remove any offensive or venemouse Matter from ye Hart or Stomach, or to be used after surfetts or in Passion of ye Mother, or for Children in fits or Convulsions, & is generally good to comfort or strengthen Nature".[6]

The list of ingredients that follows contains eleven herbs, and six roots. All are washed and dried, the roots scraped and shredded before putting them into a gallon of white wine in a glazed earthen gally pot, covered and stirred daily for two days. The detailed instructions on distilling not in an Alembic but in an ordinary still, applying a paste of rye meal, vinegar, whites of egg, and medicinal earth to close the still, before heating using a soft fire, are exemplary and rarely found for all stages of the preparation. She then gives further instructions for suitable doses and recipients for each run from the still with the most powerful first run for man or woman, even if the woman is pregnant, and the third for young children. Then, "This water to comfort is usually given luckwarm with a little sugar or sugar candy, & may be given also cold; and is most properly given when ye stomack is empty. And also it may very fittly be mix'd with any Julip where there is any infection fear'd ...." It looks as if she is familiar with Culpeper's warning on heat as she continues, "but neither this nor any other hott waters should be used ordinaryly, but where ye party hath need of such helps".[7]

The recipe tells us of the respect and confidence Anne has for this water. Her source was evidently an official one for we find in Pechey's Herbal of 1694 a recipe with the same roots and differing in only three herbs which perhaps she was unable to supply. Above is written, "The following Water was much us'd in the last *London*-Plague".[8] John Pechey recommends his work as having little curious, but most practical content. It is in fact a very useful herbal as he divides the book into a first part of herbs growing in England and a second of foreign plants. He has added an explanatory table for the lay reader and the admonition that constitutions and diseases being various, it is better to have the advice of a physician on treatments.

Stills might be made of various materials, we know of the cheaper earthen ones for a poorer household. Pewter alembics and copper or brass, even lead stills are referred to, as well as glass stills for use with roses.[9] Of conditions treated by the waters, overall, the greatest number concerned the stomach, oppression of spirits, consumption, the head, and fevers. All except those for consumption, which were largely milk waters contain predictable herbs for the expressed intention and on that basis, might be effective for that condition. In 1754, Hill wrote of milk water that it is good in fevers and to make juleps with syrup and aromatic water combined, but making recipes with milk serves no purpose.[10] However, modern herbal medicine has not investigated milk waters and we have no real understanding of them.

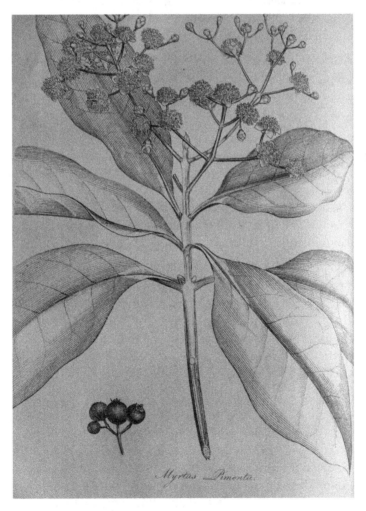

Pimento, *Medical Botany*, Woodville.

Among the 650 plus general recipes I have reviewed for the late seventeenth and eighteenth centuries many conditions are treated. They include chronic conditions, such as asthma, dropsy, rheumatism and gout; children's ailments, such as rickets, worms, whooping cough, colds and various fevers; and the results of accidents with burns and wounds. Different books have different emphasis according to the household needs. *A Collection of Receipts* published in 1746 shows the largest number are for two of our chosen conditions with eighteen mentions for coughs, and thirteen for fevers. Conditions appearing almost as often are consumptions, the stone, and convulsions. Consumption refers to a wasting disease and references may not always refer to wasting from tuberculosis of the lungs. Conditions causing wasting were also referred to as consumptions, Buchan gives a definition in his *Domestic Physician* of "a wasting or decay of the whole body from an ulcer, tubercles, or concretions of the lungs, an empyema, a nervous atrophy, or a cachexy".[11]

Cough Remedies—In these we find the long familiar hyssop, horehound, elecampane, liquorice, aniseed, fennel, and coltsfoot. Also in Smith, balsam of Tolu from Mexico and the Amazonian forest appears.[12] Squills are increasing in popularity for the chest.

Fevers—Jesuit's bark is used for fevers of various kinds.[13] Virginia snakeroot also has established use in numerous recipes. Others sound like an apothecary's dream—Mr. Gaskin's cordial powder for agues in *A Book of Simples* consists of seed pearls, red coral, hartshorn (the actual horn from a hart), white amber, the tips of crab's claws, saffron, dragon's water and crab's eyes (chalky excrescences on the heads of crayfish).[14] This appears in other works as Gascoigne's powder, and is full of expensive ingredients.

Eye Remedies—These abound, as across the centuries, many with the familiar herbs still of rue, betony, rosemary, celandine, eyebright, vervain, and rose water. Rose water also accompanies white copperas, tutty, and camphor.[15] Tutty was collected on rods of iron in furnaces where brass was being made. It is described as a recrement of mixed metals containing zinc or zinc ore.[16] The aims of the recipes cover from strengthening sight and preventing cataracts to treating them and curing other difficulties, such as broken veins, pin and web, and rheum, with gooey, runny eyes.

Boils—Seem to have receded from the list of needs as these books are for the higher level in society, where requirements are more likely to be for treatments for liver, spleen, stones, and gout if the recipes are anything to go by. Having access to plenty of rich food is not always an advantage. Joint pains, aches, and sciatica have inspired a number of ointments, probably the most effective would be of sage, rue, wormwood, and bay in sheep's suet and salad oil.[17] It was typical to use wormwood and rue externally for pain.

Burns—Treatments often contain olive oil or cream, Eliza Smith recommends an ointment containing red dock leaves, mallow leaves, houseleek, and the inner rind of elder boiled in cream with white lead added.[18] Other herbs might be rose, St John's wort, and comfrey, alternatively, white lead and camphor.

Toothache—Remedies are joined by more to clean, whiten, or preserve the teeth. Serious toothache is addressed using camphor, opium, and oil of clove made into pills to insert into the tooth. For rheum in the teeth, pills are formed of mastic, aloes, and agaric with syrup of betony.[19] Celandine juice is used to whiten teeth, or cream of tartar with myrrh, a mix we have made in workshops.

Headache—*The Book of Simples* (1700–1750) has nothing relating to headache alone, only a remedy for migraine. Anne Blencowe prescribes a laxative, diuretic wine also containing Jesuits bark.[20] Vertigo water is taken in Smith's collection. It could be that the cordial waters were generally taken to treat headaches from some of the many possible causes, certainly when they were nerve related.

In botany, the adoption of Linnaeus' binomial system of naming plants, with the second name "officinalis" to distinguish species used in medicine; aided correct identification of the herbs for use in Waters. Meanwhile in 1722, Miller's *Compendious Herbal*, or *Botanicum Officinale* described the herbs in fine botanic detail along with their uses. In his dedication to Sir Hans Sloane, he states the reason for the garden and his Botanicum for the correct identification of herbs is supported by "my own Observation of the gross Impositions frequently practised by the common Herb-folks upon their unskilful Customers, who for want of a competent Knowledge in Botany, are obliged to rely upon these People for their Dispensation of Herbs; and they make no Scruple of setting one thing for another, which may be attended with as bad Consequences, as the substituting any different Simple in the animal or mineral Kingdom".[21]

This same problem could have affected Anne Blencowe via her apothecary from whom she was obliged to buy many ingredients for the recipes in her collection. In the eighteenth century distilled simple and compound waters continued to be made by apothecaries, distillers, and private physicians as well as ladies of quality. The waters were available for rich and poor in hospitals and were used by the army, as we learn from Lewis in the appendix to his Dispensatory, *Pharmacopœia Pauperum*.[22] In the *Collection of Receipts* published in 1746, there are many good recipes, a number of which I have made and two are of particular historical interest: "Fryers Balsam",[23] a throat remedy familiar to me in childhood, although made differently by then; and "A Preservative against the Pestilence",[24] which is the famous four thieves vinegar. This early version was apparently sourced from a physician in the Duke of Berwick's Army in 1721.

In this last collection and the private household *Book of Simples* from the same period, waters make up one third of the total medicinal recipes. At this point they were clearly believed to be a necessary part of every medicine store. This is confirmed in 1754 by Hill in his herbal writing for ladies to equip them to care for their families and neighbours using readily gathered herbs, he states, "Few families are without an alembic or still, and that will be of material service. With that instrument the simple waters are to be made ... " he goes on to list those waters it will be "proper to keep".[25]

The active spirit of scientific enquiry led to an extension of knowledge in phytochemistry, which resulted in questioning whether the water coming over in the distillation actually contained active constituents from the plant. In the 1736 edition of Quincy's English Dispensatory, it is written that the number of simple waters has been greatly reduced by the College as they have now rejected all those herbs judged useless for that purpose.[26] Lewis writes in his Dispensatory twenty years later of the general complaint, that the cordials of the apothecary are less agreeable than those of the same kind prepared by the distiller. He explains this is due to the ill taste of the proof spirit base which distillers are more careful to avoid.[27]

When we come to William Buchan's influential *Domestic Medicine* in 1776, the physician includes a limited list to be made in the home, commenting that management of a still is so generally understood there is no need to give directions. His choices are to distil the simple waters of cinnamon, pennyroyal, peppermint, spearmint, rose, and Jamaica pepper. He adds two spirituous waters distilled in proof spirit, cinnamon, and Jamaica pepper.[28]

Judging by the household books many ladies seemed confident in treating serious conditions with their waters. The recipes show there would be finer flavour and keeping qualities from their base liquors compared to those of the apothecary. They also enhanced flavour infusing rosemary flowers and little bags of saffron to ensure it. Where the apothecary would use dried herbs, their guidance includes gathering and bruising each herb as it comes to perfection and mixing them with baysalt to store carefully in a well glazed earthen pot until all the ingredients can be brought together.[29] Gentlewomen continued to make simple and compound waters in their stillrooms year on year as the world changed around them with the coming of the industrial revolution.

Although many officinal waters were discontinued in the light of science, there was only one that was removed due to safety concerns. In 1753 Lewis noted the widespread use of black-cherry water for treating convulsions in children. He then observes that lately the resemblance in the taste of the kernels to the leaves of the "lauro-cerasus, which have some time past been discovered to yield, by infusion or distillation, the most sudden poison known".[30] This had prompted an animal trial with a very strong black-cherry water by a group of physicians. The Committee of the London College of Physicians repeated the trial with the same fatal result. As Lewis comments, this does not show that black-cherry water at its normal strength is poisonous to humans, but it did question its use with young children. The London College removed it from the Pharmacopoeia.

There was yet a Water to be added and pimento or Jamaica pepper, as it is also known, was to become a favourite, both the simple and the spirituous water of Jamaica pepper appear in the Pharmacopoeia of 1791, a re-print of the 1778 Pharmacopoeia.[31] This new water was especially popular with hospital staff as it could be used in place of the dearer spices it resembled. By the end of the century, it is also replacing the famed, dearer, and more elaborate Aqua Mirabilis in official medicine. Although we can still follow many waters through into the second half of this century, in the last quarter attitudes are changing fast. The attraction of the new "chemical drugs" is drawing the rich to look to the polished home medicine chest with its cut-glass containers.

References

1. Nicholas Culpeper, *Culpeper's Complete Herbal* (London: Richard Evans, 1815 edition), 203.
2. Culpeper, *Culpeper's Complete Herbal*, 283.
3. Eliza Smith, *The Compleat Housewife* (London: J. and J. Pemberton, 1739), 276.
4. J.W. Blencowe (ed.), *The Blencowe Families* (The Blencowe Families' Association, 2001), 38, 67.
5. Christina Stapley, *The Receipt Book of Lady Anne Blencowe* (Basingstoke: Heartsease Books, 2004), 130.
6. Stapley, *The Receipt Book of Lady Anne Blencowe*, 115.
7. Ibid, 116.
8. John Pechey, *The English Herbal of Physical Plants* (London: Printed for H. Bonwicke, 1694), 33.
9. Sir Hugh Plat, *Delights for Ladies* (1609) (London: Crosby Lockwood, 1948), 65.
10. John Hill, *The Family Herbal* (London: C. Brightly and T. Kinnersley, 1754), XXIII.
11. William Buchan, *Domestic Medicine* (London: W. Strahan, T. Cadell, J. Balfour & W. Creech, 1776), 187.
12. Smith, *The Compleat Housewife*, 334.
13. Ibid, 261.
14. H.W. Lewer, (ed.), *A Book of Simples* (1700–1750) (London: Sampson Low, Marston & Co. Ltd., 1908), (295) 103.
15. Lewer, *A Book of Simples*, (505) 182.
16. John Hill, *A History of the Materia Medica* (London: Longman, Hitch and Hawes, 1751), 87.
17. Lewer, *A Book of Simples*, (184) 69.
18. Smith, *The Compleat Housewife*, 304.
19. Ibid, 325.
20. Stapley, *The Receipt Book of Lady Anne Blencowe*, 127.
21. Joseph Miller, *Botanicum officinale* (London: Bell, 1722), Preface.
22. William Lewis, *The English Dispensatory Improved* (London: J. Nourse, 1753), 546–47.
23. Anon, *A Collection of Receipts*, 105.
24. Ibid, 182.
25. Hill, *The Family Herbal*, XXII.
26. John Quincy, *A Complete Dispensatory*, 10th edition (London: Thomas Longman, 1736), 362.

27. Lewis, *The English Dispensatory Improved*, 371.
28. William Buchan, *Domestic Medicine* (London: W. Strahan, T. Cadell and J. Balfour, 1776), 751–2.
29. H. W. Lewer, (ed.), *A Book of Simples* (1700–1750) (London: Sampson Low, Marston & Co. Ltd., 1908), (145) 58.
30. Lewis, *The English Dispensatory Improved*, 365–366.
31. Thomas Healde (trans.), *The Pharmacopoeia of the Royal College of Physicians of London* (London: Longman, 1791), 325.

CHAPTER 22

Meyrick and Withering—A New Approach
1721–1790

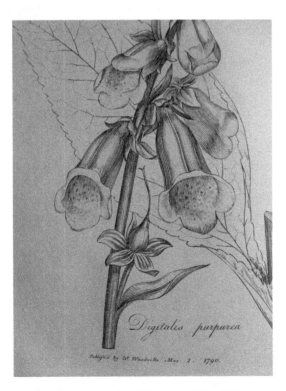

Foxglove, *Medical Botany*, Woodville.

In the last quarter of the eighteenth century, many changes took place across society. The Industrial Revolution had begun and as confidence in new ways with engineering and commerce grows, the watchword becomes progress. The general move to live and work in cities rather than the countryside reduces contact with plants and this is seen also in the reduction of their use by physicians in prescribing. The powerful calomel containing mercury, preparations of antimony, and laudanum classed later as "heroic medicines" are the order of the day. New thought in medicine is favouring a critical re-appraisal of established ways. The name of William Withering was to become well-known through his work on a powerful herb, the foxglove. His scientific approach was to provide evidence for the argument that use of prepared drugs would be safer than administering whole herbs.

Withering was far better acquainted with the botany of herbs than other physicians of the period. He had had no interest in botany whilst at University, but writing to Sir Joseph Banks later in life he dated the beginning of his interest to seeing the British Herbarium when at the house of a friend.[1] His attention had been concentrated on the foxglove when he found a herb woman using the plant to treat dropsy. Interested by her success and aware that care was required in prescribing, he decided to study the effects of the herb, but not only on his patients.

He believed in using insects and animals for testing toxic doses and carried this out, feeding foxglove to turkeys until they died. This, with his work on the vital necessity of determining the correct dose of foxglove in treating dropsy, supported by carefully recording over seventy case histories; had made him uncomfortably aware that the effects of leaves picked at different times of year did not comply with a set standard. After ten years of investigating and experimenting with digitalis he published his famous and influential *Account of the Foxglove* in 1785.[2]

The work of Carl Linnaeus in classification of plants was being appreciated and applied by enthusiasts at this time and since Withering had also written on botany describing genera and species according to Linnaeus, it is possible that he met William Meyrick through the Lichfield Botanic Society. The Society had just published a translation of Linnaeus' *Systema Vegetabilium*, something that Withering himself had earlier engaged a friend to translate but this had not come to fruition.[3] We may indulge ourselves in imagining the experienced physician and young house apothecary and surgeon coming together in discussing the finer details.

His birth date is uncertain but Meyrick was certainly under twenty years old when Withering's *Account of the Foxglove* was published and Withering appears to have taken him under his wing. It was a fruitful friendship for Meyrick as Withering was an excellent mentor, offering advice on the herbal Meyrick was working on, and allowing him to use many extracts from his late celebrated publication on botanical arrangements.[4] Trained as a house apothecary in Birmingham and subsequently as a surgeon in West Bromwich, Meyrick must have impressed Withering with his knowledge on herbs to gain such attention.

Meyrick's family herbal was clearly successful. It was first published by Thomas Pearson in 1789, with a second edition in 1790 and two more later. The title of his book is witness to the fact that medicine was still practised in the home and he stresses in his introduction that he wishes to make this practice safer and effectual. He believed that nothing was of greater importance when using plants in medicine than the ability to distinguish one from another accurately. He therefore supplies great detail in describing each herb botanically to achieve his aim and offers a glossary of necessary technical terms for the reader. In addition, there is a useful index of diseases and instructions on gathering and preserving all plant parts. For anyone at home unfamiliar with any medicinal preparations, he is eager to ensure that they have all the instruction they might need with a guide to making infusions, decoctions, syrups, pills, tinctures, ointments, and distilled waters. Here his initial training as a house apothecary shows.

Grateful for his mentor's help, Meyrick quotes freely from Withering's work on the familiar herbs, such as the red field poppy, as well as the less familiar in-home medicine, soapwort.[5,6] As well as many quotes from Withering, there are some from John Hill, and it is interesting to look at Meyrick's other sources. As we might expect, these include the work of physicians and botanists. Dr Cullen, a greatly respected Scottish professor of chemistry and medicine who was known to William Withering, is quoted with the use of coltsfoot to treat scrophula.[7] Under Broom, Meyrick quotes the medical history of a dropsical patient from the writings of Dr Mead, famous for his works on infectious diseases in the previous century.[8] We noted a prescription of his used by Anne Blencowe in the previous chapter.

He quotes the Dispensatory of Lewis, also a physician, on numerous occasions. The name of Blackwell appears after the uses of sea holly,[9] also of heartsease.[10] This is particularly interesting as it refers to her work, *A Curious Herbal*—the first herbal produced by a woman. Elizabeth Blackwell was assisted in her desire to illustrate 500 herbs in the Pharmacopoeia by various members of the Society of Apothecaries and it is no surprise to find that Blackwell used Joseph Miller's *Botanicum Officinale*, which was not illustrated, as a main source for parts of the text in her herbal.[11] In order to have each herb fresh for her study and probably to observe the plants growing at regular intervals, choosing specimens, she took a house close to Chelsea Physic Garden.

To her credit Blackwell not only drew the plants from life but also made the copper plate engravings and hand coloured them with stunningly beautiful results. Her work was doubly one of love, in that it was motivated by her desire to earn sufficient money to clear her husbands' debts. Alexander Blackwell had set up in business as a printer without serving an apprenticeship and with action brought against him went bankrupt and spent two years in prison. Alexander seems undeserving of her help, as shown by his leaving his post of planning the grounds of a mansion for the Duke of Chandos with a poor reputation. He left Elizabeth to go to Sweden where he was equally unfortunate in politics and was executed for high treason in 1747.[12] Blackwell's herbal was greeted with great acclaim and received a commendation from the President of the Royal College of Physicians in 1737.

Another source was Quincy's Dispensatory from 1721, in his preface to the third edition he writes, *"The Officinal Medicines are now entirely according to the Standard of the College; because a due Conformity thereunto in the Shops, is absolutely necessary"*.[13] Then again, at the close he refers to the sophistications by wholesale apothecaries and chemists, which have been discovered by careful inspection by the College. *"These Inconveniences are indeed as much as possible remedied in the Chymical way, by the* Care of the Apothecaries *Company; who with a joint Stock have those Medicines made at their Hall, under such careful Management and Inspection, as cannot give any possible Opportunities for Impositions of this kind."*[14] Quality control remained an important issue.

Foreign sources with a single mention include Prospero Alpinus, a Venetian physician and botanist from the sixteenth century, and Monsieur Tournefort, chief botanist to the French King whose *Compleat Herbal* was published in English in 1730.[15] This last reference book has the most exacting illustrations of plant parts I have seen and on the title page boasts that it contains additions by Ray, Gerard, Parkinson and others. I have chosen to include some of his plant illustrations in this book. It is clear, however, that the body of the text comes from personal experience and knowledge. Notable entries, each running to several pages, in contrast to the others, refer to hop and a herb we have been following, liquorice. With these he gives detailed instructions on cultivation without referencing other works.

Meyrick had also begun writing his *Miscellaneous Botany*, planned to be issued in monthly instalments, from 1794, but only the first volume was printed.[16] He signed on as surgeon on a slave ship late in 1799. If the exotic herbs he included in his *Family Herbal* were not enough to inspire him to travel in perhaps the only way open to him to see the live plants, then reading *The Natural History of Jamaica* by Hans Sloane, published earlier in the century, might have encouraged him to go. Meyrick wrote he was about to return from Jamaica in the following summer but no more was heard of him.[17]

William Woodville was a much-respected physician who had a similar motive of reforming understanding of medicinal plants. In 1791 he was appointed physician to the Smallpox Hospital at St Pancras. Four acres of grounds surrounding this imposing hospital separated contagious patients from the nearby residences. One of a number of Quaker botanists, Woodville was extremely well-informed on medicine and plants through his considerable scholarly research. He too began his elegant four volume *Medical Botany* cautiously as a serial publication in 1790 and in two of the four acres of hospital grounds he brought together a botanical garden, maintaining it at his own expense.[18] This botanic garden must have furnished many specimens used for the excellent copper-plate illustrations in his *Medical Botany*, engraved by James Sowerby detailing plants from the Pharmacopoeia. Formerly copper-plate illustrations had only been published by Blackwell and Sheldrake.[19]

Woodville points out in the Supplement volume that all the figures published, except a few where he had to resort to using plates from other studiously researched sources, were taken either from dried or recent specimens of the herbs. The care he records on finding he has made a mistake as to the source of cascarilla, in an earlier published volume, is exemplary. He has had a specimen from the correct tree and cascarilla bark sent from the Bahamas and compared these with the specimen in the herbarium of Sir Joseph Banks before publishing a correct illustration in the front of the Supplement, pointing out his mistake.[20] He apologises for being unable to obtain neither a perfect specimen nor published figure for a very few entries. These include *Piper cubeba* from Africa and *Myroxylon peruiferum* from South America.[21]

Woodville spares no pains in his investigations of the sources of foreign herbs, their gathering, and uses. He quotes from such accounts as *Travels into the Interior Parts of Africa* by Moor for Kino.[22] Unsurprisingly, he turns to the authorities on medicine familiar in his day, Scottish Dr Cullen and the materia medica of Lewis often, but the range of his quest for information was broad, spanning history, from Galen and Celsus to recent communications to the Royal Society on case histories of death from taking cherry laurel distilled water.[23]

It would be tedious to list all sources, but the standard is shown by the *Histoire de l'académie des science de Berlin*, philosophical transactions of the Royal Society 1765, Rutty's Observations on the London and Edinburgh Dispensatories, the Dutch professor of medicine, Boerhaave, along with numerous contemporary physicians, the most famous being Mayerne, Sydenham, and Mead. Culpeper is, not surprisingly conspicuous for his absence, but Gerard finds mention along with Sir Joseph Banks as the first person to cultivate certain foreign species in this country.

His chosen herbs included not only those much used, *Cassia senna* and *Papaver somniferum*, but also the now rarely used *Artemisia abrotanum* and the plainly discounted if not entirely discarded, *Betonica officinalis*. At the other end of the scale there are long quotes on use of coffee, thought good for asthmatic patients at the time, and tobacco.

This was, deservedly, to become a standard work for over fifty years. Woodville dedicated it to the President, Fellows, and Licentiates of the Royal College of Physicians, and set out to describe and provide illustrations for all those plants directed for medicinal use by the Colleges of London and Edinburgh.[24]

As a qualified physician, writing on herbs primarily for physicians, Woodville is forthright about his opinion of the value of herbal medicine as opposed to chemical. In his preface he states boldly, "Though it must be acknowledged that for some time past the medicinal uses of vegetable simples have been less regarded by physicians than they were formerly, which probably may be ascribed to the successive discoveries and improvements in chemistry; it would however be difficult to shew that this preference is supported by any conclusive reasoning drawn from a comparative superiority of Chemicals over Galenicals, or that the more general use of the former has actually led to a more successful practice".[25]

The illustrations are, as he intended, concise and accurate. Some early printed engravings of plants are superb; for example, those in Sir John Hill's *The British Herbal* of 1746, which bear the names of several engravers and were from wood-cuts. These are of similar quality if not better, but are simply labelled published by Woodville with the date. Herbals which followed in the nineteenth century show a much lower standard.

Botany is also becoming a popular pastime for ladies, and we must not forget that ladies of means continue to treat family and the poor around them. Although the golden age of the stillroom may be fading, Christian charity with visiting the neighbouring sick continues to be an expectation. Whereas Woodville was writing for the benefit of professional physicians, there was also an increasing trend by physicians to write for the general public. No doubt inspiration for this lay partly in the realisation that they would otherwise be dependent on advice from books written by housekeepers and collections of recipes sent in to publishers such as those quoted in the last chapter. Safe home medicine is the aim as judged by the professional medic.

In 1793, the Napoleonic Wars began and having collaborated with Ruth Mannion-Daniels on Georgian Herbs in Peace and War in 2010, my awareness of the continued importance of herbs in naval medicine was increased. Ruth had researched 120 surgeon's journals and the 1806 handbook for naval surgeons in addition to Woodville's *Medical Botany* for her dissertation on the subject. Responsible to the Physician of the Fleet, yet working in cramped conditions the surgeons, cared for up to 800 men on board on long voyages and in battle.

Heart-rending accounts of operating for days without sleep after battles, praying to stay awake, of almost miraculous healing of terrible injuries using simple herbs, and the differences noted between expectations from their training and actual experience, are carefully recorded in the journals. With limited space on board, the medicines were selected by the College of Physicians and supplied by the Society of Apothecaries.

William Turnbull in his handbook of 1800 made it clear that medicines must be restricted to those necessary as the most active, cheap, and useful.[26] Ship's surgeons at this time had to meet all needs with a limited medicine chest. They made their own tinctures with rum base and carried essential oil of mint, a drop of which could be shaken with water to make aromatic water.[27] This convenient method using distilled water is given in nineteenth century Pharmacopoeias. Herbs included opium, mustard, Roman chamomile, wormwood, squill, linseed oil, and seed, castor oil, guaiacum, myrrh, capsicum, peruvian bark, gentian, ginger, cinnamon, spirit of turpentine, squills, and conserve of roses. Rose honey was used with myrrh and Aqua Calais in treating ulcers, and in recipes containing antimony.[28] In Chapter 19, John Josselyn's 1668 list of supplies for his voyage also included wormwood, ginger, cinnamon, and conserve of roses, and both sources favoured lemons.

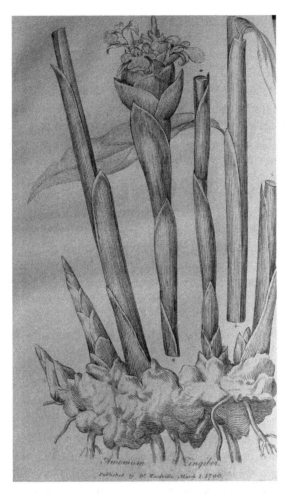

Ginger, *Medical Botany*, Woodville.

Mentions of the important role of ginger bring us to review our chosen herbs. We can now review physicians' opinions and see how this relates to their uses in household books. In 1694, Pechey writes ginger is candied in India, the candy being good for old people and the phlegmatic constitution, those of a hot disposition he warns not to use it. The root is added to protective antidotes and purges, also strengthening the brain and clearing sight. In 1722, it is being imported from Jamaica, but from there is not as strong. By 1790 Meyrick tells us that ginger is now frequently cultivated in England in heated buildings. Woodville writes it is used as syrup, often with other medicines in many compositions for colics, phlegmatic debility of the stomach and intestines.[29]

Nettle appears in household recipes in a diet drink, for itch, stopping bleeding, as a diuretic for dropsy, with honey for shortness of breath, and the powdered root for jaundice. These uses fit everything Pechey wrote about nettle in 1694. In 1722 we find the seed is used for coughs and shortness of breath.[30] Disappointingly, Woodville takes the view that little credit can be given to these uses and merely supports it for stimulant urtification of paralytic limbs to restore excitement.[31]

As early as Pechey the many actions of betony are questioned. Meyrick announces it to be formerly of great repute but disregarded in 1790; however, he goes on to list successes with betony for stubborn headaches, mentions the leaves smoked as tobacco for both head and stomach and gives many more indications for use. Woodville points out that modern writers do not allow betony to possess any considerable efficacy.[32]

Our third native herb, plantain, is most certainly appreciated in its time-honoured roles at the beginning of the eighteenth century, Miller in 1722 is also enthusiastic about vulnerary, and anti-haemorrhagic applications and more, but he notes that the only officinal preparation is the Aqua. When it comes to Woodville, seventy years later he records it as now omitted from the London Pharmacopoeia but still retained in the Edinburgh College. He states that plantain, formerly recommended as the best wound herb was commonly applied by peasants. The leaves are still applied to fresh wounds and are given internally for bleeding. He records the use of the expressed juice and root for fevers and recommends the mucilaginous seeds might be better adapted to treating the lungs.[33]

With elecampane, Pechey recommends it as excellent for the plague, and we have seen that it was included in plague waters, he tells us wine is made of the herb in Germany which improves the sight. Elecampane is praised as diuretic, and emmenagogue in addition to aiding breathing and treating coughs, convulsions and hip-gout. Meyrick agrees and adds indications for applying the juice for cutaneous eruptions and itch.[34] Woodville supports use for coughs and asthma and says spirituous liquors extract its virtue in greater perfection. Again however he hesitates on full support, saying he has no evidence of its powers in the urinary or uterine systems.

Liquorice and ginger retain their popularity in main medicine. Careful instructions are given by Meyrick for cultivating liquorice which needs deep, good soil, as well as extraction of the juice. It is recognised as helpful to the lungs, kidneys, bladder and digestion, soothing heartburn. Large quantities are imported from Spain; nevertheless, Woodville records liquorice being grown in Pontefract, Worksop, and Godalming in Surrey. Adding it is now planted in the vicinity of London to supply the city.[35] Clearly liquorice is an up-and-coming herb at the close of the century.

Henbane in Woodville's estimation was a powerful narcotic poison but while referring to dangerous and terrible symptoms from all parts of the plant, he admits that with care it can be safely employed. He writes that it seems to have been out of use in medicine for some time until interest was revived by published cases of success with treating headaches, epilepsy, spasms and chronic coughs. He quotes

Dr Cullen and concludes that as an effective substitute when opium is contraindicated it is effective in pain relief.[36]

William Buchan was also a respected physician who qualified in Edinburgh in 1758. He was particularly concerned by the need to educate the general public on health issues. The College of Physicians would rather keep such information to themselves but he strongly defended offering medical knowledge to the lay person. Unlike Meyrick who concentrated on knowledge of herbs, the emphasis of his mission is on giving sound advice on regimen in health and diagnosis of disease, with herbal recipes coming last. He hoped to reduce the fearful child mortality rates by educating mothers and gave recognition to the talents of those who cared for and nursed their families and others.

When it comes to instructions on making medicines, we are indebted to him for revealing that his expectation is that every literate household will have a still and instruction on distilling is so well known that he need not include it. His immensely popular book, *Domestic Physician* pre-dates Meyrick's work with the first edition published in 1769 and it would be strange if Meyrick and Withering were not aware of it. His scant respect for the College of Physicians shows very plainly in his introduction to his book when he makes the statement that "Very few of the valuable discoveries in Medicine have been made by physicians. They have, in general, either been the effect of chance or of necessity, and have been usually opposed by the Faculty till every body else was convinced of their importance".[37] It is a shame that even so, Buchan is true to his training. When it comes to toothache he treats by drawing off humours through scarifying the gums, and giving vomits, and he believes that few applications give more relief than blistering plasters between the shoulders. Minor headaches are relieved by a cooling regimen, intolerable pain with laudanum in a cup of valerian tea. Buchan does not approve of external applications for the eyes and again resorts to blistering plasters on the neck and bleeding.[38] For treating rheumatic pain he suggests an electuary of conserve of roses, cinnabar of antimony, and gum guaiacum brought together with syrup of ginger.[39] In instruction in the main text, however, he adds bleeding, cupping, and blistering plasters for treating such pain.

For burns, Buchan uses standard preparations from the apothecary such as Turner's cerate, according to severity. He lists the types of cough with specific remedies from teas of wild poppy petals, marshmallow root, and coltsfoot flowers for expectorating thin phlegm to the opiate paregoric for a nervous cough and that old favourite of the previous century—a maceration of woodlice in white wine for whooping cough.[40] While suggesting several cooling liquors of tamarind and other herbs for fevers, Buchan appreciates fevers are nature trying to rid the body of the disease and, therefore, believes remedies should assist this with evacuations of purging and vomiting. We should take note that he ends his comments on perspiration being a common evacuation of the body, as part of exploring the preservation of health, with a long quotation from Celsus. Boils are not mentioned as such, despite his wide range and detail of conditions, but in the chapter on diseases of children he writes of eruptions being due to improper food and lack of cleanliness. For these, which include scab and itch, he recommends sulphur in butter, oil, or hog's lard.[41]

The states of health and disease offered to the public in William Buchan's work, and the guidance on identification and use of herbs from Meyrick reveal the general concern with raising standards of healthcare. While Withering has promoted animal experiments to ensure safe dosage of powerful herbs and still supported a botanical approach, other physicians were greatly reducing herbal medications. The boldly critical statements of Buchan and Woodville on their deep dissatisfaction with the state of medicine in general give us clear indications of the challenges to be faced in a changing world as the eighteenth century draws to a close.

References

1. Blanche Henrey, *British Botanical and Horticultural Literature before 1800*, Vol. II (Oxford: Oxford University Press, 1975), 122.
2. Henrey, *British Botanical and Horticultural Literature*, 122.
3. Ibid, 124.
4. Ibid, 121.
5. William Meyrick, *The Family Herbal or Domestic Physician* (Birmingham: Thomas Pearson, 1790), 384.
6. Meyrick, *The Family Herbal*, 424.
7. Ibid, 110.
8. Ibid, 60.
9. Ibid, 159.
10. Ibid, 212.
11. Henrey, *British Botanical and Horticultural Literature*, 228.
12. Ibid, 236.
13. John Quincy, *Pharmacopœia Officinalis Extemporanea, or Complete English Dispensatory* (London: Thomas Longman 10th edition, 1736), X.
14. Quincy, *Pharmacopœia Officinalis Extemporanea*, XII.
15. Tournefort, *The Compleat Herbal*, Vol. II. (London: Walthoe, Wilkin, Bonwicke, Birt, Ward & Wicksteed, 1730).
16. Henrey, *British Botanical and Horticultural Literature*, 22.
17. Ibid, 24.
18. Ibid, 32.
19. Ibid, 30.
20. William Woodville, *Medical Botany* (London: James Phillips, 1790), Supplement, 3.
21. Woodville, *Medical Botany*, Supplement, 1.
22. Ibid, Supplement, 166.
23. Ibid, 74–76.
24. Woodville, *Medical Botany* Vol. I. Frontispiece.
25. Ibid, a.

26. Turnbull, William, John Adamson, and Warren U. Ober, *The Naval Surgeon: Comprising the entire duties of professional men at sea: To which are subjoined, a system of naval surgery, and, a compendium of Pharmacopœia* (London: R. Phillips, 1806), PART III. Naval Pharmacopoeia or Dispensary.

27. Turnbull, The Naval Surgeon, Principal and Secondary Pharmaceutical articles.

28. Ibid, Venereal Ulcers.

29. Woodville, *Medical Botany*, Vol. I. 33.

30. Joseph Miller, *Botanicum Officinale* (London: Bell, Senex, Taylor & Osborn, 1722), 460.

31. Woodville, *Medical Botany*, Vol. III, 397–8.

32. Ibid, Supplement, 79.

33. Ibid, Vol. I, 40.

34. Meyrick, *The Family Herbal*, 157.

35. Woodville, *Medical Botany*, Vol. III, 459.

36. Ibid, Vol. I. 144–145.

37. William Buchan, *Domestic Medicine* (London: Strahan, Cadell, 1776), xviii.

38. Buchan, *Domestic Medicine*, 284.

39. Ibid, 716.

40. Ibid, 312.

41. Buchan, *Domestic Medicine*, 604.

SECTION IX

SELF HELP FOLLOWING THE INDUSTRIAL REVOLUTION | 1810–1895

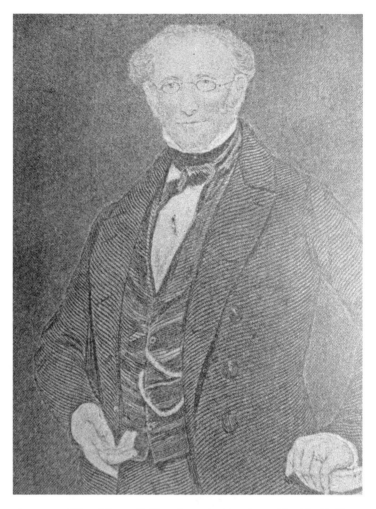

Portrait of Dr. Albert Coffin, *Botanic Guide to Health*, Coffin.

Key Figures

Samuel Thomson (1769–1843), Albert Coffin, (c1790–1866), Wooster Beech (1794–1859), Alva Curtis (1797–1881), John Skelton (1805–1880), Duncan Napier (1831–1921), Henry Potter (opened first shop in 1812).

Key Texts

Botanic Guide to Health, 1855, Coffin.
The Eclectic Practice of Medicine, 1864, Scudder.
Allopathy versus Physio-medicalism, 1870, Curtis.

Roles of Women in Medicine

Nurses, midwives, physio-medical practitioners, herbalist.

Quality Control

The Pharmaceutical Society of Great Britain was founded in 1841. Lectures on pharmacognosy were given by professors shortly afterwards to aid in correct identification of herbs. A herbarium collection was included in the Museum of Materia Medica (Pharmacy) with Theophilus Redwood as curator. Adulteration was common in medicines and food.

Herb Energetics

The classification of herbs has now changed and in place of the temperatures of herbs we find their actions given as in cathartics, nervines, antiscorbutics etc. The closest terms to heating and drying are stimulant and astringent, and with moistening herbs, mucilaginous. The coldest are termed narcotic.

Travel and Trade

Steamships, canals, and railways made transport faster. Trade was worldwide. Increased contact with America resulted in the availability of many herbs on a much larger scale. Albert Coffin was able to import herbs for his system of botanic medicine in amounts that enabled ordinary people to buy the imported herbs from his warehouse. Exploration by plant hunters increased public awareness of, and demand for, the exotics in the plant world. The slave trade was abolished by law in the British Empire in 1807, but slavery in the colonies continued until 1833 and shamefully it was the slave owners rather than the long-suffering enslaved people who were compensated.

Introduction

Once into the nineteenth century in British manufacturing areas, great numbers of people lived in squalid conditions, divorced from their familiar family traditions and simple herbal medicine which they might formerly have gathered from nearby hedgerows or fields. Home medicine in towns was obliged to fall back on whatever was to hand, herbal poultices being replaced by bread and onion if even that could be afforded. There were few physicians for the population who could afford them and the poor continued to rely on charity. Alternative herbal help arrived from America with Dr Coffin and his wholesale approach to herbal supplies. First, his largely Thomsonian system of medicine bearing traces of Native American herbal use is followed and then both an eclectic combination encompassing some orthodox treatments, and developing thought in physio-medicalism are practised in Britain. A whole new herbal medicine scene would find many followers in England and bring changes lasting into the next century.

CHAPTER 23

Wholesale Botanic Medicine | 1745–1848

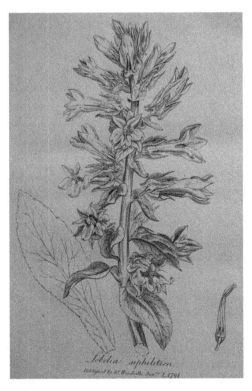

Lobelia, *Medical Botany*, Woodville.

In America, there was as much concern as that expressed in England at the allopathic approach of commonly prescribing poisonous substances such as arsenic and mercury and bleeding debilitated patients. There, this was challenged by Thomsonian medicine which began with a young man who had grown up in settler country in New Hampshire on a farm three miles from the nearest settlement, Samuel Thomson. Born in 1769, he helped on the farm from a very young age and his interest in plants was enriched by the knowledge of a friend of the family, Mrs Benton.[1] She taught him the names of the plants and their medical uses. Growing up, he wanted to be a physician but his parents found he needed to have spent more time at school even to learn from a root doctor. In time, he had his own farm and family and used his knowledge of herbs to treat them when they were sick. Neighbours noticed his success with serious conditions and began asking for help.[2]

His reputation grew until he gave up the farm and began a career as an untrained but knowledgeable physician. He was particularly interested in the properties of lobelia, labelled as a poison by orthodox medicine, but in his eyes harmless when given at the right dose. Thomson developed his ideas from the basic four elements, just as the Greeks had done before him. He reasoned that earth and water provided the solids in the body and fire and air the fluids. Obstructions to these he thought caused disease. He believed that since death exhibits the coldest state, the power of heat should be used to remove obstructions and restore the bodily systems in disease. He often added cayenne with lobelia to prescriptions as he reasoned that the heat begun by the action of the lobelia would then be continued by the cayenne.

Thomson had already established use of steaming in fevers with his own family and had devised his own system of medicine when an epidemic of yellow fever broke out in the area in 1805. His methods saved all his patients while the trained physicians using debilitating drugs and bleeding, lost many. He became famous as a success, gaining powerful supporters, physicians sought out any patients of his who had died under whatever circumstances and repeatedly accused him of murder. Imprisoned, he was helped by a judge he had cured earlier and was acquitted.[3]

After discovering one of his agents had been trying to sell his secrets, Thomson obtained a patent for his system of medicine in Washington in 1813.[4] While he was on a trip to Cape Cod collecting herbs, he treated patients in an outbreak of spotted fever and sold rights to his methods to a few people, giving lectures and supplying herbs. As his system spread, he avoided selling rights to trained physicians for as long as possible as he knew they would try to alter it. This, however, meant treatments would be carried out by those who had little, if any, medical knowledge. In various states societies grew up and education for students began. One practitioner of Thomsonian medicine was to bring it to England where the dominant theme had become one of self-treatment amongst the poor for more than simple first aid. The village cunning woman will have remained in the countryside and the lady of the manor, some of whom still dispensed medicines, as I know from the Blencowe family, were now also out of reach. Many lived crowded together in growing slums around the mills and factories unable to pay for a physician, had there even been enough of them to go round. The time was ripe for a new way offered by a middle-aged American doctor, Albert Isaiah Coffin who arrived in London in 1838.[5] He does not appear to have qualified as a physician, but was trained in Thomsonian botanic medicine.

Looking at Dr Coffin's practice, we should not think that because this was a kinder alternative to heroic medicine that it was gentle. The hot steam bath followed by a warm shower and bed looks promising. However, this was followed by a strong emetic in the form of cayenne pepper and lobelia combined with other herbs suited to the individual case. The treatment was taken at intervals until the desired effect was produced. After a period of vomiting, the patient was again steamed and showered, then given a dose of bitters.

Albert Coffin had no respect for orthodox training, disputing the right of Colleges to decide whether a man was qualified to practise on the basis of knowledge of theory. He was, however, judging from quotations in his book, very well read—from Culpeper to *The Pharmacopoeia* and *The Practice of Modern Physic*. Yet he even announces that "neither the knowledge of *astrology, astronomy, natural philosophy, nor even anatomy itself, is absolutely necessary to the quick and effectual cure of most diseases*".[6] He continues, writing that his medicine is available, "So that every man of common sense, unless in some rare case, may prescribe either for himself or his neighbour, and may be secure from doing harm even where he can do no good".[7] Coffin believed that all diseases originate in one common cause, the absence of equilibrium of heat, which should circulate through the entire system; he concentrated on regaining lost heat and restoring the stomach to healthy action.[8]

Coffin supported his constant accusations against the ignorance of general training in medicine by quoting instances from orthodox sources to support the contention that the illiterate student of nature could be better informed. One such case was of an enslaved person in Surinam who had sold knowledge of quassia wood for treating fevers to the supposedly learned world of medicine.[9] He then uses a quote from *Dr Rush's Lectures to Medical Students*. Dr Rush (1746–1813) had been an eminent physician whose extreme bleeding techniques in treating fevers eventually saw him disgraced, but he was strongly supported by Coffin because of his zeal for reform. The quote fits his case exactly as Dr Rush was apparently recommending students to take a notebook with them when abroad and record any details of efficacious herbs or recipes for medicines they might glean from old women. He also quotes the "great and good John Wesley",[10] on the power of exercise to restore health and Dr Buchan on the causes of indigestion.[11] Then, Coffin laments the enormous quantity of tobacco consumed in Britain, writing that Sir Walter Raleigh brought on this country "a severe and dangerous penance".[12]

In his guide to health Coffin writes firstly about herbs and then about specific diseases and conditions. Having described the problem and its cause, he goes on with each to detail a case where his medicine has proved successful. Lastly, he gives the orthodox treatment of the schools or faculty of medicine. This often includes a combination of potentially poisonous substances, bleeding and blistering. He has a whole chapter on the dangerous effects of physicians prescribing mercury, arsenic, prussic acid, oxalic acid, antimony, or opium. Asked whether he would remove opium from his list of medicines, since it was, after all, a herb, he answered yes as he saw it as a powerful poison. He quoted the Emperor of China who had banned sale of opium on pain of death because of the harm it did.[13]

It was certainly the case that opium was freely prescribed and had been since the eighteenth century by physicians, although some raised doubts as to safety, various forms of it could be bought from druggists without a prescription. Many were introduced to the drug through treatment for a medical condition, and since numerous physicians did not accept that addiction would follow after only several weeks of treatment, they became dependent as happens with certain drugs today. Physicians themselves became addicted and we find this illustrated in the case of the ship's surgeon in the Patrick O'Brian novels as he refers to having taken up to 4,000 drops a day.[14] He is a fictional character typical of the early nineteenth century.

Laudanum became a favourite and such was the belief in it as a ready to hand cure-all for persistent coughs, pain or diarrhoea that this included giving a freely available form to small children to quieten them. It was with this background we find Coffin writing "In the manufacturing districts, where young mothers, labouring in factories, are obliged to leave their children to the care of strangers, it frequently occurs that the children are found dead in the cradle, having been poisoned by the quantity of opium administered, in the shape of a cordial, by some ignorant old woman, in order to induce sleep and prevent the child from crying".[15]

This refers to Godfrey's Cordial, which was still being prescribed almost fifty years later in 1895. There are five recipes in *The Druggists General Receipt Book* of that year with a note that different makers produced a great diversity of strength and many accidents have arisen due to its too general use. One formula, which is not the strongest, contains laudanum which will be equal to sixteen or eighteen drops in each fluid ounce.[16]

This was the background against which his Botanic Medicine took off, but not immediately. Dr Coffin lectured first to educated audiences in London where his teachings fell on deaf ears. He then travelled north to address the poor in the manufacturing cities, Hull, Manchester, Sheffield, and Leeds where he finally settled, after living in Hull for a time. By 1850, his mass botanic medicine had branches with agents and herbal supplies in all the northern industrial cities and London. In his *Botanical Journal and Medical Reformer*, he campaigned for greater safety precautions in the factories, halting the prevalent adulteration of food, providing clean water and sanitation. His treatments for babies and young children were kinder than the orthodox, tasted better, and did not purge.

In his *Botanic Guide to Health*, he details eighty-eight herbs, poorly represented in the illustrations when compared with earlier herbals. Many were European in origin having been taken across the Atlantic by settlers, some he may have studied while living in France before coming to Britain. Coffin writes enthusiastically about ginger as a substitute for cayenne when necessary, praising it for action on the stomach, bowels, and particularly supporting chewing the root for diseases of the lungs.[17] Elecampane is illustrated but not listed in his materia medica section and our other chosen herbs are also restricted to inclusion in the list of dried herbs for sale.

The first chapter on herbs covers 'pure stimulants'—Cayenne pepper, ginger, prickly ash, black pepper, cloves, nutmeg, allspice, cinnamon, spearmint, peppermint, pennyroyal, summer savory, horseradish, mustard, American golden rod (*Solidago odora*), yarrow, may-weed, camomile, feverfew, lobelia, vervain and hyssop. His next chapters deal with astringents, tonics or bitters, diuretics, antiscorbutics, nervines—includes burdock seed, cathartics—bullock's gall, turkey rhubarb, senna, mountain flax, aloes, and butternut, mucilaginous herbs, and anthelmintics. These are followed by recipes for compound medicines and a piece on diet giving the time taken for various foods to be digested. The book ends with a section on specific diseases.

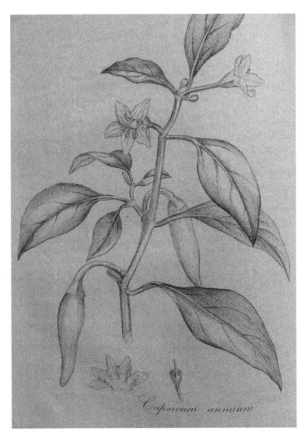

Cayenne, *Medical Botany*, Woodville.

He quotes numerous case histories and seems confident in treating diseases from hepatitis to asthma, using his simple rule of cleansing the stomach and applying stimulants to remove obstructions to the natural ordering of bodily fluids applied equally. As for his recipe for Asiatic cholera, it is typically Thomsonian. He recommends to cover the patient with a blanket, then use the vapour bath as hot as can be borne, give a strong astringent tea of raspberry leaves, tormentil root, and bayberry, made very warm with anti-cholera powder (more heat from ginger, cayenne, cloves, and cinnamon, plus bitters, pine, and bayberry with compound powder) and more cayenne pepper. He urgently encourages stopping purging or water discharges by using medicines unsparingly and when the patient is warm, give lobelia emetic every two hours as necessary, also an injection into the bowel of lobelia, cayenne pepper, gum myrrh, and valerian root, in a strong tea of oak bark, or tormentil root; and so soon as he can take it, porridge.[18]

Both cayenne and lobelia appear again and again in his remedies, as in the Thomsonian system, which he mentions in his lengthy details of lobelia. Coffin also gives us the interesting information that he obtains lobelia stocks from the religious society of Shakers.[19] This seems highly appropriate, as Ann Lee, the visionary founder of the Shaker movement was born in Manchester in 1736 and experienced the desperate conditions for the poor, first working in a mill and then as a cook at the infirmary. Her visions prompted her to go to America with members of the Wardley's society, the first home of the religious community being Watervliet. From there, they later supplied large amounts of medicinal herbs, including lobelia from 1833.[20]

As already mentioned, examples of treatments recommended by the medical faculty are often listed following Coffin's treatments. For tetanus this included opium, æther, oil of amber, camphor, musk, buckthorn syrup, and jalap, with bleeding and electricity.[21] Electricity had been introduced as a treatment for numerous conditions, including toothache in the previous century. We find the first rather alarming reports of experiments with electrifying people in that treasure trove of topical information, *The Gentleman's Magazine* in April 1745. The extract from Philosophical Transactions of the Royal Society contains the following passage, "An electrified person cannot approach an electrified tube or glass, without darting forth towards it a visible flame, attended with a small noise like the crackling of hairs set on fire".[22] At that point the idea of using the effects for medicine was still in the future, it was at first seen as good entertainment.

Returning to Dr Coffin, in the back of the forty-ninth edition of his book is a quote of a much earlier review from "*John Bull* 1864". "When a book has reached thirty-five editions, which is the case with 'Dr Coffin's *Botanic Guide to Health*,' the office of the critic is nearly superseded so far as concerns recommendation".[23]

Needless to say, the College of Physicians did not feel the same and Coffin was taken to court many times. Tired from his incredible efforts over the years, he decided to leave his botanic medicine for a time in the capable hands of a younger herbalist already working for and with him, his name was John Skelton. He had agreed a two-year contract with Coffin in 1848 and they were united in the wish to continue the flourishing botanic herbal medicine for those so much in need. He moved to Manchester to oversee agents in the north.[24]

Coffin's system was of course not the only source of advice. There was plenty of opportunity to help the poor in the industrial and other areas to care for themselves and numerous printed sources of information. This was a period when self-medical care flourished for a variety of reasons—economy being just one of them. A number of small books had already been published before and after the arrival of Coffin. He was familiar with John Wesley's work, *Primitive Physic*,[25] but that was from the previous century and contains a blend of homely remedies such as warm lemonade for a bilious colic, with some equally objectionable ideas—applying goose dung and celandine beat together for cancer in the breast, and others sounding very like the physician's approach, with quicksilver for the green sickness. He is not against purging and a definite supporter of cold bathing, and when all else fails, he recommends the patient should be electrified for curing earache, headache, epilepsy, toothache, eye problems, dropsy, or obstructed menstruation.

Albert Coffin had herbal treatments for these problems, but they are mainly different to those we have recorded so far.

Headache—His approach to curing a headache, through opening the bowels, does relate to some we have seen. Constipation has been recognised as a possible cause for headaches before. Reasons for derangement of digestion he believes are sedentary habits, excess eating and drinking, or being overwrought by severe application to business. He offers a recipe using first a decoction of barberry bark and agrimony. Then, Turkey rhubarb with ginger root to ease any griping and his favourite cayenne pepper for added heat.[26]

Eye Conditions—Coffin gives a wince inducing cure for ophthalmia of blowing a little cayenne pepper into the affected eye every other day. The patient suffered brief agony, and this was followed by a vapour bath. Treatment was continued for two months, when the patient was cured.[27]

Rheumatism—He identifies the cause as cold, leading to deranged circulation and so mustard foot baths at night and a strong decoction of yarrow, centaury, agrimony, ginger, and cayenne is suggested, again following a pattern of heat and stimulating digestion. Vapour baths and regulating the bowels and stomach with a necessary lobelia emetic and laxative complete the treatment.[28]

Toothache—It does not appear in his book although there are several pages on dentition with a strong denial that teething should produce any symptoms in a healthy child.[29]

Burns—Treatment naturally depends on the severity, beginning with cold, wet applications left on to avoid blistering and leading on to a burn salve of Burgundy pitch with half the amount of Hog's lard and half again of beeswax for where the skin is open and the area sore.[30]

Coughs—For chronic and spasmodic asthmatic coughs, Coffin uses pills of equal parts of lobelia and valerian with half the amount of cayenne made into a mass with gum Arabic.[31]

Fevers—An important subject as Coffin spends considerable effort on admonishing physicians for debilitating patients to no purpose. He takes an opposite view of treatment, looking upon the fever as nature trying to deal with the cause and therefore assisting by adding heat and preparing a decoction of vervain, centaury, cleavers, and raspberry leaves and after straining this, adding a powerful tablespoonful of cayenne pepper to two pints, now boiled down to less than a litre of decoction. This he gives to a typhus fever patient with positive results.[32]

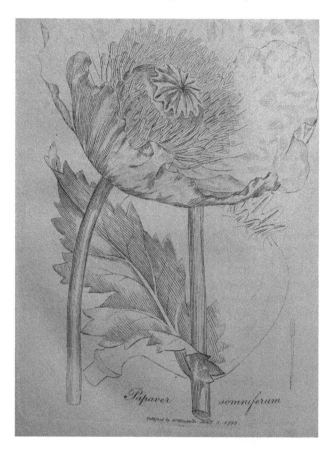

Opium poppy. *Medical Botany*, Woodville.

The Key and Companion to the Poor Man's Friend by Samuel Thompson M. B. had reached its twelfth edition by 1848. This small, highly concise guide contains information on sixty-six herbs, mostly available from the English countryside or garden. There is a marked absence of American plants and readers are encouraged to apply to an address in Halifax if they have questions on any plant or disease with a remittance of eighteen postage stamps. This would cover advice and a prescription. For those who could read there would be many familiar herbs their granny might have picked and used.

Dried herbs are also offered for sale. There is no lobelia, and vapour baths are replaced by cold sponging, exercise, and air. As for diet, there is a table showing the amount of earthy, indissoluble matter in fruits, vegetables, animal food, dairy, and fish. It is stated that chemists affirm premature old age to be due to an excess of calcareous matter taken in with food.[33] Study of botany is recommended. Recipes for specific treatments include liquorice root in a medicine for coughs and colds, elecampane and marshmallow for whooping cough, ginger in an indigestion mix, and nettle for stopping bleeding and in a drink with fennel and mallows for nervous diseases. Plantain and betony do not enter the recipes. A sick headache is treated with a decoction of rosemary, lavender and feverfew.[34] It all looks very innocent until the recipe for making laudanum is noted; "Take of hand purified Opium powdered, ten drachms; proof spirit of wine, one pint, digest for ten days, then strain it".[35]

It is hard for us to imagine the scale of opium use but in *Thomson's London Dispensatory* of 1826 we find, "Opium is more generally used than any other remedy …. consumption in Great Britain alone being upwards of 16,500 lbs".[36] Anyone could readily buy opium in the form of laudanum, paregoric or syrups from the druggists, and we find it recommended as of considerable efficacy in many spasmodic diseases. Paregoric has always struck me as an emotive title for a medicine. It is named from the Greek "paregoricon" meaning soothing. Originally applied to a soothing speech, the word had been in use for a long time as applied to pain relievers. Paregoric was widely prescribed and first appeared in the 1721 Pharmacopoeia.[37]

At the end of the previous century, some druggists had formerly been trained as apothecaries, now this was no longer the case. In *The Westminster Magazine* for 1782 a question to the editor asks what is the difference between an apothecary and a druggist? The answer reads, … "the same that subsists betwixt a Breeches-maker and a Taylor".[38] Danger associated with druggists being in charge of selling poisonous substances caused much concern, particularly among apothecaries, but was not stopped. Syrups for children were especially cheap. The formulation of laudanum had varied over centuries as we see from the Pharmacopoeias. At the end of the eighteenth century, it was rendered more powerful. Also, not all opium was the same.

Laudanum had been properly entitled *Tinctura Thebaica*, a reminder that from the sixteenth century onwards a superior opium had been imported from Cairo, prepared in the district of Thebaid, near Karnak. However, the 1751 history tells us that Thebaic opium is no longer distinguished from that of Asia Minor.[39] Healde's 1791 translation of the *Pharmacopoeia* records the new, stronger recipe.[40] Earlier *Tinctura Thebaica* also contained heating, stimulant spices—cinnamon and clove—to offset the cooling, sedative effect of opium and the tincture liquor had been wine. With the stimulants removed and proof-spirit that had replaced wine extracting a higher proportion of opium, the tincture was potentially more dangerous.

Thornton's Herbal of 1810 gives us a typical list of when opium was used, chiefly to mitigate pain, diminish morbid sensibility (delirium and tremors), procure sleep, allay spasms, check diarrhoeas, and other excessive discharges. Also, in fevers, small-pox, dysentery, cholera, colic, gall-stones, tetanus, asthma, dyspepsia, hysteria, syphilis, sometimes in childbirth and for external problems such as wounds, skin problems, and burns.[41] From other sources we can add coughs, teething babies, almost every childhood illness, neuralgia of all types, recurrent headaches or migraine, toothache, insomnia, internal bleeding, for after effects of being bled by a physician, and rheumatism. It was commonly believed, even by physicians, that addiction only happened after the patient had taken it for a long period.

Taking laudanum was regarded very differently to smoking opium. Many patients who found themselves addicted, however, were not thankful for what had been done to them by prescribed medicine. Heroic medicine administered by physicians turned opinion towards the botanic medicine available. At a time when life was extremely hard for so many who were often left helpless in the face of diseases that were encouraged by the miserable conditions in which they lived and worked, Coffin provided another option to the oblivion of cheap opium.

References

1. William Fox, *The Working Man's Model Family Botanic Guide* (Sheffield: William Fox & Sons, 1909), 22.
2. Fox, *The Working Man's Model Family Botanic Guide*, 23.
3. Ibid, 28.
4. Ibid, 28.
5. Barbara Griggs, *Green Pharmacy* (London: Jill Norman & Hobhouse, 1981), 198.
6. A. I. Coffin, *Botanic Guide to Health*, 49th edition (London: Haynes, Coffin & Co., c1900), 74.
7. Coffin, *Botanic Guide to Health*, 74.
8. Ibid, 67–68.
9. Ibid, 136–139.
10. Ibid, 69.
11. Ibid, 253.
12. Ibid, 255.
13. Ibid, 53.
14. Patrick O'Brian, *H.M.S. Surprise* (London: Harper Collins, 1993), 374.

15. Coffin, *Botanic Guide to Health*, 53–54.
16. Henry Beasley, *The Druggist's General Receipt Book* (London: J. & A. Churchill, 1895), 182.
17. Coffin, *Botanic Guide to Health* 79–81.
18. Ibid, 315–316.
19. Ibid, 103.
20. Amy Bess Miller, *Shaker Herbs. A History and a Compendium* (New York: Clarkson Potter Inc., 1976), 1–4, 198.
21. Coffin, *Botanic Guide to Health*, 307.
22. Urban Sylvanus, *The Gentleman's Magazine and Historical Chronicle*, Vol. XV. (London: Edward Cave, 1745), 194.
23. Coffin, *Botanic Guide to Health*, (penultimate page of the book).
24. Griggs, *Green Pharmacy*, 214.
25. Tarl Warwick, ed, Wesley *Primitive Physic* 1743 (South Carolina: CreateSpace Independent Publishing Platform, 2016).
26. Coffin, *Botanic Guide to Health*, 263.
27. Ibid, 289–290.
28. Ibid, 294.
29. Ibid, 220–223.
30. Ibid, 205.
31. Ibid, 202.
32. Ibid, 375.
33. Samuel Thompson, *The Poor Man's Friend*, 12th edition (Halifax: Thompson, 1848), 21.
34. Thompson, *The Poor Man's Friend*, 15.
35. Ibid, Section Two, Key and Companion, 20.
36. A. T. Thomson, *The London Dispensatory*, 4th edition (London: Longman, Rees, Orme, Brown, and Green, 1826), 462.
37. Barbara Hodgson, *In the Arms of Morpheus* (New York: Firefly Books, 2001), 48.
38. The Proprietor, *The Westminster Magazine*, Vol. X (London: John Walker, 1782), 30.
39. John Hill, *A History of the Materia Medica* (London: Longman, Hitch & Hawes, 1751), 779.
40. Thomas Healde, trans, *The Pharmacopoeia of the R.C.P. of London* (London: Longman, 1791), 104.
41. Robert Thornton, *A New Family Herbal* (London: Richard Phillips, 1810), 526–527.

CHAPTER 24

Reform and Change | 1847–1899

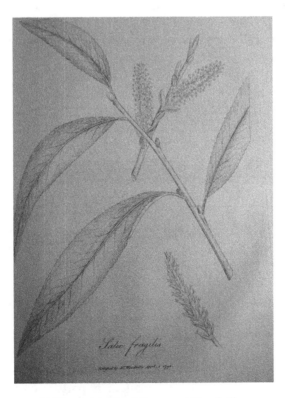

Willow. *Medical Botany*, Woodville.

Having set the broader English scene at this time with options available for the working population and treatments prescribed, we return to following the progress of Coffin's business. Returning to the north of England from America, having left John Skelton in charge, between winter 1847 and autumn 1849, Coffin found that Skelton had proved very popular. He began to see Skelton, who had set up a private business in Edinburgh at the end of his two-year agreement with Coffin, as a formidable rival. Where Coffin sought a monopoly of botanic medicine Skelton welcomed new ways, even warmly greeting the establishment of a homoeopathic doctor in Sheffield. Reconciliation was tried but it was soon evident to Skelton that Coffin still expected supremacy in the botanic market, whereas Skelton promoted self-help with native herbs.[1] By 1852 Skelton had established a herbal import business with a growing number of agents, rivalling Coffin.[2]

Their differences only grew with the arrival of Dr Wooster Beach from America preaching Eclectic medicine and reform. Although equally horrified by heroic allopathic methods, and filled with zeal to change matters, Wooster Beach had very different ideas of how reform should be approached. After learning gentler herbal medicine from a German doctor in New Jersey, using only medicinal plants, he had deliberately studied orthodox medicine, to be accepted by the New York Medical Society, hoping to reform medicine from the inside. This did not go well.

On moving to the more liberal State of Ohio, success rewarded his perseverance and he began training more Eclectic practitioners and writing to advertise his methods.[3] According to Priest, he was responsible for the initial concept of equalising the circulation, which was further developed later by Cook in *Science and Practice of Medicine*, 1879.[4] His reformed medicine did not depend on the heroic poison of mercury or on debilitating bleeding and purging, but on herbal treatments. Arriving in England he was welcomed by Skelton, although they did not entirely agree on all treatments. Matters between Coffin and Skelton came to a head in Bradford at a public meeting in 1852 when Coffin tried to demand his agents used only herbs recommended by him. Skelton challenged Coffin to a discussion and won a decided victory.

In America, Alva Curtis, who had initially worked for Samuel Thomson, had set up his own botanico-medical school and infirmary in physio-medicalism. This included a female medical college where students would be taught everything that they needed to know in just twenty weeks. The fee, he wrote, was less than the cost of a piano and five months practice on it. He regarded the long training of orthodox medical schools as proof that what was called medicine was not a science.[5]

At this point it will be useful to determine the difference between physio-medicalism and Eclectic practice. Physio-medicalism is set out very clearly by Curtis and he boasted that he could cure ninety-nine out of one hundred cases and treat virtually every disease using a single method. Curtis said that in thirty-eight years he had not lost a patient to smallpox or parturition and had performed surgical operations safely using chloroform as an anaesthetic. He did not use any poisonous substance. He believed that the human body is formed and maintained in health by the invisible vital force. In essence, all disease was caused by obstacles to the free flow of this force. Disturbances of this equilibrium caused inflammation and a host of other conditions, including destruction of the tissues. In order to restore health, no treatment should be harmful to organic tissues, or the vital force. This ruled out not only poisonous narcotics, but blistering, cupping and many of the orthodox treatments. Poisons he defines as substances known to have destroyed life in authorised medicinal doses.[6]

While Eclectics gave medicines opposing the action of the disease, Physio-medicalism worked in harmony with the body, recognising indications from the vital force. In order to relax constricted tissue, water treatments from applying cold wet cloths to vapour baths were aided by antispasmodics, often lobelia, which in the face of contradiction by the medical profession, he maintained was harmless. In order to stimulate tissues to health as necessary, heat was applied by giving capsicum, ginger, xanthoxyllum, cloves, and pennyroyal along with lubrication from mucilages. Finally, to restore healthy tone, a healthy lifestyle was recommended as regards diet, fresh air, and so on.[7]

The indications for treatment required, it was maintained, could be discerned promptly by the practitioner noting irregular actions of the nervous or circulating systems or both. Much of the treatment plan is reminiscent of Dr Coffin's methods and Alva Curtis gives due credit to Samuel Thomson who he styles doctor.[8] Emetics and bathing are strongly and frequently recommended.

While equally scathing about orthodox practice, John Scudder in his book *The Eclectic Practice of Medicine* gives a very different picture. In this the practices of dry cupping, cupping with scarification, and particularly irritant plasters used even to promote suppuration, feature in treatments. Eclectic medicine was, therefore, using treatments forbidden in physio-medicalism due to their damaging effects on the vital force.

The patient is given an emetic before other treatments in many cases and this is often followed by a purgative. The potentially poisonous herbs such as belladonna, stramonium, conium, and opium are prescribed fairly often, and gelsemium almost invariably where pain is concerned.[9] Stramonium, conium, and opium are, however, also accepted in botanic and physio-medicalism and the price list at the back of my edition of Coffin's *Botanic Guide to Health* includes belladonna root and leaves, gelsemium root, hemlock leaves and seeds, henbane leaves, and stramonium leaves and seeds.[10] Robinson in his *New Family Herbal and Botanic Physician* wrote of *Datura stramonium* that it was sold for smoking to relieve spasmodic asthma but internally was "a deadly poison, exercising much the same influence as *belladonna*".[11] Robinson pronounces that administration ought to be restricted to persons of medical skill.

The principles of science, based on botanic medicine were enlarging the field of knowledge. The chemist's isolation of active principles was started by a German apprentice pharmacist, Friedrich Wilhelm Serturner in 1803, with the extraction of an alkaloid called morphine from opium. In 1818 the name alkaloid was given to more narcotic substances from plants. It was applied to atropine from belladonna, quinine from Peruvian bark, conine from hemlock, and strychnine from nux vomica. In 1852 salicylc acid was prepared synthetically but the action of the acid had highly irritant effects on the stomach. Nevertheless, doctors were happy to prescribe it, appreciating the therapeutic effects. The milder form, aspirin (acetylsalicylic acid) did not relieve the situation until 1899.[12] Skelton, along with other herbal practitioners, was completely opposed to administering isolated constituents.

In 1854, Mr Brady's medical reform bill was presented to Parliament. The Bill was intended to stamp out quackery, leaving only those in practice who had qualified from an orthodox medical school. At the time it was estimated that the partially trained practitioners outnumbered the licensed medical doctors. The outcry from Coffinites and other botanic medicine supporters was so huge that with friends in parliament, the bill was defeated.[13] The British Medical Association was formed in 1856 and the Medical Act of 1858 established the position of the General Medical Council (GMC) as the authority controlling central registration of physicians and surgeons.

The Pharmacopoeias of Edinburgh, Dublin, and London were now merged. The role of Dispensatories had formerly offered insight into considerations when prescribing and Thomson's dispensatory of 1826 retained a humoral view with cautions on stimulants more readily affecting the sanguine patient, which required lower doses. The phlegmatic temperament is contrasted as having torpid bowels requiring doses of purgatives which would produce alarming results if given to the sanguine.[14] By 1882, this has been reduced to a mere mention of temperament with sex, climate, custom, and age as affecting dosage. In the same paragraph there is a note on the great care required when administering opium to children. A table following of the proportions of the more important drugs of the Pharmacopoeia contained in officinal preparations begins with antimony (tartar emetic), followed by arsenic, mercury and belladonna and ending with many preparations of opium.[15]

In the Medical Act setting up the GMC clause XXXII directed that from the first of January 1859 no person not registered would be entitled to recover charges for medical or surgical procedures or attendance to a patient in a Court of Law. (The GMC policy was to refuse entry on the register to women). Chemists, druggists, and licentiates of The Society of Apothecaries were exempted. However, there was no clause that specifically criminalised unlicensed practitioners. Provision was also made for new charters for physicians in Scotland and Ireland to be granted by the Crown.[16]

The National Association of Medical Herbalists was founded in 1864. In the 1870s the British botanic movement tried a link with the Eclectic practitioners in America. The idea proposed by the Eclectics of being given a "qualification" and allowed to use the letters 'M.D.' after their names by a Medical University in Pennsylvania was enticing.[17] With all the American-inspired herbal factions and their supporters, one herbalist stands out as claiming his own discovery of pure herbalism, firstly in America and then once again bringing it to England.

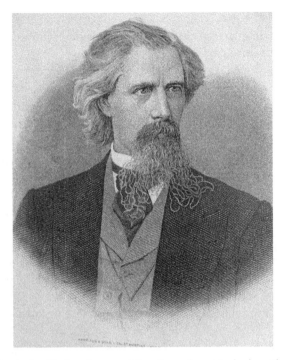

Portrait of Prof. O. Phelps Brown, *The Complete Herbalist*, Phelps Brown.

Professor Phelps Brown's *The Complete Herbalist or the People Their Own Physicians by the use of Nature's Remedies*; was published in London in 1878. In the preface he gives a brief, succinct history of medicine, addressing the main points in a few pages from the Egyptian goddess of healing, Isis, through to Paracelsus, who he calls a Prince of Quacks for introducing mercurial and antimonial practice. Commenting on the lack of progress in medicine so that none of the eminent new schools and sects is more successful than Hippocrates, Galen, or the famed Dr Sydenham of the previous century, he concludes simple herbal medicine is best.

Disillusionment with the ordinary routine of therapeutics led him to reject the many changes in medical doctrines and practice in order to begin his own investigation of the mineral and vegetable Kingdoms.[18] Chemical analysis and experiment convinced him that the materia medica of herbs alone was sufficient without further addition of minerals. As with Culpeper and Paracelsus before him, Professor Phelps Brown came to appreciate the microcosm in man and its relationship within the macrocosm of the universe.

Extensive travel and many years of medical experience and research in the physiology of plants, qualified him to present the system of medication in his book. The Professor cautions readers to take heed of the difference in plants when they are cultivated in a climate foreign to them. He also notes the importance of gathering at the correct season while understanding the chemical constituents of each plant and their medicinal qualities. Using in part the doctrine of signatures, but also their internal biology, he deduces specific uses. He states that plants can be destroyed by minerals and/or poisons just as we can.

Phelps Brown believed that chemical constituents such as iodine should be given through administering the whole plant containing it, rather than isolating the substance and giving that alone. He prescribed mainly North American plants and comments under lobelia, "It was used in domestic practice by the people of New England long before the time of Samuel Thomson, its assumed discoverer".[19] He writes that great skill and caution are necessary when treating such conditions as epilepsy, cramps, and hysteria internally with lobelia or it will cause as much harm as good. In his opinion, it is best applied in an ointment. In fact, he is remembered for his ointments as he had special containers made bearing his name. These are now collectables.

Phelps Brown gives numerous recipes for all manner of treatments and supplied fluid extracts of 143 of the 207 herbs included. His American practice became international when he set up another practice in London and was happy to dispense advice by mail. His wide-ranging approach involves discussion of diseases, treatments, diet, drinks, sleep, air, clothing, hygiene, regulating the passions, and longevity. Additional subjects are urine analysis, advice on the basis of a happy marriage, sexual philosophy and comments on divorce.

Professor Phelps Brown appears to have worked alone and been extremely successful. However, the hoped-for arrangement between English herbalists and the American Eclectic movement was doomed. Many herbalists in Britain could not afford to import and use the concentrated formulas the Americans were prescribing, and were not willing to dispose of much of their familiar materia medica to do so. Of the few degrees that did materialise, one was challenged in court and this did not go well for the herbalist in question who was shown to be a fraud.[20] It was seen that the physio-medicalists in America prescribed in a much more acceptable way.

At this time, Jesse Boot (founder of Boots Chemists) was president of one of the associations involved—the Midland Botanic and Eclectic Association. Another respected member of an English Medical Reform Society and prominent member of the Edinburgh Botanical Society was Duncan Napier. Having treated himself successfully with lobelia sourced from Coffin's herbal warehouse in London, he began by treating family and friends. In 1860 he founded Napiers' the Herbalists in Edinburgh and in 1868 achieved registration as Chemist and Druggist. Napiers was to become a highly successful herbal business, continued by his sons who went into the countryside gathering herbs with him before training as herbalists.[21]

With the added history of Plough Court Pharmacy where William Allen became a partner in 1795, we can see the origins of three paths herbal pharmacy was to take, as chemists, herbalists, and pharmaceutical manufacturer. William Allen was a founding member of the Royal Pharmaceutical Society in 1841 and Allen and Hanbury's Pharmacy was later acquired by Glaxo Pharmaceuticals. A young man who had trained with Jesse Boot, Henry Potter, bought his uncle's business in Fleet Market, London on his retirement in 1846. The elder Henry Potter had moved south from Yorkshire in 1812 to continue as a supplier of herbs and dealer in leeches. Retaining the approach of their founder in combining herbs in medicines to take advantage of their synergistic effects brought great success. Henry Potter the third, with his partner Charles Clarke, expanded the business nationally, supplying, amongst other places the manufacturing centres in the north in the 1880s and 90s. R. C. Wren became a partner in 1896, writing the first Potter's Cyclopaedia of drugs in 1907.[22] Potters began growing, grinding, and distilling herbs, adding laboratories to keep up with the times.

In 1881, a royal commission was appointed to suppress unlicensed practitioners. The National Association of Medical Herbalists made a representation that their members were not simply sellers of herbs but were trained and examined in herbal medicine, materia medica, therapeutics, anatomy, and physiology and must show themselves to be of good character before practising as a member. They also pointed out the large numbers of dependent patients in the manufacturing areas and succeeded in averting suppression.

Interest in herbal drugs would not seem to have died away when Friedrich Flückiger professor in the University of Strassburg and Daniel Hanbury, fellow of the Linnean and chemical societies of London wrote *Pharmacographia. A History of the Principal Drugs of Vegetable Origin met with in Great Britain and British India*. This considerable work, written for pharmacists, is made fascinating by their wish to record new facts about the plants and trees from painstaking research, rather than simply repeating what has been said in herbals over the centuries.

This remains a valuable secondary source on herbal history, filled with plants familiar to herbalists—the comment under *Lobelia inflata* is telling, "In America it has long been in the hands of quack doctors, but its value in asthma was set forth by Cutler in 1813. It was not employed in England until about 1829, when, with several other remedies, it was introduced to the medical profession by Reece".[23]

In 1886 a proposed Amendment to the Medical Act threatened herbal medicine by making it actionable to practise medicine unless professionally qualified. Once again, the bill was defeated. The year of 1887 saw the publication of a regular Journal of the National Association, *The Botanic Practitioner*. This was followed in 1891 by David Younger establishing a College of Herbal Medicine in London with a clinic and free dispensary for the poor of the surrounding area. In the 1890s what was to become a familiar battle to be awarded the status of registered practitioners was lost for the first time by the Association. Eventually they formed a limited company in which they were amalgamated with the United Society of Herbalists and the Midland Botanic Society in 1895, as the National Association of Medical Herbalists.[24]

A general updated work had appeared in 1892, Cooley's Cyclopaedia of Practical Receipts, designed as a comprehensive supplement to the Pharmacopoeia and general book of reference. In the two volumes we find a reassuring number of herbs. It is stated in the preface that "in no instance has any formula or process been admitted into this work, unless it rested on some well-known fact of science, had been sanctioned by usage, or come recommended by some respectable authority".[25] With this in mind, we find over one hundred herbal decoctions listed, among them avens root, elecampane, figs, guaiacum wood, horehound, liquorice root, root and herb of marshmallow, mugwort root, myrrh grains, sarsaparilla, turmeric, green bark of walnuts, and yarrow. Herbs also appear under extracts, oils, pills, plasters, syrups, tinctures, and more.

Use of herbs and herbalist practice lived on into the followig century having faced many challenges. Not only from legislation but more fundamentally to the use of native herbs in time honoured fashion, as well as the personal relationship between practitioner and patient in the face of over-the-counter medicine.

References

1. Graeme Tobyn et al., *The Western Herbal Tradition* (London: Churchill Livingstone, 2011), 31.
2. Barbara Griggs, *Green Pharmacy* (London: Jill Norman and Hobhouse, 1981), 215.
3. Griggs, *Green Pharmacy*, 183.
4. A. W. and L. R. Priest, *Herbal Medication* (Essex: C.W. Daniel Co. Ltd, 2000), 2.
5. Alva Curtis, A. M., *The Provocation and The Reply; or, Allopathy versus Physio-medicalism*: (1870), (Miami: HardPress, 2019), 144.
6. Curtis, *The Provocation and The Reply*, 132.
7. Ibid, 133.
8. Ibid, 137.
9. John Scudder, *The Eclectic Practice of Medicine* (Madrid: Hardpress publishing, 2020), Chapter II, Diseases of the Respiratory Apparatus—See Diphtheria & Quinsy.
10. A. I. Coffin, *Botanic Guide to Health*, 49th edition. (London: Haynes, Coffin & Co., c1900), 402–410.
11. Matthew Robinson, *The New Family Herbal and Botanic Physician* (Halifax: William Nicholson and Sons, c1872), 272.
12. Griggs, *Green Pharmacy*, 221.
13. Ibid, 224.
14. Anthony Thomson, *The London Dispensatory*, 4th edition (London: Longman, Rees, Orme, Brown, and Green, 1826), Appendix III, 1019.
15. Alfred Baring Garrod, *The Essentials of Materia Medica and Therapeutics* (London: Longman, Green, and Co., 1882), 484, 497–498.
16. The National Archives. UK Public General Acts. Medical Act 1858. Clauses III, IV, XIV, XV, XXXII. Legislation.gov.uk. https://www.legislation.gov.uk/ukpga/Vict/21-22/90/enacted Medical Act 1858 accessed August 22nd 2022.
17. Griggs, *Green Pharmacy*, 240.
18. O. Phelps Brown, *The Complete Herbalist* (London: Published by the Author, 1878), 8.
19. Phelps Brown, *The Complete Herbalist*, 116.

20. Griggs, *Green Pharmacy*, 241.
21. Tom Atkinson, *Napiers History of Herbal Healing, Ancient & Modern* (Edinburgh: Luath Press Ltd., 2007), 111, 114, 116.
22. R. C. Wren, *Potter's New Cyclopaedia of Botanical Drugs & Preparations* (Saffron Walden: C. W. Daniel Co. Ltd., 1998), XII–XIII.
23. Friedrich Flückiger and Daniel Hanbury, F.R.S. *Pharmacographia. A History of the Principal Drugs of Vegetable Origin met with in Great Britain and British India*, 2nd Edition, (London: Macmillan & Co., 1879), 399.
24. Hananja Brice-Ytsma and Frances Watkins, ed, *Herbal Exchanges* (London: Strathmore Publishing, 2014), 4.
25. W. North, *Cooley's Cyclopaedia of Practical Receipts and Collateral Information* (London: J. & A. Churchill, 1892), Vol. I, 576–586.

SECTION X

THE FIGHT FOR SURVIVAL OF HERBAL MEDICINE | 1901–2021

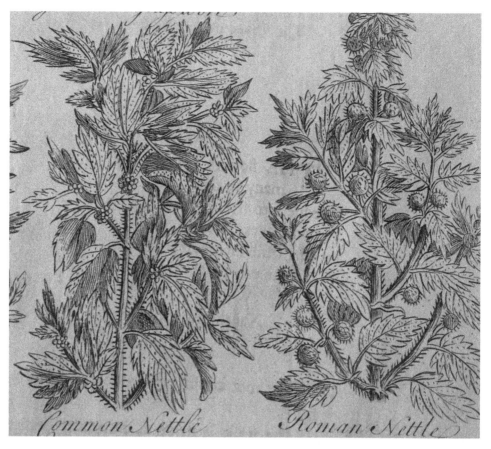

Roman and Native Nettles, *The British Herbal*. Hill.

Key Figures

William Webb (dates unknown), Maud Grieve (1858–1941), Ada Teetgen (1879–1957), Albert Orbell (1901–1986), Fred Fletcher-Hyde (1911–2004), Albert Priest (c1920–2001), Sarah Webb (dates unknown), Hein Zeylstra (1928–2001), Michael Mcintyre, Anne McIntyre, Simon Mills, Graeme Tobyn.

Key Texts

National Botanic Pharmacopoeia, 1905, Scurrah.
The Science and Practice of Herbal Medicine, 1869/70, Skelton.
Profitable Herb Growing and Collecting, 1916, Teetgen.
Standard Guide to Non-Poisonous Herbal Medicines, 1916, Webb.
A Modern Herbal, 1931, Grieve.
Physio-Medical Therapeutics, Materia Medica and Pharmacy, 1932, Lyle.
British Herbal Pharmacopoeia, 1983.

Roles of Women in Medicine

Nurse, midwife, pharmacist, herbalist, physician, surgeon.

Quality Control

Even with constant efforts by all controlling bodies this remains an issue. Practical pharmacognosy is an important part of herbalist training. The currently proposed joint BHMA/EHTPA Herbal Medicine Quality Testing program with availability of testing of small samples of herbs for herbalists is seen as a valuable step forward.

Herb Energetics

Knowledge of the importance of herb energetics is increasingly put into practice again.

Introduction

The twentieth century saw extensive social change, heightened by the after effects of two World Wars. In the first, 1914–18, the importance of national self-sufficiency in growing medicinal herbs was highlighted, but by the second, 1939–45 this was seen as less of an issue by government. Medical science as a whole progressed rapidly in new understanding of physiology, surgery, and laboratory testing. Pharmaceutical companies developed powerful drugs and the National Health Service raised patients' expectations of treatment.

Herbalists also progressed in their standards of education and practical training with a new emphasis on science that enabled some to work alongside physicians and healthcare professionals, gaining respect. Phytotherapy was taught as a degree course and the fight for registration continued into the twenty-first century. Use of herbs broadened, including more from other cultural systems. Endobiogenics provided a new approach.

CHAPTER 25

The 20th Century—Herbs in Wartime | 1901–1945

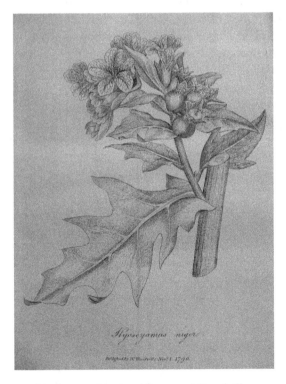

Henbane, *Medical Botany*, Woodville.

With the death of Queen Victoria in 1901 the lengthy Victorian age ended and the Edwardian age began with social changes already being demanded as the suffragette movement gained in strength. Women had made great strides in the way their role in nursing was perceived, as Elizabeth Fry and then Florence Nightingale opened this as a respectable vocation for ladies, but setting training standards with a uniform curriculum and examinations only began in 1916 with the establishment of the College of Nursing.[1]

When we moved into an old cottage in Hampshire and I was seen gathering herbs, I was told of a previous occupant of the house who had made comfrey ointment from the plants still growing in a nearby ditch, seventy years before. I have heard stories about so many others, the great aunts and grandmothers of people coming round my herb garden in the 1970's. One remembered a cupboard for herbs used to treat people on one side of her grandmother's room and another for animal treatments on the other. Then there were the wealthy families who helped the poor around them, Anne Blencowe's descendants still had a queue of locals who came once a week for free treatment to the big house until the coming of the National Health Service in 1948.

Herbalists as a group had already experienced almost half a century of struggle in the face of what might be described as persecution by 1900. The initial aim of the National Association of Medical Herbalists formed in 1864 had been to promote and protect medical herbalism, giving patients their right of choice in treatment. It was hoped that by increasing knowledge of herbal medicine through study and research, with a growing emphasis on training, herbalists would achieve the status they needed to survive continued challenges from orthodox, allopathic medicine. In this, the standard for drugs was set by the Pharmacopoeia, a formulary of recipes pharmacists and physicians were expected to adhere to. A major step for herbalists was the formulation and publication, *The National Botanic Pharmacopoeia*, intended as a textbook and compiled for the National Association of Medical Herbalists by James Scurrah. This was issued in 1905 after many requests from prospective association members. A main aim to keep cost low unfortunately leaves much to be desired from this slim volume recommended as containing "all that the modern well-informed practitioner needs to know".[2]

While apparently saving new practitioners the expense of buying many herbals, readers still needed more background information. One aim of the Pharmacopoeia was to discard "lengthy formulæ, adorned with astrological and superstitious fancies, and give to Herbalists rational and practical preparations".[3] It was an ongoing ambition for herbalists to keep up with new information on constituents and actions from science.

This publication was seen by herbalists as particularly important in the face of developments in the growing drug industry. A strong need was felt to direct attention to the cause of taking safe herbal preparations rather than the irritating and poisonous mineral products, serums and coal-tar derivatives offered by druggists. The materia medica includes approximately 200 herbs. While details of uses of many are adequate, some entries are only four lines long. This is a guide for herbalists who are buying herbs in, rather than gathering, for there is no botanical information and there are no illustrations.

In searching for our chosen herbs, we find elecampane given as expectorant, carminative, diaphoretic, and tonic. It is recommended as having been valued for many years for treating chronic lung diseases and asthma. Elecampane is also eaten as a confection for piles.[4] Ginger root is described, and indicated for cold states and debility of digestion. It is principally to accompany medicines that produce pain and unpleasant symptoms, and is preferred as an infusion.[5] Liquorice extract or root is recommended as demulcent, expectorant, nutrient and slightly laxative and is generally indicated for coughs.[6] Nettles are seen as an astringent tonic, largely to arrest bleeding. Use to act on the kidneys is doubted.[7] Plantain of any kind has been omitted while wood betony on the other hand appears as a whole herb nervine tonic, more frequently combined with other herbs. It is recorded as being used extensively as a substitute for tea in many areas.[8] Henbane is listed as used to reduce nervous excitement and aid sleep in cases of neuralgia, rheumatic and joint pain and asthma. Where with other herbs the part of the plant used is indicated, with henbane it is simply labelled as poisonous.[9]

American herbs include notably the beautiful Beth root, blue cohosh, black cohosh, fringetree, yellow jasmine, lobelia, American mandrake and slippery elm. Appendices contain necessary guidance on the current Patent Medicines Act passed in 1904. There is a list of non-dutifiable titles to guide the practitioner and the exemptions from the Act, which must have been welcomed by herbalists, as they included herbs, simple or mixed.[10] Also, the Schedule of Poisons restricted to sale by a registered chemist and the conditions under which they could be sold. Aconite and Savin join atropine and strychnine with other preparations in Part I. Belladonna and its preparations are included in Part II, which only carries the conditions of the word *poison* being written with the name and the name and address of the seller on the label. They were also restricted to sale by a registered chemist. Arnica root and tincture and digitalis leaves were in a separate unscheduled list, free to be sold by unqualified dealers.[11] It is noticeable that although labelled as a poison in the earlier section henbane does not appear in either list.

The section on preparations is thorough, making it a useful manual in the dispensary. Both crude and fine powders are required and in the back are advertisements by two wholesale druggists and drug grinders, one a manufacturing chemist, Hirst, Brooke and Hirst, the other, W. H. Blunt & Son dealing in botanics, and manufactured Eclectic preparations. There is an illustrated advertisement headed

"To Asthma Sufferers, a Potter & Clarke remedy",[12] I remember this being used by my grandmother. Potter & Clarke are thanked in the front of the book for availability of their various publications.

A further list of publications by the National Association begins with *The Science and Practice of Herbal Medicine* by John Skelton. Of equal interest in our history is an advertisement complete with picture of the Botanic Sanatorium & Training College for Herbalists at Southport offering a change of air and special attention to diet prescribed by their own herbalist. The training college was set up by the American physio-medicalist William Webb, initially in 1901, and after a time of closure, again in 1911 under the auspices of the National Association to further the cause. By 1907 the National Association published a directory of 152 members.[13] Herbalists looked set to make progress towards registration but this was interrupted by the First World War.

At the beginning of the twentieth century, Britain was already heavily dependent on importing herbs for use in making mainstream drugs by pharmaceutical companies, and for supplying vets, homoeopaths, and herbalists, as well as distillers, tobacconists, confectioners, and perfumiers. We are reminded that herbs still play an important part in the officinal Pharmacopoeia in 1914 by the swift response from government to the situation now facing mainstream medicine. Not only was England dependent on German grown herbs, but also on herbs from other parts of the world which were bought through the German suppliers. Such was this dependence that within two months of the outbreak of war in 1914 the Board of Agriculture and Fisheries issued a leaflet on *The Cultivation and Collection of Medicinal Plants in England*.[14] This appeal was not specific to herbalists or druggists but to the general public. The herbal industry had waned as heroic medicines had taken over and there was now a rush to regain knowledge and cultivation.

Mr E. Holmes, an authority on medicinal plants and Curator of the Pharmaceutical Society read a paper on cultivation and collection before the Royal Horticultural Society and this was collated with other material. Although of no help, *The Botanic Pharmacopœia* has honourable mention in the guide below, which describes it as an interesting compilation that shows how common plants are still used, compounded, and esteemed in this particular system of medicine.[15] Potter & Clarke's Cyclopaedia was considered too technical for the man or woman in the street. It became clear that the whole project needed good organisation of co-operative effort and this led to the foundation of the Herb Growers Association.[16]

In 1916 Ada Teetgen's *Profitable Herb Growing & Collecting* was published with all the advice one could hope for, ranging from clear guidance on identification with some good line drawings, herb families, tools needed, and drying herbs—including specified times and methods for the parts of the plant. Much fascinating detail on the contemporary situation is given including the recommendation for the would-be herb gatherer to make his or her list a comprehensive one, including official, non-official, homoeopathic, veterinary, and herbal drugs—as some paid better than others. She wrote, "Even in these days of the Insurance Act the Herbalists flourish, especially in the country districts of the north, and many consult them … It is this large unrecognised herbalist practice which furnishes his best market for the herb collector".[17]

Against this, we must place the depressing statement only two pages later— "Few people except the Society of Apothecaries, the wholesale herb dealers, and their own particular clients, seem to know much about present-day herbalists".[18] Botanical practitioners had no recognised standing, and while there was nothing in the National Insurance Act of 1911 to prevent an insured person obtaining the services of a qualified herbalist, there had been no authoritative statement as to what constituted a qualified herbalist.[19]

Ada Teetgen had written earlier works and on her return from a stay in Canada helping her pregnant sister, she served for a time as a matron for prison services and then as a nurse. She was enthusiastic also on the subject of herbs and pharmacy, and hoped for the revival of the herb industry and possibly even the domestic stillroom after the war. Reflecting how far the average person was from that prospect, she recalled her own astonishment on learning that many of the commonest weeds of lanes and fields have valuable medicinal properties and a price in the drug market. She relates present itinerant root gatherers working for manufacturing chemists to the green men in the previous century carrying their distilling apparatus with them.[20]

Some herbs are best from cultivated stock as with aconite, which has about twenty-four wild varieties, not known to be equally active. This is an example of a herb where because the German root was cheaper the cultivation in England had almost died out. Even though the German root was not pure and had given unreliable results, and this had lessened use of the plant. Pharmaceutical companies such as Burroughs & Wellcome did have a limited supply of herbs from their own medicinal farms. Some of these were sited at Mitcham, Carshalton, Hitchin, Ampthill, Long Melford, Steppingley, Market Deeping, and Wisbech.[21] Herbalists listed around thirty species of North American plants they were using at this time for possible cultivation here. The most difficult to grow being *Hydrastis canadensis*.[22]

Herbalist Maud Grieve had set up the Whins Medicinal and Commercial Herb School and Farm at Chalfont St Peter some years earlier, in 1905. A Fellow of the Royal Horticultural Society, President of the British Guild of Herb Growers and Fellow of the Science Guild, Mrs Grieve dispensed her encyclopaedic knowledge of plants with courses on growing, collecting, drying, and marketing medicinal herbs. When it came to the First World War, she also published helpful pamphlets on cultivation of specific herbs which included the uses of herbal medicines to aid the war effort.[23]

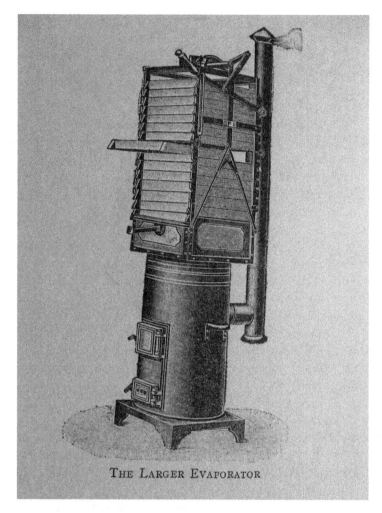

THE LARGER EVAPORATOR

Herb Dryer, *Profitable Herb Growing and Collecting*, Teetgen.

Ada Teetgen paid particular attention to those herbs regarded as essential to mainstream medicine. She noted that by 1916 Continental supplies of foxglove leaves had stopped. The wild plant could however, be collected. Great care was needed in correct gathering and drying but Ada confidently confirmed that she has been able to dry the leaves so that they retained their colour and their activity for eleven years. She also noted that one British firm exported large quantities of the leaves to the United States that had been physiologically tested after drying. Best practice was to dry them in the shade and then store in closed barrels or boxes.[24]

Five more herbs from the Solanaceae family were required by the Board of Agriculture to be grown in greater quantities for officinal drugs. Belladonna, henbane, and datura were already grown on herb farms, but details were now given for others to grow them. Much of the belladonna had come from Germany, one grower there exporting 30,000 lb of it every year to England. A shortage was therefore expected for some years. Necessary to supply atropine and hyoscyamine, belladonna was a particular concern as it should not be harvested until the fourth year of growth, although the third was suggested in the circumstances. It was recorded that British belladonna yields more atropine than the German and that Mr Beetham Wilson, a Dorking analytical chemist, had obtained wild belladonna roots at the outbreak of war. He now had 3,000 plants still a few inches high in their second year.[25]

A letter of appeal is reproduced in Ada's book asking for all those working for the benefit of horses at the front to gather elderflowers and either to dry them to be sent with directions for making a cooling lotion, or to make elderflower ointment for veterinary use. Ointment and bags to be sent to the Blue X hospitals.[26] Gertrude Jekyll organised gardeners to grow Calendula and shipped the herb to France for men in the trenches. As may be imagined many dressings were needed for the horrific wounds encountered in the war and there were problems supplying cotton wool. Sphagnum moss was gathered in huge amounts as a superior substitute. Ada wrote of a new works opening in Edinburgh for cleaning and treating the moss in readiness. She suggested gathering from the Wye Valley, Lake District, and Wales, in addition to Scotland.[27] Sphagnum moss is able to absorb twenty to twenty-two times its own weight in liquid, making it superior to the cotton wool as a wound dressing. By the end of the war up to a million dressings per month were being sent to military hospitals.[28]

The War ended in 1918 and the hoped-for return of the British herbal industry did not appear. Although after the war there was disappointment for many who had set out to grow herbs for profit during those dark days, interest in herbs had been re-vitalised. Meanwhile, although their political ambitions had been thwarted by the war, herbalists had not been idle. In 1916, The *Standard Guide to Non-Poisonous Herbal Medicines* was published, edited by William Webb. This contained chapters by physio-medicalists from America as well as England. The Materia Medica containing thirty-one American herbs was written by Alva Curtis and includes American herbs familiar to us today, such as *Hydrastis canadensis, Lycopus virginicus, Eupatorium purfoliatum, Baptisia tinctoria,* and *Phytolacca decandra*. Almost the same number of native British plants was detailed by physio-medicalist Richard Lawrence, President of the Bolton Linnean Society. This Society met regularly, going on country rambles in summer, gathering specimen herbs and holding discussions and lectures on symptoms, pathology, and treatments in the evenings.[29] Of the British plants, plantain is represented possibly owing to the quoted note from John Skelton who recommended it particularly for making an ointment to treat piles. Use to treat thrush in children is also given, along with the herb's past high reputation. Wood betony is given the praise it deserves with the comment that it cannot be over-rated as a stomachic. And there are recipes for headache, neuralgia, and bilious complaints.[30] Webb himself contributed several chapters to the book including Formulae for Compound mixtures.

His American wife, Sarah Webb who later taught for the National Association School in London contributed the therapeutics section on the nervous and sympathetic nervous system in relation to the abdominal brain.[31]

The effects of the legal position of herbalism in England, and challenging recent history show in the vitreolic rhetoric in Webb's contributions against doctors and the growing interference from Parliament. He also regarded herbal medicine in England as having sadly lapsed since the time of Culpeper. While admitting physio-medicalism had rejected what he termed as Culpeperism, presumably referring to astrology, although far more was involved, he saw America as taking up the abandoned cause.[32] Herbalism was already receiving growing interest due to the focus on herbs in the experience of the general public during the war. An encouraging number of students were signing up to the tutorial course of the National Association with 112 students accepted in 1922.[33]

It was decided once again to lobby for registration. The Medical Herbalists' Registration Bill was introduced into the House of Commons in 1923, and passed the first reading. However, that session of Parliament had a short life and the Minister did not give time for a second reading. Under Parliamentary Notes in the first issue of *The Medical Herbalist*, August 1925 members were urged to interview their parliamentary representatives and it was recorded with satisfaction that there were already over 100 supportive MPs. The bill provided for registration of medical herbalists who had passed an exam to prove their fitness for practice.[34] *The Medical Herbalist* journal is explained by the President of the Society, Joseph Watmore, as fulfilling the advice of the chief secretary to Lloyd George in educating the public and creating a public demand for herbalist treatment.

Herbalists were also advised to improve their training facilities and programme. In 1925 the Postal Tuition Course available offered a thorough groundwork in anatomy and physiology, materia medica and therapeutics, pathology and physical diagnosis, diseases of women and children and chemistry in the first year. The second year's course consisted of an advanced study of the above subjects and medical jurisprudence.[35] Clearly nothing was happening to extend this training, for an editorial comment in *The Medical Herbalist* of October 1930 reads "For many years now our Education Scheme has done great and valuable service in teaching the principles and practice of Herbal Medication, but for many years it has also remained stationary, and it has not as was intended, blossomed out into its full growth as a school and teaching centre for Herbal students ... Are we as an Association devoid of all ideas and plans for the furtherance of education in this country?".[36]

By December of that year real worry is expressed about the numerous free clinics, school welfare services, and baby welfare centres providing competition to herbalists who charged fees. With the GMC proposal to the government for a state medical service catering for every man, woman, and child on the lines of health insurance it is clearly seen that people will not choose to pay if they have free treatment from a doctor on offer. This is followed by the strong suggestion that what was needed was a medical herbalists' trade union to fight for the rights of members.

While there were concerns in the National Association about the future of members, the College of Botanic Medicine was opened in London in 1931. This was, of course not the only source of herbal education. Mrs Grieve had continued with teaching and writing. Hilda Leyel, author of many books on herbs herself, including a history, *The Magic of Herbs* worked closely with her.[24] Hilda inspired the work that was to make Mrs. Grieve famous, *A Modern Herbal*. This was a compilation of information leaflets printed during the war with additional material. Having taken on the gargantuan task of editing the whole book, in response to the request from the publisher, Hilda also added North American plants.[37] The final result was published in 1931 and contains many references to our history and knowledge gained from centuries of traditional practice. It has been an exceedingly popular and influential herbal.

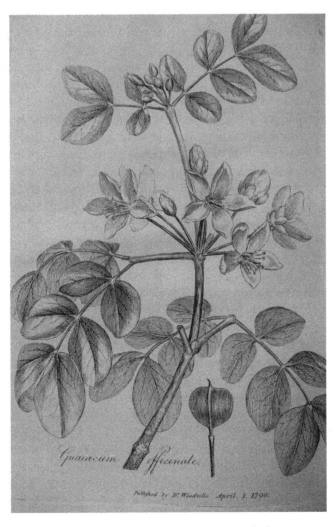

Guaiacum, *Medical Botany*, Woodville.

In 1932, it is clear that the mood of many of the National Association members was to turn finally away from their long heritage of practice and identify themselves as a group with physio-medicalism, cementing their links with their colleagues in America. This is evidenced by a number of articles that appeared in *The Medical Herbalist* relating to physio-medicalism including on Samuel Thomson's favourite herbs of *Lobelia inflata* and *Capsicum*. The National Association also reprinted an important physio-medicalist textbook from 1897 written by the professor of therapeutics at the Chicago Physio-Medical College, Lyle.[38] In the new edition, it was stated that herbs for which there is doubt in efficacy had been removed and some new ones added. The opening synopsis and pharmacy treatise were left as written forty years earlier.

This re-inforced the rule of respecting the evident condition of the vital force of the patient as guiding the herbalist in diagnosis, prognosis, and treatment, with the emphasis on physiology as understood in physio-medicalism. Opposed to the stance of science as they were, they yet looked upon urinalysis and microscopy as valuable in diagnosis. The materia medica is large but with little detail for many herbs. This was a textbook for the school and the editor of *The Medical Herbalist* in September 1932 states, "We are Physio-Medicals by education and training".[39]

In the presidential address from the 1932 sixty-eighth Annual Conference of the National Association, Mr Wilson is quoted saying he hoped that great progress would be made in respect of entrance of students for the diploma. He predicted that the time would come when membership must be restricted to those who qualified by examination.[40] A new edition of *The National Botanic Pharmacopoeia* is hot off the press. This time edited by Alfred Hall and Arthur Barker. Hall taught chemistry on the postal tuition course, while Arthur Barker taught pathology and physical diagnosis. There are marked changes in this new Pharmacopoeia, with some detail of the part of the plant used, appearance of the herb, individual constituents, actions, and uses.

Of eighty-one herbs, half are native British plants, with almost as many American herbs. Some herbs had long been established in British use from India, Africa, and the Mediterranean. Recipes include vinegars and waters; most of these—dill, anise, caraway, clove, cinnamon, fennel, peppermint, and spearmint—were now made by the inferior method of shaking the essential oil with water and filtering as in the British Pharmacopoeia. Due to their delicacy, elder flower, chamomile, orange flower, rose, and meadowsweet are each distilled with ten pounds of flowers to the gallon.[41] Other items relating to historical pharmacy are confections, with rose sugar and honey. Insufflations include hydrastis snuff and menthol snuff. Under nebulae are benzoin, eucalyptus, and camphor spray. Bringing the Pharmacopoeia up to date are the assay methods of standardisation for liquid extracts of Cinchona and Hydrastis, together with a list of articles used in testing and preparations of the pharmacopoeia. Also, a supplementary list of drugs including such items as agar-agar, galbanum gum resin, hydrastine from golden seal, and lycopodium spores of the clubmoss.[42]

High hopes dwindled as there were not enough students to make the College a continued success in spite of the enthusiastic support of Fred Fletcher Hyde. He was a successful second-generation herbalist whose graduation in botany with first class honours at London University was announced in *The Medical Herbalist* September 1931 with a photo of him.[43] This was his third degree. He planned physics and chemistry courses to add to the training scheme. Sadly, as numbers fell the enterprise became a night school and splinter herbalist groups had divided the National Association, even before bombing in the Second World War closed the College in 1940.[44]

At the end of the First World War Albert Orbell had been assisting with surgery and planned a career as a surgeon. However, a bout of rheumatic fever left him unable to continue on that path. After visiting Mr Purdue's herb shop for a purchase, he became friendly with this knowledgeable herbalist and learned herbal practice from assisting him. He had set up in practice after Mr. Purdue's death, having joined the National Association.[45] After some years of successful practice, Orbell brought together a group of interested people to form the Association for Natural Healing. Countryside rambling identifying and gathering herbs and other activities brought in subscriptions to pay for herbal medicine for the poor. An in-patient clinic was a long-term aim and in 1935 the Hospital for Natural Healing was opened in London.[46]

Orbell's charitable work received the support of both West Ham Borough Council and the Minister of Health who had, after negotiation, approved the opening of his clinic as the Hospital for Natural Healing. Five herbal practitioners gave their time voluntarily on particular days of the week, largely to treat the poor. Funds continued to be raised by grateful patients, as members of the Association of Natural Healing and many seriously ill patients were treated. Methods were Eclectic, and Orbell sought and quickly obtained permission from the health minister to treat cases where the doctor was unwilling for him to do so.[47]

The success of the hospital was such that there were plans for an extension and a School of Reform Medicine to be linked with it. Unfortunately, the outbreak of war ended hopes for opening the school. The hospital continued to function and made a valuable contribution to the war effort, as did many other practitioners, Fred Fletcher Hyde among them, in a time when the shortage of doctors was pressing.

In 1941, the Pharmacy and Medicines Act was passed with speed, depriving herbalists of the legal right to supply medicines directly to their patients. Herbalists objected and continued to practise, supplying medicines to patients as members of the Association.[48] World War II saw a very different reaction to that in World War I as once again access to herbs from the re-established German suppliers was cut. The Ministry of Agriculture and Fisheries, Kew Gardens, the Herb Growers, and

Pharmaceutical Society appealed to schools, Girl Guides, Scouts, Women's Institutes, and the Women's Royal Voluntary Service to gather specific herbs.

Best remembered are rose hips and haws to supply vitamin C as citrus fruits were not getting through to England. Horse chestnuts were eagerly gathered and produced glucose for making Lucozade and acetone needed for explosive cordite.[49] Other herbs were asked for—dill, caraway, foxglove, limeflowers, horehound, coltsfoot and valerian, as well as the predictable henbane, and stramonium. With collection of foxglove, it was found that cardiac glycoside levels were highest in July. Conditions in Wales produced the best results.[50] A nurse who had worked at St Barts Hospital in London at the time told me many years later that the gardens were dug over to grow poppies for a safe supply of opium as any from a foreign supply could not be trusted.

Herbs were also needed by the wholesale druggists who appealed for home gathering. One such booklet issued by Brome and Schimmer of London covers sixty-one herbs, from agrimony, thuja, and belladonna to wood-sage, wormwood, and yarrow. Barbara Keen and Jean Armstrong give clear, concise instructions on collection, harvesting, and drying.[51] Where Ada Teetgen had illustrated drying machines in the last war, this time a shed not less than twelve by thirteen feet with a lofty roof is recommended.[52] In 1942, 250 drying sheds were in use nationwide.[53]

Hanging sacks, tea chests, or potato barrels were listed as acceptable containers for dried herbs. Seeds once dried were stored in tins. Sphagnum moss needed a different approach, being collected as tufts and left to dry on the spot in the sun and wind. Partly dried clumps could be shaken and picked clean before finishing. Collection of long-stemmed species was encouraged.[54]

Elecampane is described as found growing in moist meadows and pasture land. The root to be dug in autumn after the flowers have died down and dried. It is listed as diaphoretic and diuretic.[55] The whole nettle herb is to be cut in May for drying as an anti-asthmatic. When cut in June, it is directed to remove the leaves from the stem for drying. Wood betony found in thickets, woods, and road-sides was to be pulled when the flowers are at their best in July and August and dried.[56] There are also neat line drawings of each herb to help with identification. The whole is given approval in the foreword by W. O. James of the Department of Botany, Oxford, dated April 8th 1941.[57] Barbara Keen was still growing an acre of herbs in the early 1970s in Shropshire when I went to buy herbs from her for my first herb garden. On that visit she gave me a copy of the booklet and said that she had been growing an acre of herbs for forty years and was just beginning to really know about them. When I had been growing herbs for the same time, I knew what she meant.

We have followed the attitudes to herbs and herbalists in the twentieth century through two World Wars and seen the challenges met with determination for herbal medicine to survive in a much-changed world. In 1945, the National Association was renamed the National Institute of Medical Herbalists (NIMH) and a smaller group, the British Herbal Union had sprung into existence. Put together they did not represent even half the herbalists in practice and several groupings were tried in advance of asking again for government recognition. When the National Health Service was formed in 1948, members of NIMH were offered a subordinate place within it by Aneurin Bevan, which they refused. In America, the last Eclectic School closed in 1938 and the future looked bleak. Concern that the ease with which patients would now be able to access free medical care would discourage patients from consulting herbalists, painted a dark picture.

References

1. G. Barry and Lesley Carruthers, *A History of Britain's Hospitals* (Lewes: The Book Guild Ltd., 2005), 348.
2. James Scurrah, *The National Botanic Pharmacopœia* (Bradford: National Association of Medical Herbalists, 1905), Preface.
3. Scurrah, *The National Botanic Pharmacopœia*, IX.
4. Ibid, 31–2.
5. Ibid, 40.
6. Ibid, 53–4.
7. Ibid, 65.
8. Ibid, 94.
9. Ibid, 45.
10. Ibid, 195–197.
11. Ibid, 214–217.
12. Ibid, penultimate page of the book.
13. Hananja Brice-Ytsma, and Frances Watkins, ed, *Herbal Exchanges* (London: Strathmore Publishing, 2014), 5.
14. Ada Teetgen, *Profitable Herb Growing & Collecting* (London: George Newnes Ltd., 1916), 1.
15. Teetgen, *Profitable Herb Growing & Collecting*, 11.
16. Ibid, 3.
17. Ibid, 11.
18. Ibid, 13.
19. Ibid, 13.
20. Ibid, 13.
21. Ibid, 8.
22. Ibid, 8.
23. Peter Ayres, *Britain's Green Allies. Medicinal Plants in Wartime* (Leicestershire: Matador, 2015), 35–7.
24. Teetgen, *Profitable Herb Growing & Collecting*, 141–142.
25. Ibid, 149.
26. Ibid, 170.
27. Ibid, 115.
28. Ayres, *Britain's Green Allies*, 45.
29. William H. Webb, ed, *Standard Guide to Non-Poisonous Herbal Medicine* (Southport: Webb, 1916), XX.

30. Webb, *Standard Guide to Non-Poisonous Herbal Medicine*, 211.
31. Ibid, 17–25.
32. Ibid, VI–VII.
33. Barbara Griggs, *Green Pharmacy* (London: Jill Norman & Hobhouse, 1981), 272.
34. J. Whatmore, "Parliamentary Notes", *The Medical Herbalist*, Vol. 1, No. 1 (London: NAMH, August 1925), 28.
35. H.R.G. Skelton, "Postal Tuition", *The Medical Herbalist*, Vol. 1, No. 2 (London: NAMH, September 1925), inner back cover.
36. The Editor, "Editorial", *The Medical Herbalist*, Vol. 6, No. 3 (London: NAMH, October 1930), 38.
37. Maud Grieve, *A Modern Herbal* (Adelaide: Jonathan Cape. Saavas, 1984), XIV.
38. T. J. Lyle, *Physio-Medical Therapeutics, Materia Medica and Pharmacy* (London: The National Association of Medical Herbalists, 1932).
39. The Editor, "Editorial", *The Medical Herbalist*, Vol. 8, No. 2 (London: NAMH, September 1932), 21.
40. W. T. Dawes, "68th Annual Conference: Presidential Address", *The Medical Herbalist*, Vol. 8, No. 2 (London: NAMH: September 1932), 25.
41. Alfred Hall, & Arthur Barker, *The National Botanic Pharmacopoeia* (London: National Association of Medical Herbalists, 1932), 43.
42. Hall & Barker, *The National Botanic Pharmacopoeia*, 119.
43. The Editor, "Leicester Man's Exam Success", *The Medical Herbalist*, Vol. 7 (London: NAMH, September 1931), 26.
44. Griggs, *Green Pharmacy*, 274.
45. Brice-Ytsma, and Watkins, *Herbal Exchanges*, 31.
46. Ibid, 34.
47. Ibid, 32.
48. Griggs, *Green Pharmacy*, 275–6.
49. Ayres, *Britain's Green Allies*, 84.
50. Judith Sumner, *Plants Go to War* (North Carolina: McFarland & Co. Inc., 2019), 188.
51. Barbara Keen and Joan Armstrong, *Herb Gathering* (London: Brome and Schimmer, 1941), 9–16.
52. Keen and Armstrong, *Herb Gathering*, 11.
53. Ayres, *Britain's Green Allies*, 67.
54. Sumner, *Plants Go to War*, 188.
55. Keen and Armstrong, *Herb Gathering*, 28.
56. Ibid, 46.
57. Ibid, 7–8.

CHAPTER 26

Peace, Politics, and Phytotherapy | 1947–2023

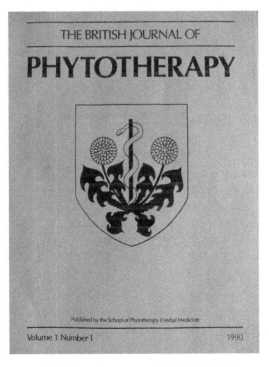

The British Journal of Phytotherapy, Vol. 1. 1990. Courtesy College of Practitioners of Phytotherapy.

After the war, there was still a hard road to economic recovery. Food rationing continued for several years on some items, such as sugar, which as it happened was helpful to health. The population as a whole had deep trauma and loss to recover from and there was a need for re-building in every sense of the word. The Hospital for Natural Healing, funded by charity and run with dedication and goodwill had survived. Albert Orbell the herbalist founder and head had taken an Eclectic approach using a mix of orthodox and herbal treatment before and during the war. In 1947 Orbell declared the Hospital for Natural Healing would give fundamentally herbal treatments. NIMH helped with funds as education began again.[1]

One of Albert Orbell's students had been Albert Priest who began practice in 1948. He was later Director of Education for NIMH. Working with his wife who was a homoeopath, they wrote *Herbal Medication: A Clinical and Dispensary Handbook* published in 1959 and again in 1983, promoting physio-medicalism. Although basically a handbook in the later chapters, Thurston's focus on reassessment of anatomical and physiological values results in chapters on eliminative functions, circulatory dynamics, nervous equilibrium, and alterative changes.[2]

In the 1950s, pharmaceutical companies began a brief enthusiasm for exploring plant drugs but by the following decade, it had passed. Thalidomide was a widely prescribed drug produced by molecular synthesis rather than being a synthetic copy of a plant constituent—it was intended to lead a new way. The results of the tragedy which accompanied use of thalidomide and more unfortunate side effects with eraldin, which blinded some angina patients, coupled with the devastating effects of chemotherapy of the time turned the public attention back to safer herbal treatments. Thalidomide was prescribed for thousands of pregnant women to reduce morning sickness and caused mutations in the foetus. Many babies were born with severe defects such as malformed arms and legs, deafness, or paralysis of certain muscles. Recognition of what was happening and removal of the drug was painfully slow, taking years. The government was also to react to public concerns about what was now called iatrogenic disease and harmful side effects of drugs by drafting a fresh Medicines Bill in 1964, restricting who was entitled to prescribe and dispense medicines.

Fred Fletcher Hyde led the movement with other herbalists against this new, possibly lethal threat to herbal medicine, which would have restricted herbal prescribing to doctors. Members of Parliament were deluged with letters from grateful patients and the sheer force of public opinion once again saved the cause of choice for patients in their medical treatment. The British Herbal Medicines Association (BHMA) was formed in 1964 to defend the right of the public to choose herbal medicines, while promoting high standards of quality and safety through advancing the science and practice of herbal medicine by modern techniques. It also aimed to encourage wider knowledge of herbal medicines.

Fletcher Hyde chaired the Scientific Committee of the BHMA and through negotiations with the Government a vital exemption was inserted in the Bill. This allowed for remedies to be given if prepared on practitioner's premises where the public could be excluded, but only when requested following a private consultation, or to those asking on behalf of another such person. In the 1968 Medicines Act, exemption was also given for remedies made by drying, crushing, or commuting them, with a label simply describing the contents.[3] Legislation was not as simple for those manufacturing herbal medicines in the following exemption applying to them. The Traditional Herbal Medicine Products Directive would have a seven-year implementation plan meaning any over the counter remedies medicinal by sale and description would need to be licensed through verifiable research. In 1972, Product Licences were introduced which depended on quality, safety, and satisfying traditional use.

While there was a rise in general interest in herbs in the 1960s and 1970s, there was not a corresponding rise in students wishing to train. Potential legal restrictions had done a lot of damage to confidence. At the Clinic for Natural Healing, no longer termed a hospital, ageing practitioners had no-one to take their place.[4] Training continued in other areas, including postal courses with additional seminars, which had been ongoing since 1969 from Hyde's Herbal Clinic in Leicester. Fred Fletcher Hyde was also Director of Research for NIMH from 1965.

Hyde worked with the BHMA committee to update the herbal pharmacopoeia. The Committee of seven members each contributed on their specialised knowledge. For instance, Professor Shellard carried out chromatographic examination of the herbs while Mrs. Robinson contributed, pharmacy as well as researching literature with Mrs Hyde who also advised on botany and chemistry.[5] The Committee was also able to call on a further three well-qualified advisory members. The resulting 1983 British Herbal pharmacopoeia published by the BHMA brought together previously published Volumes I, II, and III with 233 monographs and reproduced the 1974 preface to Volume I giving details.

In 1973, Hein Zeylstra made contact with Fletcher Hyde. Zeylstra had a background that included growing herbs, organic farming, and studies in pharmacy and plant analysis. He subsequently trained with Fletcher Hyde in a class of three students and by 1980 had opened a full-time school of herbal medicine in his clinic in Tunbridge Wells.[6] These two very different men were to play important parts in developing education for NIMH. Medical herbalism could not afford to be complacent about survival in this constantly developing pharmaceutical world.

Further threats loomed from the European Union directives. In 1980, the BHMA became a founder member of the European Scientific Co-operative on Phytotherapy (ESCOP) together with comparable organisations in Belgium, France, Germany, the Netherlands, and Switzerland. More countries subsequently joined. Their aims were to advance the status of phytomedicines throughout Europe and assist harmonisation of regulatory status at the European level.

During the 1980s in Britain, public appreciation of herbs and health gradually became better informed. Later in the decade, there were many articles appearing in popular as well as health magazines offering information. Health food shops were busy and, as well as writing for a wide range of magazines on herbs, I had a role in educating on diet (including herbs) at a local comprehensive school. Meanwhile, interest in training had been rising in the south. From the membership lists of NIMH, it can be seen that where of 189 members in 1937/38, 106 of them practised in the industrial midlands and the north, in 1983 of 113 members, northern practitioners had dwindled to thirty-six with sixty-three south of Birmingham and a much smaller number in the regions.[7] Changes were also noted in the social class of the most likely patients for the herbalists. The Welfare State now cared for those in poverty, an aspect of herbalism that had been ever present and one which was highlighted during the Industrial Revolution.

Zeylstra and Fletcher Hyde worked together to restore professional and educational standards to meet the growing interest from the public. Zeylstra re-wrote the NIMH course as parts of it dated back to the 1920s. He remained on the NIMH council until the end of the 1980s but increasingly introduced the European view of the role of practitioners who could work with other healthcare professionals and preferred the term *phytotherapy*.[8]

Some herbalists went on to train in other herbal systems. Michael McIntyre, who trained in the 1970s had been brought up in Malaysia and developed a strong interest in Chinese culture from living amongst Chinese people. After meeting another herbal practitioner, Giovanni Maciocia, soon after starting to practise, McIntyre decided to take an acupuncture course with him at the Nanjing College of Traditional Chinese Medicine to integrate with his herbal practice. Searching for a prescribing system, he followed this with two further courses and clinical training in TCM at Nanjing, qualifying in 1987. He then opened the first British School of Chinese herbal medicine with Giovanni, importing Chinese herbs to serve the school.[9] Michael McIntyre was principal of the school with Mazin Al Khafaji until 2000.

One pupil, Dedj Leibbrandt joined the two-year course with clinical hours in China because, as she told me, after qualifying in Western herbal medicine she felt she did not have sufficient guidance on dermatology treatments. Chinese herbal medicine, she understood, had a high reputation for treating the skin.[10] Numerous budding practitioners have looked at the long established systems of medicine in the East that have apparently not changed over centuries and felt the lack of guidance from a strong Western philosophy that applies to treatment of the individual patient, offering guidance. This issue has come up as a common question from first-year students in my experience.

The more recent history in the preceding pages, with changes in direction of herbal medicine in England, made under constant threat from legislation to end freedom to practise, has quite covered any traces of the humoral system practised here which was comparable to the philosophies from the East. It is, therefore, not surprising, as we follow events in the twentieth century, that we see a continued divergence of approach mirrored by the formation of associations and registers to cater for all needs. While the Association of Master Herbalists was formed in 1995 keeping a strong bond with the North American Eclectic movement through Dr Christopher, with more herbalists qualifying in Chinese and Ayurvedic systems of medicine, The Unified Register of Herbal Practitioners, soon followed. This Register was founded in 1997 from a coalition of small independent herbal schools, bringing together highly trained practitioners in Ayurvedic, Unani t'ibb, Tibetan, Western Traditional and Traditional Chinese Herbal Medicine. They are unified by recognition of the vital force and energetics within herbs and patients, which requires individual prescriptions.

Prescribing herbs simply on the basis of their chemical constituents does not take into account that they will act differently in different types of people. I mentioned that in 1826 this was still acknowledged to an extent with reference to traditional humoral medicine in Western allopathic prescribing. When, or whether, during the Industrial Revolution, this was entirely lost to herbalism is difficult to trace. Specialised research is needed at the end of the eighteenth century and into the nineteenth to discover the answer, as I do not believe that our traditional herbalism had died out before the North American Thomsonian system arrived. We simply do not have the written evidence to prove it. Physio-medicalism has a system different to the humoral and was one some practitioners could not relate to.

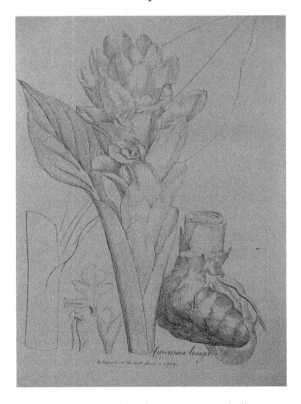

Turmeric, *Medical Botany*, Woodville.

A merging of prescribing herbs from different traditional systems continued. The inclusion of a number of Chinese and Indian herbs, such as andrographis, astragalus, and curcuma, within the materia medica of phytotherapy is evident in the following decade. The College of Ayurveda was established in Milton Keynes in 1997 headed by Maroof Athique. Herbalist Anne McIntyre had already become deeply interested in the philosophy of Ayurveda, taken a shorter course and with other healthcare practitioners benefitted from visiting teachers. She studied with the College, as did Sebastian Pole, graduate of East West Planetary School who later set up Pukka Herbs to ensure a reliable supply of Indian organic herbs. In 2005, the college developed a collaborative partnership with Middlesex University. They were the first British institution to accept Ayurvedic medicine taught as a University degree course.[11]

Practitioners of Ayurvedic and Chinese systems have made the strong point to me that Western practitioners need understanding of the place of both herb and patient within that system of prescribing, before including Ayurvedic or Chinese herbs. The progress of science has been so overwhelming in the past decades leading to an ever more microscopic view, that we are losing the value of, and respect for, ancient wisdom linking the natures of the herbs with our own at the microcosm/macrocosm level. In different parts of the world various cultural approaches have evolved for defining wholistic treatment for individual patients using knowledge of energetics in the plants suitably matched to understanding of the corresponding inner needs and energetic balance within the patient. These are expressed according to that culture and include terms such as vital force, chi, heat, vitality, and so on. These considerations have traditionally been the basis for all treatment and as such need to be respected and understood.

When I trained in phytotherapy I already had a thorough knowledge of the classification of herbs and patient temperaments from the Western humoral tradition in history. I practised this after spending many clinical training hours with Dedj Leibbrandt, where I was exposed to informed Chinese and Western prescribing. The writer I found of most help during this time was Peter Holmes on *The Energetics of Western Herbs*, which seeks to relate Eastern and Western thought and includes aspects of Native American medicine.

The first copy of the British Journal of Phytotherapy was published in 1990 with a distinguished editorial board including members of the original scientific committee from 1965, including Fletcher Hyde and Professor Shellard. It published articles on scientific and clinical studies. Phytotherapy had replaced physio-medicalism as a main teaching at the school. The editorial sets out aims and ideals for phytotherapy, one of which was to promote the philosophy of herbal medicine re-evaluating the meaning of health and disease. In the following article, *What is Herbal Medicine?* It is made clear that assessing plants on their total complex of constituents rather than isolated pure principles would be a step forward.[12] In 1991, ESCOP added to the European debate on safety and regulation of herbal medicines by providing a clear definition, restricting plant medicines to the active ingredients of plants, parts of plants or plant materials, or crude or processed combinations.[13]

In that same year, Simon Mills' book *Out of This Earth* was published and I will never forget my astonishment, steeped in historical herbals as I was at the time, in reading this ground-breaking scientific, thoroughly medical book. It totally changed my conception of herbal medicine and was the first catalyst to my decision to train as a practitioner. By the time I joined students with the College of Phytotherapy in 1999, then located at Bucksteep Manor, an impressive country house with a physic garden, first the full-time training course and then my own distance course had been validated by the University of Wales as BSc (Hons) courses in phytotherapy. The College of Practitioners of Phytotherapy was already a professional body, acting to self-regulate standards of education among practitioners and giving ongoing professional development through regular seminars.

In 1992, the Scottish School of Medicine was set up as an independent charity to promote research and education. In later years, courses would include those on Ayurveda taught by Anne McIntyre, and BSc and MSc courses in herbal medicine. The umbrella organisation, The European Herbal and Traditional Medicine Practitioners Association was established in 1993 and the BHMA brought out the *British Herbal Compendium Vol. 1* as a handbook of scientific and regulatory information on the eighty-four plant drugs contained in volume one of the *revised British Herbal Pharmacopoeia* (1992), bringing the knowledge of fast-moving research up to date for the practitioner and student. Fletcher Hyde, now with Hein Zeylstra and Simon Mills contributed to the sections on therapeutics.[14] Connection with the European community was emphasised and Volume II was to follow in 1996. The editor, Peter Bradley, was responsible for the scientific information in both volumes.

In the 1990s raised awareness of the increasing use of herbal medicines and a number of concerns raised about the safety of particular herbs led to consideration of further action to ensure safe practice. Concerns were recognised across the European community and greater pharmacovigilance was a focus of attention with the idea of bringing the UK into line with the EU. The term traditional use, as applied to herbs, suggests widespread use without documented serious side-effects over a long period of years, in many cases actually centuries. The term begins to be applied as an indication of safety for herbs at this time as use of certain herbs is increasingly questioned before being accepted by the E.U. The growing interest in scientific studies and clinical research on recommended herbs directed attention to available sources of information. Sadly, the British government has never seen the need to fund projects on researching medicinal plants. The pharmaceutical giants of the West were also reluctant. The Chinese government on the other hand has been willing to invest in traditional herbal knowledge. In response, the European Herbal and Traditional Medicine Practitioners (EHTPA) was formed in 1993 as an umbrella organisation to protect practitioners' access to herbs.

Kerry Bone's book *Clinical Applications of Ayurvedic & Chinese Herbs* was published in 1996. *The British Herbal Compendium* and the *Principles and Practice of Phytotherapy* written by Simon Mills and Kerry Bone were used as student guides at the College of Phytotherapy soon afterwards. In the preface of the latter, it is stated that the new NIMH school had decided to adopt phytotherapy following the pattern of established herbal medicine in Germany and France where modern pharmacists and physicians still prescribed herbs.[15] Phytotherapy is described as a successful blending of tradition with science and the work adds a therapeutic context for prescribing.[16] Simon Mills and Kerry Bone have continued to lead in the educational field. The publication of the expanded Commission E monographs added more scientific herbal information. For a more traditional approach Thomas Bartram distilled his long and valued experience into his *Encyclopaedia of Herbs*.

A further inspirational book, published in 1999, was *Herbal Medicine in Primary Care*. An account of a herbalist working within a GP practice where patients could self-refer or be referred by any of the healthcare team, including doctors, and their cases discussed between them.[17] A number of herbalists had varying experiences working within health centres, Graeme Tobyn briefly describes his in the NIMH publication, *Herbal Exchanges*.[18] Anita Ralph, inspired by a menopause study, initially made contact with a local GP, surgery which led to giving talks to practice managers and nurse practitioners. During her Masters study she was contacted by a gynaecologist and a working relationship between them for educating the public on the decision between taking HRT or opting for herbal management of menopausal symptoms has helped many women.[19]

During training, I spent thirty-six hours mostly with experienced herbalist Alex Laird in her clinic within the Dermatology Department at Whipps Cross Training Hospital in London. Time spent learning her approach to skin conditions in the mornings contrasted to the afternoon sessions with the consultant. Sessions with the chest consultant in his outpatient clinic were another valuable learning experience. One of my first actions on setting up in practice was to contact the nearest surgery and give a talk on my training and approach to the doctors there. This stood me in good stead later when I referred a patient for tests and a previously sceptical doctor told our very surprised patient that he knew my training and was happy for him to see me.

In 2001, the editorial in the British Journal of Phytotherapy reported the transformation of education since the middle of the previous decade. Six universities now offered or validated courses and more were being considered. An advanced diploma was available for medically qualified healthcare professionals with the College and increasing awareness of phytotherapy was encouraged within healthcare. The prediction was for 150 practitioners qualifying by mid-decade. University courses varied in content and practical instruction. Some did not teach pharmacy.

Dr. Graeme Tobyn, senior lecturer at the University of Central Lancashire recalled a local agricultural college teaching botany, and some cohorts studied with physiologists.[20] Alison Denham taught pharmacy. NIMH set up a series of seminars, one of which was tutored by Salim Khan, a respected authority on Unani t'ibb medicine and Principal of the College of Medicine and Healing Arts, to explore humoral temperaments.[21]

Alongside this the drive for statutory regulation, which had come so close long before in 1923, had been revived by the combined energies of herbal associations through the European Herbal and Traditional Practitioners Association, formed in 1993 to protect access to herbs for practitioners. A crisis in 1994 when the Medicines Control Agency decided to sign up to the European Directive, which had twenty-five to thirty commonly used herbs on a restricted list stimulated a campaign to save herbal medicine. Help from Paul McCartney through use of his PR company resulted in thousands of letters of support being received by the government. A way out was found by stating that formulations of traditional medicines would not be subject to the ruling.[22] The Labour Health Secretary Alan Milburn appointed Professor Michael Pittilo as Chair of the Herbal Medicine Regulatory Working Group set up to begin the detailed process of herbal Statutory Regulation.[23] A recent decision by the Medicines Control Agency to withdraw several herbs from sale over safety issues, brought concern over maintaining herbalists' rights to access certain herbs. That this might be retained for recognised practitioners with protected title brought further urgency to negotiations.

In the first document about Statutory Regulation, the Department of Health advised that herbal practitioners of all systems, whether Western, Chinese, Ayurvedic, Tibetan, or Unani Tibb would be treated as one body. The EHTPA was given funding for a scoping study as a first step. Alison Denham, the NIMH representative at meetings shared with me an Interim report on the Herbal Medicine Regulatory Working Group (HMRWG) from November 2002. This shows that considerable work went into the effort to gain a consensus with Ayurvedic and Chinese practitioner groups who were not already members of the EHTPA, which had recently set up an Accreditation Board. This had been a major achievement. Concerns of imposing unworkable relationships and costs as part of regulation had to be balanced against the need for the general public to gain safety in knowing the standard of qualification of herbalists when consulting them.[24]

By 2008 the smaller Steering Group was able to show that all the professions were able to agree to the Standards and Code of Practice of the Health Professions Council. This included a common core curriculum across all traditions, ensuring minimum standards of knowledge and safety in prescribing. An independent accreditation board was to verify standards of education. As a result, the Health Professions Council recommended that medical herbalists, acupuncturists and traditional Chinese medicine practitioners should have Statutory Regulation.

In 2011, the government announced that statutory regulation would be in place in autumn 2012. It did not happen. In 2013 the Conservative government reversed the decision, stating a new investigation led by Prof David Walker was to look at state regulation of herbal practitioners. The resulting report in 2015 recommended regulation should not go ahead and this was ratified two years later.[25] The extraordinary dedication of herbalists such as Andrew Chevallier, Peter Conway, Michael McIntyre, and Emma Ferrant, former President of the Register of Chinese Herbal Medicine and others involved in the years of discussions and committees, working on behalf of herbal medicine, had come to nothing. Under the Human Medicine Regulations 2012, the 1968 Medicines Act exemptions no longer applied. The former restricted Schedule 3 herbs were replaced by the new Schedule 20 herbal practitioners only list, with permitted dosages, and herbalists were now not allowed to use third party dispensing arrangements.

As the door on regulation of practitioners closed, university courses also began closing, partly due to the raised tuition fees and lack of support from government affecting mature students from 2012 onwards. The time was right for new provision with the established high standards in herbal education. That some herbal degree courses did not cover the more extensive pharmacy practised by herbalists in the past had been evident for several years. Those qualifying from the School of Natural Medicine, the East West School, the University of Central Lancashire, and Lincoln College had wider teaching in this area. However, poultices, ointments, foot and hand-baths, use of juices and administering powders in troches, conserves, or electuaries were no longer familiar to many newly qualified herbalists.

As a result, after demonstrating historical pharmacy at the annual NIMH gathering in 2009, I was asked by NIMH to tutor a postgraduate course, *Stillroom to Dispensary Hands On*. At the end of a day in 2010 when groups of herbalists had experienced making several historical recipes illustrating different preparations, we then discussed whether any of these recipes might be valuable today and how they might be incorporated into modern practice. There was an enthusiastic response.

That same year the Herbal History Research Network (HHRN) was founded by a group of academic researchers who were also medical herbalists. The aim of the group was and remains to promote and encourage accurate research into the history of herbal medicine, particularly in the Western tradition. The network still flourishes, offering seminars and a website with numerous scholarly blogs on subjects ranging from ancient Greek medicine with a translation *of Galen Simple Medicines Books I–XI*, by John Wilkins, professor of Greek culture, Department of Classics and Ancient History, University of Exeter, through many on the intervening centuries to *A Survey of Deletions of Plant Products From the British Pharmacopoeia Between 1864 and 1993*, by Hilary Mifflin. An online academic mailing list links active researchers, encouraging contact and exchange of queries and knowledge.[26]

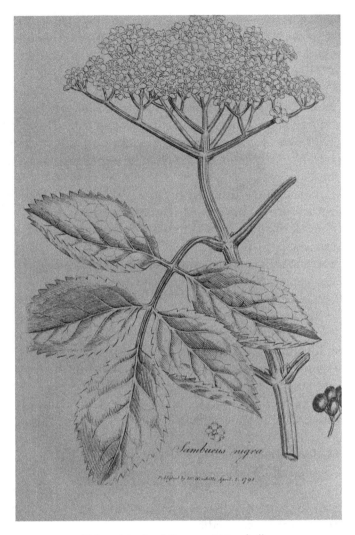

Elder, *Medical Botany*, Woodville.

Two herbalists who had attended the NIMH Stillroom to Dispensary day, Susan Vassar and Maggie Pope, had been working towards a vision for a school offering a longer, six-year training course for several years already. This would include 150 days of face-to-face teaching and hands on experience in botany, pharmacognosy, and pharmacy. They opened a new School of Herbal Medicine in the south west in 2015, with an advanced diploma requiring rigorous training in all core subjects and 500 face-to-face clinical hours. The Betonica Herbalist training programme followed the next year with a blend of online and face-to-face teaching also requiring 500 clinical hours, some of which could be online. A third recently opened school offers the Heartwood Professional course with online learning in either four or six years depending on time available to the student, and again 500 clinical hours. Up to half of these may be online. All three courses are accredited by NIMH. Accreditation of professional standards of education is also granted by the other largest self-regulating body, the College of Practitioners of Phytotherapy as well as the EHTPA.

In the last three years repeated Covid restrictions have affected the ability of herbalists to come together in person and at times their ability to have face-to-face consultations with patients. This restriction on necessary physical observation of the patient, which normally begins with noting how they walk into the consulting room and involves physical examination, has been detrimental. Careful observation of the patient has, I hope, been shown by this history to sit at the heart of successful diagnosis and herbal practice. The present challenges in the health system mean patients are all too often unable to see a doctor in person or obtain simple physical examinations, which might either put their mind at rest or indicate immediate referral. It is an area where herbalists can show, along with the time they give to listening to the patient, the full benefits of a truly patient-centred approach.

The recent history of herbalism in Britain has been dominated by reactive moves to try to ensure the survival of herbalist practice. Science, safety, and monographs have become the watchwords during a time of stark realities. This increased knowledge is another illustration of herbal medicine speaking to the current time. However, if we lose physical and emotional connection with our native plants along the way we will have lost the craft of herbalism which without experience cannot grow.

If anyone is in doubt of what this re-connection with nature involves, they only need to read Christopher Hedley on the inspiration to be found simply walking in the countryside to find the answer. He was a much-loved wise practitioner, who taught many students about plants with emphasis on their being, rather than their chemistry. He centred on "producing the well-rounded herbalist".[27] The award for significant contribution to herbal medicine set up in honour of his memory in 2021 by NIMH, prizes supported by Joe Nasr with Avicenna products, underlines his personal contribution to herbal medicine.

References

1. Brice-Ytsma H. & Watkins F. (ed.), *Herbal Exchanges* (London: Strathmore Publishing, 2014), 37.
2. A. W. and L. R. Priest, *Herbal Medication A Clinical and Dispensary Handbook* (Saffron Walden: C. W. Daniel Co. Ltd., 2000), 7–57.
3. Medicines Act 1968. Part II. Licences and Certificates relating to Medicinal Products. Clause 12. *Exemptions in respect of herbal remedies.* The National Archives, UK Public General Acts. https://www.legislation.gov.uk/ukpga/1968/67/enacted accessed August 4th 2023.
4. Brice-Ytsma & Watkins, *Herbal Exchanges*, 38.

5. Evans et al., *British Herbal Pharmacopoeia* (British Herbal Medicine Association, 1983), 7.

6. Simon Mills, *"A Remembrance of Hein Zeylstra"*, *The British Journal of Phytotherapy*, Vol. 5, No. 4, (East Sussex: The School of Phytotherapy, 1991), 218–219.

7. P. Brown, *The Vicissitudes of Herbalism in Late Nineteenth-and Early Twentieth-Century Britain: Part 1*, The British Journal of Phytotherapy Vol. 2. Spring 1991. (East Sussex: The School of Phytotherapy, 1991), 32.

8. Simon Mills, *"A Remembrance of Hein Zeylstra,"* 218.

9. Personal communication, Michael McIntyre.

10. Personal communication, Dedj Leibbrandt.

11. Personal communication, Anne McIntyre.

12. The Editor, *"What is Herbal Medicine?"*, *The British Journal of Phytotherapy*, 1990. Vol. 1. No. 1. (East Sussex: The School of Phytotherapy, 1990), 8.

13. The Editor, *"Editorial"*, *The British Journal of Phytotherapy*, 1991. Vol. 2. No. 1. (East Sussex: The School of Phytotherapy, 1991), 38.

14. P. Bradley (ed.), *British Herbal Compendium* Vol. 1. (Bournemouth: BHMA, 1992), 7.

15. Simon Mills & Kerry Bone, *Principles and Practice of Phytotherapy* (London: Churchill Livingstone, 2000), XII.

16. Mills & Bone, *Principles and Practice of Phytotherapy*, XIV.

17. Sue Eldin & Andrew Dunford, *Herbal Medicine in Primary Care* (Oxford: Butterworth-Heinemann, 2000), 3.

18. Brice-Ytsma, & Watkins, *Herbal Exchanges*, 102–5.

19. Personal communication, Anita Ralph.

20. Personal communication, Graeme Tobyn.

21. Personal communication, Graeme Tobyn.

22. Personal communication, Michael McIntyre.

23. The Editor, *"Editorial"*, *The British Journal of Phytotherapy.* Vol. 5. No. 4. (East Sussex: The School of Phytotherapy, 2001), 163.

24. Personal communication, Alison Denham.

25. U.K. Parliament. Written questions, answers and statements. Statement by Nicola Blackwood, "Government Response to Professor Walker's advice on Regulation of Herbal Medicines and Practitioners." February 2017. http://www.parliament.uk/business/publications/written-questions-answers-statements/written-statement/Commons/2017-02-28/HCWS505/. Accessed 4th August 2023.

26. https://www.herbalhistory.org

27. Brice-Ytsma & Watkins, *Herbal Exchanges*, 119–122.

CHAPTER 27

Looking Back—Herbs and Treatments Through Time

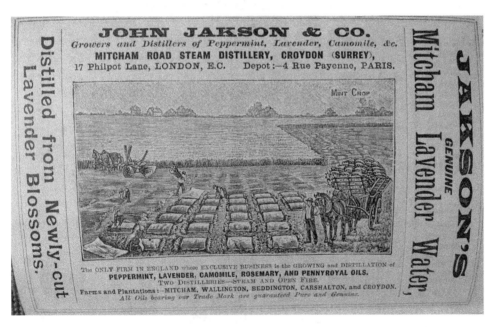

Jakson's Advertisement, *Pharmaceutical Formulas*, MacEwan.

Having reached the present day in our account of herbal medicine we can now look back at the use of our chosen herbs that represent the hundreds of others that would form a complete British pharmacopoeia. Choosing which of the many possible herbs to follow was difficult. My choice is a deliberate balance of native and introduced herbs, with betony, plantains, nettle, and henbane grown in Britain from very early times, and then elecampane, ginger and liquorice. Between them, these herbs have provided treatment for each of the conditions we have also followed. In the concise details from current pharmacy below, it should be understood that although certain main constituents have been highlighted, other constituents in the whole herb and synergy between them should also be regarded as important in their healing role. The parts, dosage, and indications given for each herb are those used in current practice today.

Plantain (*Plantago major, P. lanceolata*)

Including plantain was an easy decision. Long entries on plantain began with Dioscorides giving styptic and anti-inflammatory actions in treating dog bites and ulcers, tuberculosis of the lungs, and dysentery. The cooling juice was applied to burns and both plantains were associated with treating lymph glands in the neck and throat. Ribwort was always looked upon as less powerful than the broad-leaved herb. Plantains have eighteen to twenty-two different uses across the medieval and stillroom periods, including for fevers, in ear and eye drops, for abscesses and wounds. It is extraordinary that Woodville in 1790 can only say that despite a reputation as the best wound herb, plantain is now omitted from the Pharmacopoeia.[1]

Part Used: Leaf
Dosage: 6–12 g, 6–12 ml, 1:5 tincture per day.[2]
Constituents: Glycosides, including aucubin, tannins, flavonoids, apigenin, baicalin, allantoin, steroids.
Actions: Diuretic, anti-haemorrhagic, antibacterial, anti-inflammatory.
Indications: Cystitis, haemorrhoids, especially with bleeding.
Contraindications and Warnings: Toxicity is low but allergic contact dermatitis is possible.[3]
Research: Efficacy has been shown for chronic bronchitis in clinical trials and Commission E approved plantain in respiratory catarrh.[4]

Betony (*Stachy betonica*)

The second native herb, betony, sits alongside plantain for reputation and was originally in Celtic use and adopted by the Romans. It has attracted some impressive folklore. With successive counts over time reaching numbers even higher than those for plantain from Roman to stillroom periods, it has been held as more essential than a coat. Predominantly used for treating the head and stomach, remedies are largely for the eyes, ears, sinuses, wounds, brain function and vomiting, particularly vomiting blood. As pharmacy goes through a metamorphosis in the late eighteenth century, once again we see a hugely popular herb discarded in favour of chemical medicine. It is as if vested interest has picked out the two greatest rivals to new practices. In 1790 after a period when there had been enthusiasm for critically reviewing individual herbs and their preparations, Woodville made the telling statement that "Modern writers do not allow the Betony to possess any considerable efficacy."[5] In later periods wood betony is often specified to distinguish it from water betony.

Part Used: Aerial parts
Dosage: 6–12 g by infusion, 6–12 ml, 1:5 tincture per day.[6]
Constituents: Tannins, alkaloids, betonicine, and stachydrine and the iridoid glycoside harpagide.[7]
Actions: Sedative, stomachic, bitter, general tonic.
Indications: Headache, vertigo, anxiety, loss of memory, weak digestion, sciatica, Myalgic encephalitis. chronic rheumatism, nightmares.[8]
Contraindications and Warnings: None found.
Research: There is little research on betony.[9]

Nettle (Urtica dioica)

For many centuries the uses of nettle have been consistent, with the seeds taken internally to benefit the lungs and treat coughs from the earliest references to being regarded as anti-asthmatic in the First World War. The astringency of the leaf as a styptic and anti-haemorrhagic, stimulating, heating, and cleansing properties of nettle have also been applied in treating wounds and internal medicines. The seeds in oil applied to heat and ease rheumatic pain is still valued. Nettle has filled a role as a diuretic for dropsy, urinary gravel, cleansing the skin, and use in diet drinks. A single mention of the root for jaundice confirms some use and in recent times the root has a new application in treating benign prostatic hyperplasia.

Parts Used: Leaf, seeds, and root
Dosage: 6–12 g or by infusion, 6–12 ml tincture 1:5 per day. Juice 10–15 ml 3 times daily[10]
Constituents: Acetylcholine, histamine, flavonoids, organic acids, amines and up to 20% minerals. The rhizome contains six lignans and lectins.[11]
Actions: Diuretic, anti-inflammatory, re-mineralising, styptic and anti-haemorrhagic, anti-rheumatic, anti-allergic.

Indications: Inflammatory urinary tract conditions, rheumatism and gout, internally and externally, chilblains, Raynaud's disease, anaemia, and benign prostatic hyperplasia (with the root). Osteoarthritis, eczema, nosebleeds, burns, and wounds.
Contraindications and Warnings: Allergic reactions are rare.[12]
Research: Clinical trials have provided some evidence for diuretic and anti-inflammatory effects and the German Commission E approved nettle for internal and external rheumatic treatments and for inflammatory urinary tract conditions.[13] Clinical evidence has given support to use of the root for reducing difficulty in urination in benign prostatic hyperplasia.[14]

Elecampane (Inula helenium)

Use of elecampane as a warming expectorant for asthma and coughs is consistent throughout recorded history. The tonic digestive properties also follow from early references and are still used today. Poultices of the root or leaf for sciatica and hip pain are now discontinued but had support over centuries. The antibacterial aspects are highlighted by use in plague waters and treatments for infectious diseases. Diaphoretic, emmenagogue, and diuretic properties are mentioned as well as use of the juice for skin conditions and chewing the root to fasten loose teeth, which may relate to scurvy or gum infections.

Part Used: Root, rhizome
Dosage: Dried root decoction 4.5–9 g per day. 3–6 ml of 1:2 liquid extract per day.[15]
Constituents: Volatile oil with sesquiterpene lactones, mainly alantolactone, inulin, triterpenes, and sterols.[16]
Actions: Digestive, bronchial dilator, expectorant, antitussive, diaphoretic, bactericidal, and anthelmintic.[17]
Indications: Bronchitis, bronchial catarrh, asthma, colds.
Contraindications and Warnings: Elecampane may give allergic reactions in those sensitive to sesquiterpene lactones in Asteraceae. Caution in pregnancy and lactation.[18]
Research: Alantolactone, another term for the extract, has been reported to show high antibacterial properties in vitro, as well as hypotensive and hypoglycaemic properties in animal trials.[19]

Henbane (Hyosycamus niger)

Henbane has always proved its worth as a sedative and analgesic, especially valued for treating toothache and sufficiently strong to be part of early anaesthetics. Applied in salves, poultices, or plasters or taken internally it has been used to treat all manner of inflammatory conditions and trauma. The white-flowered *Hyoscyamus niger* is consistently specified and seed, root, or juice used. Warnings on dosage as the cooling strength may endanger reasoning and ultimately life, began early.

Currently henbane is is included on Schedule 20. Part 2 as a restricted herb, pharmacy only, with exemption for qualified herbal practitioners.

Parts Used: Leaf, flowering tops, or fruits
Dosage: Maximum single dose allowed 100 mg or 19 drops 1:10 tincture in 45% alcohol. 21 ml per week.
Constituents: Tropane alkaloids, hyoscyamine and hyoscine, flavonoid glycosides.
Actions: Antispasmodic and sedative effects acting on smooth muscle, the autonomic and central nervous systems.[20]
Indications: Toothache or pain of any kind, spasms, and tremors.
Contraindications and Warnings: Arrhythmia, tachycardia, glaucoma.[21]
Research: More detail on use and effects of black henbane can be found in the publication by Alizadeh et al.[22]

Ginger (Zingiber officinale)

Dioscorides recommends ginger as a digestive and ingredient of antidotes. In Britain the herb is not appreciated until used in medieval cookery. Absent from the Welsh collections, ginger appears in others as digestive and heating, sometimes partnered with elecampane in cough and digestive remedies. In a powder for migraine, stimulation of the brain is noted, and contributes to recommendations for the elderly and longevity. Helpfully providing heat ginger has relieved rheumatic pain. Difference in action of the fresh and dried root has been observed.

Part Used: Fresh or dried rhizome
Dosage: Daily dose 2 g. 0.7–2 ml 1:2 liquid extract per day.[23]
Constituents: Essential oil containing zingiberene and pungent gingerols, which are dominant in the aroma of fresh ginger. Shogaols are mainly formed in the drying process giving different actions between the two forms.
Actions: Anti-emetic, inhibits inflammatory prostaglandins, peripheral circulatory stimulant and support to the digestive system.[24]
Indications: Nausea, vomiting, colic, fever, osteoarthritis, poor circulation.
Contraindications and Warnings: Ginger may increase absorption of drugs. Large doses may increase bleeding, interacting with blood thinners. May cause contact dermatitis.[25]
Research: Numerous studies have been carried out on ginger, including for anti-inflammatory action, inhibition of platelet aggregation and for motion sickness and nausea. ESCOP recommends ginger for prophylaxis of nausea and vomiting in motion sickness and as an antiemetic after minor surgical procedures.[26]

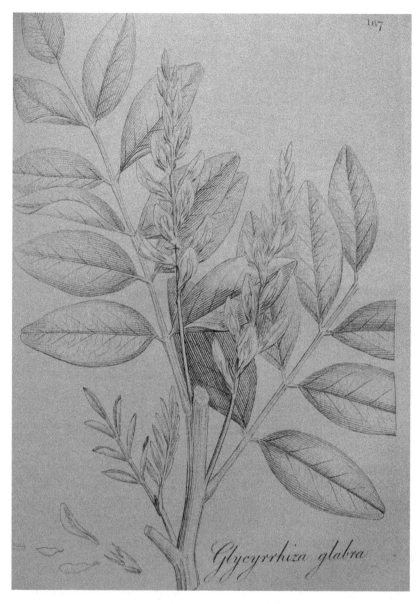

Liquorice, *Medical Botany*, Woodville.

Liquorice (*Glycyrrhiza glabra*)

Dioscorides recommends use of the root and extracted juice for quenching thirst and comforting the organs. The soothing and moistening qualities have always centred on use for the lungs and throat. It is repeatedly portrayed as a benign, sweet herb and was given to counteract problems from sharp and salty humours. Also, as a gentle laxative comforting the stomach.

Part Used: Root and stolon
Dosage: 1.5 g, infused or decocted or 2–5 ml liquid extract, three times daily.[27]
Constituents: Triterpene glycosides, especially glycyrrhizin.
Actions: anti-inflammatory, demulcent, expectorant.
Indications: Bronchitis, gastritis, rheumatism, polycystic ovary syndrome, adreno-corticoid insufficiency.
Contraindications and Warnings: Excessive dosage can cause metabolic distur-bance. Contraindicated in hypertension, hypokalaemia, cirrhosis of the liver, and pregnancy.[28]
Research: Many clinical studies are available for liquorice in treating numerous conditions. In Germany Commission E supports liquorice for treating catarrh of the upper respiratory tract and gastric and duodenal ulcers.[29]

It has been seen that some herbs pass in and out of favour in a way that equates to their perceived, rather than actual efficacy. There are often other factors in the history of individual herb use such as imported plants as with elderberry, for example, being overshadowed by echinacea in modern thought. Foreign herbs are perceived as more effective—this has always been true all over the world.

Treatments

Treatments for several common conditions, have also been followed through the centuries. The summary below shows the most popular herbs used individually or in combinations, taken from personal analysis of sources used throughout this book. We can also review how treatments of common ailments have evolved and judge whether they show continuity, are possibly evolving with a growing under-standing of the condition, or being influenced by other factors such as introductions of more popular herbs.

Some of these, headaches, fevers, and coughs, may also actually be bodily responses to a range of diseases which widens the range of therapeutic approach.

First century treatments are from Celsus. The Anglo-Saxon Leechbooks and the *Macer Floridus* reflect treatments from the second half of the first millennium. In the post Norman period household and Leechbooks supply information. Household recipes and published herbals were used for the stillroom period to 1785. Herbals and self-help books were consulted for the last period, plus recent publications. The information below reflects those herbs with the most mentions found. More detail is given in the last period as changes have been considerable.

Coughs

Herb choices have been consistent, taken into account whether the cough needs to be productive or not, and proven the efficacy of those herbs beyond doubt. They are brilliant examples of herbs with strong traditional use.

First Century—Horehound, plantain juice, garlic, hyssop, myrrh, castory, poppy tears, pepper, mallows, and fig.
600–1066—Sage, horehound, elecampane, fennel, comfrey, hyssop and mullein. Liquorice, betony and nettle.
1066–1485—Garlic, mallows, sage, horehound, elecampane, and fennel. Liquorice, hyssop, betony.
1485–1785—Coltsfoot, elecampane, horehound, hyssop, liquorice, marshmallow. Water of elecampane, hyssop or saffron.
1785–2000—Lobelia and cayenne enter in the nineteenth century. Forms of opium as paregoric or laudanum also feature, then, comfrey and coltsfoot were popular in the Victorian period. Wild cherry was used by 1905 for nervous coughs, and henbane for asthmatic coughs. Horehound, hyssop elecampane, mullein and fennel have continued in frequent use. Marshmallow, thyme and liquorice are popular today.

Headaches

Headaches arise from numerous causes and we can see from the herbs used that the emphasis in treatment may be on nervous or digestive symptoms. When constipation may be a cause then laxatives are used. We can see that betony and chamomile are strongly indicated for traditional use, as is feverfew, which may long have had a link with treating migraine. Limeflower and lemon balm seem only to become popular later in history.

First Century—Warm rose oil, or, at the other extreme, mustard is used to cause ulceration over the pain site.
600–1066—Betony, greater plantain, wormwood, rue, dill, pennyroyal, or mint, wild thyme.
1066–1485—Betony remains herb of choice, vervain, chamomile, wormwood and fennel.
1485–1785—Betony, mint, pennyroyal, feverfew, lavender and rosemary. In waters, hyssop or saffron.
1785–2000—Betony fell largely out of use but is returning. Chamomile was particularly popular in the Victorian era. It remains in every dispensary either as *Anthemis nobilis*, or *Matricaria recutita* depending on the herbalist choice. Feverfew is now associated particularly with migraine headaches. Turkey rhubarb and ginger, or cayenne were given in the nineteenth century. Valerian, lemon balm, and limeflower are used. Rosemary and lavender continue in popularity in the last 200 years.

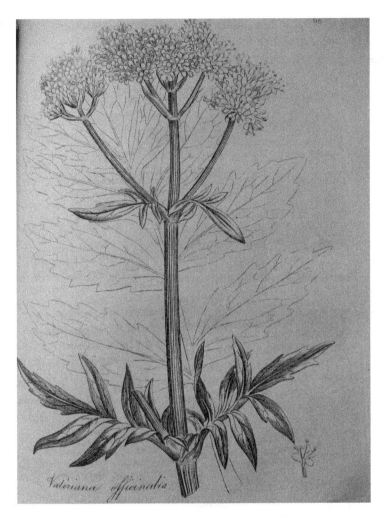

Valeriana officinalis

Valerian, *Medical Botany*, Woodville.

Eye Conditions (painful ophthalmia to cataracts)

Eye treatments have been consistent from the second half of the first millennium onwards. The greatest change comes with those that were unavailable for a time after the Romans left. Then native herbs with some they have introduced such as rue dominate prescribing. With the possible exceptions of greater celandine, rue and agrimony they are the herbs still used by modern practitioners.

First Century—Celsus treats with saffron, myrrh, poppy tears, mandrake, hemlock, frankincense, rose, acacia, or quince.
600–1066—Greater celandine, fennel, rue, agrimony, elder, and betony show preference for native herb use.

1066–1536—Greater celandine, fennel, and rue have continued use along with ground ivy, houseleek, and eyebright.

1536–1785—Greater celandine, elder, eyebright, fennel, houseleek. Waters of fennel and rose.

1785–2000—Greater celandine continued in use for treating cataracts until the last century Eyebright, fennel, chamomile and elderflower.

Toothache

Heating, astringent, and analgesic herbs dominate. Henbane is the most consistently used.

First Century—Cinquefoil, henbane, poppy, mandrake, pomegranate rind, oak galls, and pine bark.

600–1066—Garlic, yarrow, betony, henbane, rosemary, or elecampane.

1066–1485—Rose and shepherd's purse. There is use of a peppercorn or ivy berry to extract teeth.

1485–1785—Pellitory of Spain is the only herb mentioned repeatedly as specific for toothache. Rosemary, betony, hyssop, and elder have brief mentions. Reference to the problem is much less than before.

1785–2000—By Victorian times we see the common use of essential oil of clove. Oil of capsicum, lobelia seeds and prickly ash berry appear briefly, yarrow and henbane remain. For the gums and inflammation in the mouth, cinquefoil, sage, and myrrh feature.

Boils

These were a common problem in periods when there was widespread malnutrition, but often they may be hidden under different terms for the problem; it has not been as easy to follow their history as with other conditions and so the results are less reliable.

First Century—Treatments for superficial abscesses included galbanum, myrrh, frankincense, caper root bark, calcined murex, and vinegar. For slow boils, we find sulphur, soda, myrrh, frankincense soot, ammoniac salt, and wax.

600–1066—Waybroad (greater plantain), houseleek, and elecampane.

1066–1485—Sage, mallows, and greater plantain.

1485–1785—Burdock and dandelion.

1785–2000—Burdock, figwort and nettle with laxative herbs as necessary.

Fevers

Fevers relate to many diseases and so we find a great many herbs used. Marigold and saffron have associations with eruptive conditions such as measles and smallpox. We find other herbs labelled specifically for recurrent fevers such as tertian or quartan, returning on the third or fourth days. Willow was laid round the bed in early times and later, to cool the room. I have not included that aspect in the table below as these are vague references. Some, such as angelica were regarded as specifics for plague. Numerous antibacterials are used.

First Century—Treated largely through regimen—diet, bathing and vomits. We therefore do not have a list of herbs.
600–1066—White horehound, wormwood, betony, liquorice, yarrow, waybroad and ribwort.
1066–1485—Betony, feverfew, sage, rue, garlic, cinquefoil, elderflower, greater plantain, mugwort and wormwood.
1485–1785—Angelica, betony, chamomile, marigold, sage, rue, ribwort. Water of sorrel saffron, marigold or borage. Peruvian bark, (*Cinchona* spp.) used late in this period.
1785–2000—Peruvian bark (*Cinchona*) features in the nineteenth century becoming more expensive, so that willow is popular in the search for a substitute, Lobelia, capsicum and virginian snakeroot from the nineteenth century. Vervain, occasionally used throughout becomes more popular. Chamomile and yarrow.

Joint Pain

Joint pain includes symptoms from a number of causes—these are mostly arthritic or rheumatic. Not surprisingly there are many heating herbs in this list, along with analgesics and some, such as burdock and nettle that also remove toxins from joints. Colchicum stands out as a herb that has been developed as a modern treatment for gout. Henbane and nettle are the most consistent and we see a wider interest in using introduced herbs from the Victorian period onwards.

First Century—Treated with dried fig and catmint, black bryony berry (no seed), pennyroyal, or pounded henbane and nettle seeds in fat. Elecampane root was applied for the hip.
600–1066—Poppy, nettle, colchicum, waybroad, marshmallow, or elderberry.
1066–1485—Betony, coltsfoot, burdock, feverfew, hemlock, henbane, nettle and wormwood.
1485–1785—Burdock, chamomile, comfrey, white lily, nettle, sage and rue.
1785–2000—Burdock and opium are each used in the Victorian period. Henbane, nettle, colchicum, comfrey (now restricted), and horseradish. For rheumatic pain buckbean, guaiacum, ginger, cayenne, prickly ash, *Gelsemium*, willow, and juniper have been popular. There is occasional use of meadowsweet. Turmeric and Frankincense enter the picture in more recent times.

Burns

In the list below although treatment changes a number of herbs are used for a considerable period of time. The white lily stands out as a herb of interest. Houseleek may be seen as a fore-runner of aloe vera in that it has similar cooling and healing properties.

First Century—Lily, hound's tongue, or beet leaves. Sometimes lentil meal and honey are applied following rue, leek, or horehound.

600–1066—Woad, woodruff, lily bulbs, yarrow, elm inner bark, mallow, wild thyme.

1066–1485—Mallow, white lily bulbs, linseed, houseleek, greater plantain.

1485–1785—Burdock, elder inner bark, houseleek, marshmallow, mallow, plantain, rose, red dock leaves, St. John's wort.

1785–2000—Elder leaf was used in Victorian times. Lily leaf survived until recently in folk cures. Lavender essential oil is recent as a first aid treatment. St John's wort oil, marigold, aloe vera and ti-tree are now also used.

Influential imported herbs in these lists have been largely from America and many of these herbs came into use in the context of an American system of prescribing. At present, the picture is changing and more Chinese and Ayurvedic herbs are taking the place of native herbs. With the exception of turmeric, I have felt it too early to reflect this. It will be interesting to see what the future holds.

References

1. William Woodville, *Medical Botany*, Vol. I (London: James Phillips, 1790), 40.
2. *British Herbal Pharmacopoeia* (Bournemouth: British Herbal Medicine Association, 1983), 164.
3. Joanne Barnes et al., *Herbal Medicines* (London: Pharmaceutical Press, 2002), 376–377.
4. Mark Blumenthal et al., *Herbal Medicine* (Austin: American Botanical Council, 2000), 308.
5. Woodville, *Medical Botany, Supplement*, 79.
6. *British Herbal Pharmacopoeia*, 42.
7. James A. Duke, *Handbook of Phytochemical Constituents of GRAS Herbs and other Economic Plants* (London: CRC Press, 2001), 576.
8. Thomas Bartram, *Bartram's Encyclopedia of Herbal Medicine* (London: Robinson Publishing Ltd., 1998), 55.
9. *British Herbal Pharmacopoeia*, 225.
10. Barnes, *Herbal Medicines*, 360.
11. Kerry Bone, *A Clinical Guide to Blending Liquid Herbs* (Missouri: Churchill Livingstone, 2003), 343–348.
12. Bone, *A Clinical Guide to Blending Liquid Herbs*, 345.
13. Barnes, *Herbal Medicines*, 362.
14. Bone, *A Clinical Guide to Blending Liquid Herbs*, 193.
15. Peter Bradley, ed, *British Herbal Compendium*, Vol. I (Bournemouth: British Herbal Medicine Association, 1992), 88.
16. Barnes, *Herbal Medicines*, 190.
17. Bone, *A Clinical Guide to Blending Liquid Herbs*, 193.
18. Barnes, *Herbal Medicines*, 190.
19. Bradley, *British Herbal Compendium*, 131.
20. James A. Duke, *Handbook of Medicinal Herbs*, (Florida: CRC Press, 2nd edition, 2000), 374.

21. Bone, *A Clinical Guide to Blending Liquid Herbs*, 228.
22. Alizadeh A, Moshiri M, Alizadeh J, Balali-Mood M. "Black henbane and its toxicity – a descriptive review", *Avicenna J Phytomed*, Vol. 4, Issue 5 (September 2014): 297–311.
23. Bradley, *British Herbal Compendium*, 112–113.
24. Bone, *A Clinical Guide to Blending Liquid Herbs*, 227.
25. Ibid, 313.
26. Bone, *A Clinical Guide to Blending Liquid Herbs*, 230–231.
27. Bradley, *British Herbal Compendium*, 146.
28. Ibid, 146.
29. Bone, *A Clinical Guide to Blending Liquid Herbs*, 317.

CHAPTER 28

Towards the Future—Points to Consider

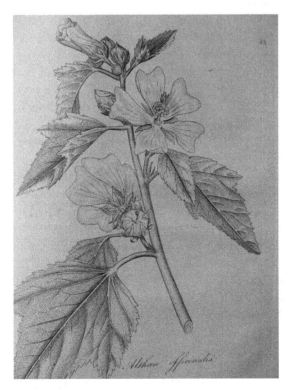

Marshmallow, *Medical Botany*, Woodville.

361

Successive generations have learnt to adapt to cultural changes, so that our medicine has and continues to respond to the needs of the times. Western herbal medicine has its source in Ancient Greece and I believe that the Hippocratic tradition of patient-centred practice still underpins Western herbal medicine. Reaching more than a superficial diagnosis of immediate symptoms requires knowledge of elements of balance in diet, exercise, and rest. as well as establishing sufficient restorative sleep, regular evacuations of bodily toxins, and a healthy environment of clean air. These keys to health and longevity have appeared in instructions since the beginning and are part of the philosophy behind plant medicine.

As we leave history and prepare to consider the way ahead, we look briefly at those truths that have remained over the centuries and also at inevitable changes. Emphasis is placed on those elements of tradition that still unite Western herbalists. Finally, the metaphor of the living, evolving tradition of herbal medicine in Britain as a river, presented in the foreword, is once again thought provoking. Over the two thousand years of medicine portrayed in these pages, the potentiality within herbs for healing has remained constant in empirical terms. It is our understanding of medicine and therefore the wording of our description of the plant that has evolved and altered most. Understanding of the physiology of the physical body has also changed beyond recognition since the time of Galen. However, understanding of the emotional involvement in health has been a tortuous maze with many wrong turns. The scientific view is now rediscovering lost knowledge by translating it into the currently acceptable term of psychoneuroimmunology. This is surely just as mysterious and possibly as impressive to the general public as a Celtic or Anglo-Saxon ritual charm. With the complex involvement of the endocrine and immune systems, endobiogenic medicine offers modern herbalists a possible credible way forward in this area.

The greatest factor in separating the main stream of medicine from herbal practice has been our different conceptions of causes of disease. This, in turn, has governed the way in which medics have responded as they have designed treatments. It has been gradual as science has moved forward by consistently proving its former truth to be wrong, with whole systems of belief overturned by a single discovery. In herbal medicine, historically the emphasis was on the nature of a plant rather than its chemical constituents. Prescribing the whole plant shows due respect for the clear superiority of synergy of multiple constituents in nature when it comes to chemistry. This acknowledgment and understanding have been another main marker for herbalism.

Involvement of the patient in the remedy necessitates a confident, face-to-face working relationship between practitioner and patient. This is a traditional key to success that has always been evident and is now supported by modern trials. Traditional herbal medicine adds another dimension to this, in the relationship between the herbalist and the herbs. As Dioscorides pointed out, a good herbalist knows the plant from seed to maturity. This was the case in the past, even for some physicians, such as William Woodville, who took especial care in growing and examining the plants themselves and made a bold stand for herbal versus chemical medicine. It has also been the case for those outstanding herbalists in the last century, who gathered herbs with the aid of their families for their prescriptions.

Respectful, sustainable gathering at a time when familiar observation has confirmed the best time for harvest and a deep relationship with the herbs themselves, which informs synergistic combining in a prescription, is at the heart of all indigenous practice. This is the basis of the craft of herbalism. It is my belief that although the science can be taught, the craft cannot. It comes from experience in working with the herbs themselves. From coming to know their individual preferences, the challenges they have to meet to survive, and learning what makes their healing potential, or in modern language, chemical composition stronger.

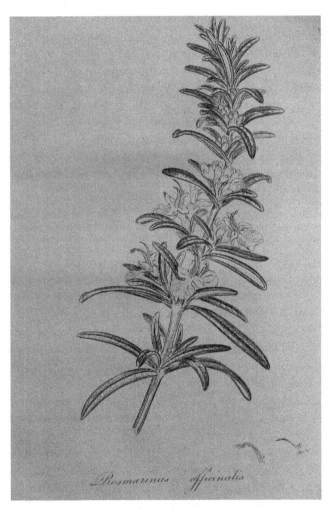

Rosemary, *Medical Botany*, Woodville.

Science is beginning to penetrate a fascinating area only formerly available through intuition and keen observation. This is one of plant relationships and chemical communication between plants, threatening insects and foraging animals, and friendly pollinators and protectors. Humans fall into both categories and the way in which our chemistry interlocks points to evidence for a deeply dependent relationship on other levels. The benefit of horticultural therapy, forest bathing, and simple appreciation of plants, to physical and mental health is now widely accepted.

Herbalists able to introduce patients to herbs in their prescription, whether in a garden with their practice or on herb walks can foster the ancient circle of practitioner–patient–herb interactions, which is physically, emotionally, and potentially spiritually effective in promoting health. In encouraging wild foraging, however, we must also be aware of the challenge to respect and care for our countryside. The modern notion of "hedge-witch" plays to the romantic ideal of survival of indigenous medicine and is a predictable reaction back towards emotional contact with plants, following a diet of soul-less scientific monographs. I would suggest that a combination of approach offers the best way forward. Herbalists today are needed as guardians of our native herbs to ensure their protection from unsustainable gathering, something herbal medicine has been responsible for in other countries.

We have followed a long journey downstream along our metaphorical river, noting the tributary streams of influence in introduced herbs and practices, the calm wide stretches where there is little disturbance and the rock-strewn rapids of persecution. In returning to the source, we can see that certain practice, understanding, and knowledge was lost along the way. Whether the very different understanding and knowledge gained in the past fifty years is a fully evolved replacement will be seen in time.

The present adoption of many herbs from the Ayurvedic and Chinese traditions and the increasing dependence on imported herbs and scientific interpretation of them may be seen by some as a threat to our tradition. Evidence from history however, points to this being a continuation of it. The present emphasis on scientific validation rightly speaks to the mindset of the present day and has enabled herbalists and physicians to work together in the best interests of the patient. It is the latest adaptation of British herbal medicine enabling it to survive and serve.

Herbal knowledge was once far more widespread. At the present time the river is in a narrow gorge where the contribution of every herbalist matters. In order to take traditional herbal medicine into an uncertain future unity is needed. The importance of holding to teaching an informed understanding of patients and maintaining a strong, practical relationship with native herbs and with the past is vital for the true survival of tradition. There will be twists and turns to come as climate change and the consequences unfold. Human connection with the plants runs deep in the psyche of the human race and far more than 2,000 years of history assures us that the river will flow on through the generations to come.

LIST OF ILLUSTRATIONS

TIMELINE

BC

1,534	Ebers papyrus lists herbal medicines
6th century	Anaximander wrote *On Nature*
c 433	Hippocrates flourished
c370	Theophrastus is born
339	Pytheas—writes first account of Britain
331	Alexander the Great campaigns into India. Greek influence from Punjab to Karnak and the Danube
2nd century	Asclepiades of Bythnia flourishes
1st century	Crateuas first illustrated herbal

AD

c70	Dioscorides' Materia Medica
50	Invasion of Britain leads to military hospitals in Britain
79	Pliny's works published

1st century	Celsus 8 books on Medicine
131	Galen born, writes c160 onwards
407	Main body Roman troops leave Britain
5th century	Herbarium of Pseudo-Apuleius often combined with work of Dioscorides
597	Augustine's mission to convert King Aethelbert of Kent
598	First Monastery in Britain
670	Bishop Theodore's school at Canterbury
c700	Bede writes first History of the English Church and People
754	First pharmacies Baghdad under Abbasid caliphate
c800	School at Salerno founded
777–857	Mesue Senior head of the medical school in Baghdad. His pharmaceutical formulary influenced first London Pharmacopoeia
849–1112	Macer Floridus written
854	Rhazes born. Dioscorides translated into Arabic in Baghdad
871	Alfred the Great rules and encourages learning and medicine. Rhazes heads hospital in Baghdad
900–950	Leechbook of Bald written
10th century	Translation of the Lacnunga Leechbook into Anglo-Saxon
10th century	Old English Herbarium Leechbook

1010	Avicenna writing *Canon of Medicine*
1016	Famine throughout Europe
1066	Norman rule, William the Conqueror
11th century	Arabic manuscript Taqwim al-Sihha bi al-Ashab al-Sitta by Ibn Botlan. Text used as the basis for The *Tacuuinem Sanitatis*, in 14th century
1095	Salerno becomes base hospital for crusaders
1096	Oxford University no definitive date founded, but teaching known there
1123	St Barts hospital is founded in London
1137	Montpellier University has faculty of medicine

1193–1280	Albertus Magnus writes a good description distillation
12th century	Physicians of Myddfai
1209	Cambridge University founded
1303	Small Faculty of Medicine Oxford University
1337	Hundred Years War with France begins
1348	Black Death in England
1362	Emma Huntyngton, apothecary mentioned
1382	Earliest suggested date for Welsh Red Book of Hergest
14th century	*Agnus Castus* written
1403	Bernard of Gordon writes *Lilium Medicinae*, core text of medicine
1405	Astrology required for medicine, Universities Paris and Bologna
c1408	Joan de Sutton, a practising leche appeared before the Westminster court of pleas
1415	Latin manuscript using the Circa Instans as primary source translated from Latin into Irish, also includes herbs from Irish tradition
1421	Act to stop foreign physicians and women practising in England
1435	Guild of Surgeons formed
1455–71	Wars of the Roses
1476	Caxton sets up printing press in Westminster
1484	Pope Innocent VIII authorizes inquisition on witchcraft
1485	Sweating sickness
1488	Sweating sickness, returns at intervals till 1552
1498	First official Pharmacopoeia in Florence
c1500	Licensing of midwives by bishops
1517	Syon Herbal written
1518	Royal College of Physicians formed, begin regulation of physicians practising within seven miles of London
1525	Banckes Herbal taken largely from earlier *Agnus castus*
1527	*Virtuose book of Distyllacion* translated into English
1533	First botanic garden at Padua. Luca Ghini begins assembling the first Hortus siccus (herbarium) record of plants
1536	Paracelsus appointed to lecture in Basle. His work on Surgery published

1537–38	Paracelsus writes *Astronomia Magna*
1536–39	Dissolution of monasteries
1540	*Birth of Mankind* popular book on midwifery published
1542	Parliament passes Witchcraft Act, now punishable by death
1543	Vesalius *Fabrica* published, transforms understanding of anatomy
1543	Herbalists Charter
1547	Witchcraft Act repealed
1548	Turner, *Names of Plants* published
1553	College of Physicians given power to survey stocks of apothecaries, druggists and distillers
1558	St Thomas, Hospital, Southwark re-opens with resident apothecary
1562	Witchcraft Act restored
1577	Frampton's *Joyfull newes out of the newe Founde Worlde*
1581	*Opera de Medicamentorum* printed
1597	Gerard's *Great Herball*
1599–1607	Diary of Lady Margaret Hoby includes tending the sick poor
1604	Act re-inforces 1562 Act transferring trial of witches from jurisdiction of the Church to ordinary courts
1609	Sir Hugh Platt *Delights for Ladies* published
1612	Pendle witch trials
1618	First London Pharmacopoeia. Amended in second edition same year
1618	Charter of the Royal Society of Apothecaries
1620	Pilgrim fathers take herbals to New Plymouth
1621	Oxford Botanic garden founded
1631	John Winthrop Jnr. Governor of Connecticut
1635	Thomas Parr died supposed age, 152
1638	Worshipful Company of Distillers
1640	Parkinson *Theatrum Botanicum*
1642	Culpeper accused of witchcraft – acquitted
1649	Culpeper's translation of the Pharmacopoeia

1651	*History of Life and Death* Francis Bacon
1651	Culpeper *Directory for Midwives*
1652	Culpeper *Herbal and English Physician Enlarged*
1670	Edinburgh Botanic garden founded
1670	Henry Jenkins dies, supposed age 169
1672	*Josselyn's New England's Rarities Discovered* written
1673	Chelsea Physic garden established
1681	Royal College of Physicians of Edinburgh founded
1685	Last known execution of a witch
1694	Pecheys *English Herbal of Physical Plants*
1699	Edinburgh Pharmacopoeia
1718	First revision of Pharmacopoeia
1722	Miller *Botanicum Officinale*
1735	Irish Herbal by John K'Eogh
1736	Witchcraft Act repealed, fines for those claiming magical powers
1736	Quincy's *English Dispensatory*
1737–39	Elizabeth Blackwell *A Curious Herbal* published
1746	Sir John Hill *British Herbal*
1747	Wesley's *Primitive Physic*, medicine for the poor
1776	Buchan *Domestic Medicine*
1785	Withering's work on foxglove published
1790	Meyrick *The New Family Herbal*
1790	Woodville *Medical Botany*
1790	Royal Dublin Society receives funds to establish a botanic garden
1800	Willich *Lectures on Diet and Regimen*
1803	Extraction morphine from opium
1806	*The Naval Surgeon* by William Turnbull
1807	Dublin Pharmacopoeia
1810	Thornton's *Family Herbal*
1818	Word alkaloid coined
1832	British Medical Association formed

1836	Alva Curtis opens Botanico-Medical College in America (Physio-medicalism)
1838	Arrival of Albert Coffin in Britain bringing Botanic Medicine
1852	Skelton and Coffin part
1854	Mr Brady's Reform Bill. Medical Freedom League formed
1858	Medical Act establishes General Medical Council as authority granting register of practitioners
1859	No person not registered by GMC could now recover charges for medical or surgical procedures, or attending a patient from now on. Entry refused to women
1864	National Association of Medical Herbalists formed
1870	*The Science and Practice of Herbal Medicine.* John Skelton MD
1880s	Henry Potter's herbal cures expanded into the northern manufacturing districts in this decade and the next
1881	Commission to suppress unlicensed practitioners, defeated
1887	Regular journal of National Association. *Botanic Practitioner* published
1891	David Younger establishes College of Herbal Medicine in London
1895	Herbalists form amalgamated Ltd. Co. National Association of Medical Herbalists after battle for state registration of herbalists
1904	Patent Medicines Act
1905	*National Botanic Pharmacopoeia*
1911	National Insurance Act
1911	Teaching College re-opens under auspices of NAMH
1914–18	World War 1 brings herbal medicines to attention of the nation
1916	Ada Teetgen *Profitable Herb Growing and Collecting* for war effort
1916	Webb publishes *Standard Guide to Non-Poisonous Herbal Medicine*
1922	Postal Tutorial course of NAMH has 22 students
1923	Medical Herbalists' Registration Bill passed first reading in the House of Commons
1925	First issue *The Medical Herbalist* journal
1931	College of Botanic Medicine
1931	Mrs Grieve's *A Modern Herbal* published

1932	National Association reprinted *Physio-medical Therapeutic Materia Medica and Pharmacy* by Lyle from 1897
1935	College of Botanic Medicine opens in London
1938	Last Eclectic School in America closes
1939	Start World War II
1940	Bombing closes College
1941	Medicines and Pharmacy Act
1945	National Association re-named National Institute
1947	Hospital of Natural Healing opened in London by Albert Orbell
1948	National Institute offered place in new NHS. Refused
1965	British Herbal Medicines Association formed
1968	Medicines Act. Fred Fletcher Hyde negotiated 250 herbs for approved use
1972	Product Licences introduced
1976	*British Herbal Pharmacopoeia* Part 1 is published
1978	Hein Zeylstra opens School of Medicine in Tunbridge Wells
1979	*British Herbal Pharmacopoeia* Part 2 is published
1980	The BHMA became a founder member of ESCOP the European Scientific Co-operative on Phytotherapy
1983	*British Herbal Pharmacopoeia*. New edition
1987	Michael McIntyre opens School Chinese Herbal Medicine
1989	Bucksteep Manor provides physic gardens, laboratory and school facilities for live-in course
1990	First edition of *The British Journal of Phytotherapy* published
1991	BSc courses validated by University of Wales
1992	Scottish School of Herbal Medicine founded. *British Herbal Compendium*. Part 1
1993	European Herbal and Traditional Medicine Practitioners Association founded
1994	Crisis caused by Medicines Control Agency on access to herbs. Health Secretary sets up a working group towards Statutory Self-Regulation
1996	Vol. II *British Herbal Pharmacopoeia*

2000	Botanic Garden in Wales
2001	Six Universities either offer or validate courses
2002	All forms of herbal medicine come together for regulation
2011	Statutory Self-Regulation announced by government as imminent
2015	Report recommends regulation should not go ahead
2012–15	Several University courses close
2015	School of Herbal Medicine opens in the West
2016	Betonica School and Heartwood Education open
2019–20	Covid pandemic begins, lockdowns affect seeing patients

BIBLIOGRAPHY

Alcock, J. (2001). *Food in Roman Britain*. Stroud: Tempus.

Adams, J., and Forbes, S. ed. (2015). *The Syon Abbey Herbal. A.D. 1517*. London: AMCD Publishers Ltd.

Afnan, S. M. (2009). *Avicenna*. Kuala Lumpur: The Other Press.

Amr, Samir, S. and Abdulghani Tbakhi. "Abu Bakr Muhammad Ibn Zakariya Al Razi (Rhazes): Philosopher, Physician and Alchemist." *Annals of Saudi Medicine* 27, no. 4 (2007): 305–7. https://doi.org/10.5144/0256-4947.2007.305.

Anon. (1746). *A Collection of Receipts*. London: Printed for the Executrix of Mary Kettilby.

"Apothecaries and Physic Gardens: An Early History of the Royal Hospital's Grounds." Royal Hospital Chelsea, October 23, 2020. https://www.chelsea-pensioners.co.uk/news/apothecaries-and-physic-gardens-early-history-royal-hospital%E2%80%99s-grounds.

Arano, L. C. ed. (1976). *The Medieval Health Handbook. Tacuinum Sanitatis*. New York: George Braziller.

Arber, A. (1912). *Herbals Their Origin and Evolution*. Cambridge: University Press.

Aston, M. (2000). Monasteries in the Landscape. Stroud: Tempus.

Atkinson, T. (2007). *Napiers History of herbal Healing, Ancient & Modern*. Edinburgh: Luath Press Ltd.

Ayres, P. (2015). *Britain's Green Allies. Medicinal Plants in Wartime*. Leicestershire: Matador.

Bacon, Francis, Lord Verulam, Vis-Count Saint Alban. (1650). *History Naturall and Experimentall, of Life and Death or Of the Prolongation of Life*. William Lee and Humphrey Moseley.

Bakhtiar, L. adapt., (1999). *The Canon of Medicine. Avicenna*. Great Books of the Islamic World Inc.

Baldick et al., ed. (1968). *Bede A History of the English Church and People*. London: Penguin Classics.

Barker, J. *History, Philosophy and Medicine*. Kent: Winter Press, 2007.

Barnes, J. et al., *Herbal Medicines*. London: Pharmaceutical Press, 2002.

Barry, G. and Carruthers, L. A. (2005). *A History of Britain's Hospitals*. Sussex: Book Guild Publishing Ltd.

Beasley, H. (1895). *The Druggist's General Receipt Book*. London: J.A. Churchill.

Berlin, M. (1996). *The Worshipful Company of Distillers*. Chichester: Phillimore & Co. Ltd.

Bernhold, J. M. *Compositiones Medicamentorum. Scribonius (Largus)*. 1786. Franklin Trade Press. Scholars Select.

Best, M. R. ed. (1986). Gervase Markham. *The English Housewife*. London: McGill-Queen's University Press.

Black, M. (1996). *The Medieval Cookbook*. London: British Museum Press.

Black, R. III. (1966). *The Younger John Winthrop*. New York: Columbia University Press.

Blackburn, E. and Epel, E. (2017). *The Telomere Effect*. London: Orion Spring.

Blackwood, N. "Government Response to Professor Walker's Advice on Regulation of Herbal Medicines and Practitioners." Written questions, answers and statements, 2017. https://questions-statements.parliament.uk/written-statements/detail/2017-02-28/HCWS505.

Blencowe, J. W. ed. (2001). *The Blencowe Families*. The Blencowe Families Association.

Blythe, R. ed., George Herbert. *The Country Parson*. Norwich: Canterbury Press, 2003.

Bos, G. and McVaugh, M. ed. (2015). *Al-Razi, On the Treatment of Small Children*. (De curis puerorum). Leiden: Brill.

Bowman, A. (2003). *Life and Letters on the Roman Frontier*. London: The British Museum Press.

Bradford, W. (1981). *Of Plymouth Plantation 1620–1647*. London: Random House.

Bradley, P. ed., *British Herbal Compendium*. Vol. 1. Dorset: British Herbal Medicine Association, 1992.

Brice-Ytsma, H. and Watkins, F. ed. (2014). *Herbal Exchanges*. London: Strathmore Publishing.

British Herbal Pharmacopoeia. Bournemouth: British Herbal medicine Association, 1983.

Britten, et al., intro. (1965). William Turner. *Libellus de Re Herbaria* 1538 *The Names of Herbes* 1548. Facsimiles. London: The Ray Society.

Brock, A. J. (1971). *Galen On the Natural Faculties*. London: Harvard University Press.

Brodin, G. ed. (1950). *Agnus castus*. Cambridge Mass: Harvard University Press.

Brown, P. *The Vicissitudes of Herbalism in Late Nineteenth-and Early Twentieth-century Britain*: Part 1, British Journal of Phytotherapy V Spring 1991.Vol. 2.

Browne, E. G. (1921). *Arabian Medicine*. (A Series of Lectures). Reprint. Cambridge: University Press.

Bruton-Seal, J. and Seal, M. *The Herbalist's Bible*. New York: Skyhorse Publishing Inc., 2019.

Buchan, W. (1776). *Domestic Medicine*. London: W. Strahan & T. Cadell.

Buhner, S. H. (1998). *Sacred and Herbal Healing Beers*. Boulder: Siris Books.

Campbell-Culver, M. (2001). *The Origin of Plants*. London: Headline Book Publishing.

Card, N. et al., ed., (2020). *The Ness of Brodgar, As it Stands*. Orkney: Kirkwall Press.

(Cascino, A. et al., Medicine and Surgery). Ciarallo, A. & De Carolis, E. ed., (1999). *Pompeii Life in a Roman Town*, Milan: Electa.

Chapman G. and Tweddle, M. ed., (1989). *A New Herball*. William Turner 1551. Manchester: Carcanet Press.

Cholmeley, H. P. (1912). *John of Gaddesden and the Rosa Medicinae*. Oxford: Clarendon Press.

Cockayne, Oswald. (1864–66). *Leechdoms, Wortcunning and Starcraft in Early England*. London: Longman, Green, Longman, Roberts, and Green. Vol. 1 & 2. Facsimile.

Cockayne, O. (2012). *Leechdoms, Wortcunning, and Starcraft of Early England*. Vol. 3. Cambridge: University Press.

Coffin, A. I. (c.1900). *Botanic Guide to Health*. 49th ed. London: Haynes, Coffin & Co.

Coghill, N. trans. (1975). *Chaucer The Canterbury Tales*. Middlesex: Penguin Books.

Coles, J. and Minitt. (1995). *Industrious and Fairly Civilized*. Somerset Levels Project.

Columella, J. M. (1745). *Of Husbandry in Twelve Books*. London: A. Millar.

Culpeper, N. (1649). *A Physical Directory*. London.

Culpeper, N. (1815 edition). *Culpeper's Complete Herbal and English Physician enlarged*. (1652). London: Richard Evans.

Culpeper, N. (2005). *Astrological Judgements of Diseases from the Decumbiture of the Sick*. Bel Air: Astrology Classics.

Culpeper, N. (2022). *A Directory for Midwives*. 1762. Gale ECCO Print Editions.

Curtis, A. (1870). *The Provocation and The Reply; or, Allopathy versus Physio-medicalism: Cincinnati*: published for the proprietor.

Davies, J. (2007). *A History of Wales*. London: Penguin Books.

Dawson, W. ed., (1934). *A Leechbook of the XVth Century*. London: Macmillan & Co.

De Bairacli-Levy, J. (1991). *The Illustrated Herbal Handbook for Everyone*. London: Faber and Faber.

Dobson, A. intro. (1905). *The Diary of John Evelyn*. London: Cassell and Co.

Duke James, A. *Handbook of Phytochemical Constituents of GRAS Herbs and other Economic Plants*. London: CRC Press, 2001, 576.

Edelstein, E. J. and L. (1945). *Asclepius. A Collection and Interpretation of the Testimonies*. II. Baltimore: The John Hopkins Press.

Eldin, Sue and Andrew Dunford. *Herbal Medicine in Primary Care*. Oxford: Butterworth-Heinemann, 2000.

Evans, D. M. et al. (2003). *Rebuilding the Past. A Roman Villa*. Methuen.

Fitch, J. G. trans. (2013). *Palladius The Work of Farming*. Devon: Prospect Books.

Fitzgerald, R. trans. (2008). *Homer. The Iliad*. Oxford: Oxford University Press.

Fletcher, H. and Brown, W. (1970). *The Royal Botanic Garden Edinburgh*. Edinburgh: Her Majesty's Stationery Office.

Flückiger, F. and Hanbury, D. (1998). *Pharmacographia. A History of Drugs*. London: Macmillan & Co., 2nd Edition. 1998.

Fox, R. (2022). *The Invention of Medicine from Homer to Hippocrates*, London: Penguin Books.

Fox, W. (1909). *The Working Man's Model Family Botanic Guide*. Sheffield: William Fox & Sons.

Francis Adams, The medical works of Paulus Aeginata, the Greek physician translated into English: Vol. I, 1834. https://wellcomecollection.org/works/xe48qeu8. accessed May 2023.

Frisk, Gösta. ed. (1949). *Macer Floridus de Viribus Herbarum*. Cambridge Mass: Harvard University Press.

Garmonsway, G. N. (1953). *The Anglo-Saxon Chronicle*. London: J.M. Dent & Sons Ltd.

Garrod, A. B. (1882). *The Essentials of Materia Medica and Therapeutics*. London: Longman, Green, and Co.

Geber. *Geber's Best Writings on Alchemy*. Kessinger's Legacy Reprints.

Godwin, Sir, H. (1975). *History of the British Flora*. (2nd edition). London: Cambridge University Press.

Goodrick-Clarke, N. trans. (1990). *Paracelsus Essential Readings*. Northants: Crucible.

Green, M. ed, trans. (2002). *The Trotula*. Philadelphia: University of Pennsylvania Press.

Greenhill, W. A. trans. (1843). *Rhazes. A Treatise On The Small-pox And Measles*. London: The Sydenham Society.

Grieve, M. (1984). *A Modern Herbal*. Adelaide: Jonathan Cape. Saavas.

Griggs, B. (1981). *Green Pharmacy*. London: Jill Norman and Hobhouse.

Grocock, C. and Grainger, S. (2007). *Apicius*. Devon: Prospect Books.

Gunther, R. T. (1922). *Early British Botanists*. Oxford: University Press.

Gunther, R. T. ed. (1968). *Dioscorides Greek Herbal*. London: Hafner.

Hagen, A. (1998). *A Handbook of Anglo-Saxon Food*. Norfolk: Anglo-Saxon Books.

Hagen, A. (2007). *A Second Handbook of Anglo-Saxon Food and Drink*. Norfolk: Anglo-Saxon Books.

Hall, A. and Barker, A. (1932). *The National Botanic Pharmacopoeia*. London: National Association of Medical Herbalists of Great Britain.

Harington, Sir, J. (1957). *The School of Salernum. Regimen Sanitatis Salerni*. Rome: Ente Provinciale per Il Turismo. Salerno.

Harris, S. A. Oxford Plant Systematics, *What's in a date?* Oxford: Department of Plant Sciences, University of Oxford, 2021.

Harvey, J. (1972). *Early Gardening Catalogues*. Chichester: Phillimore & Co.

Harvey, J. (1990). *Mediaeval Gardens*. London: Batsford.

Hatfield, G. (1999). *Memory, Wisdom and Healing*. Stroud: Sutton Publishing.

Haycock, Daniel, B. (2008). *Mortal Coil*. London: Yale University Press.

Healde, T. trans. (1791). *The Pharmacopoeia of the Royal College of Physicians of London*. London: Longman.

Heaton, V. (1980). *The Mayflower*. Exeter: Webb and Bower.

Henrey, B. (1975). *British Botanical and Horticultural Literature before 1800*. Vol. II. London: Oxford University Press.

Henslow, G. (1972). *Medical Works of the Fourteenth Century*. New York: Burt Franklin.

Herbert, G. (2003). *The Country Parson*. Norwich: Canterbury Press.

Hicks, R. D. trans. (1972). *Diogenes Laertius. Lives of Eminent Philosophers*. Vol. 1. London: Harvard University Press.

Hill, C. P. (1965). *Who's Who in History*. Vol. III. 1603–1714. Oxford: Basil Blackwell.

Hill, J. (1751). *A History of the Materia Medica*. London: Longman, Hitch & Hawes.

Hill, J. (1754). *The Family Herbal*. London: Bungay edition, C. Brightly and T. Kinnersley.

Hobby, E. ed. (2009). *The Birth of Mankind*. (1560). Farnham: Ashgate.

Hodgson, B. (2001). *In the Arms of Morpheus*. New York: Firefly Books.

Hogáin, D. Ó. (2002). *The Celts. A History*. Woodbridge: The Boydell Press.

Hort, A. trans. (1980 & 1999). *Theophrastus Enquiry into Plants*. Volumes I, II. London: William Heinnemann Ltd.

Ireland, S. (1996). *Roman Britain A Sourcebook*. London: Routledge.

Jackson, R. (1988). *Doctors and Diseases in the Roman Empire*. London: British Museum Publications.

James, P. and Thorpe, N. *Ancient Inventions*. Great Britain: Michael O'Mara Books Ltd., 1999.

Johnson, T. ed. (1975). *The Herbal*. John Gerard. (1633 edition). New York: Dover Publications.

Johnston, I. and Horsley, G. (2011). *Method of Medicine*. Books 5–9. London: Harvard University Press.

Jones, E. A. (2015). *England's Last Medieval Monastery*. Leominster: Gracewing.

Jones, M. (2001).*The Molecule Hunt*. London: Allen Lane, The Penguin Press.

Jones, W. H. S. trans. (1931). *Hippocrates*. Volume IV. London: Harvard University Press.

Josselyn, J. *New-Englands RARITIES Discovered*. 1672. Bedford Mass: Applewood Books.

Kahl, O. (2015). *The Sanskrit, Syriac and Persian Sources in the Comprehensive Book of Rhazes*. Leiden: Brill.

Keen, B. and Armstrong, J. (1941). *Herb Gathering*. London: Brome and Schimmer.

Keller, F. trans. Lee, E. (1878). *The Lake Dwellings of Switzerland &c*. London: Longmans Green and Co.

Kingston, R. (2021). *Ireland's Hidden Medicine*. Lewes: Aeon Books.

Labarge, M. W. (1965). *A Baronial Household of the Thirteenth Century*. London: Eyre and Spottiswoode.

Largus, S. *Compositiones Medicorum*. (1786). Scholar Select. Franklin Classics Trade Press.

Larkey, S. V. and Pyles, T. ed. (1941). *An Herbal* (1525), New York: Scholars Facsimiles and Reprints.

Latham, R. ed. (1985). *The Shorter Pepys*. London: Penguin Books.

LaWall, C. H. (1927). *Four Thousand Years of Pharmacy*. Philadelphia: Lippincott Company.

Lawson, W. (1656). *A New Orchard and Garden*. London: Brewster and Sawbridge.

Leighton, A. (1970). *Early American Gardens*. Boston U.S.A: Houghton, Mifflin Company.

Le Rougetel, H. (1990). *The Chelsea Gardener*. London: Natural History Museum Publications.

Le Strange, Richard. *A History of Herbal Plants*. London: Angus and Robertson, 1977.

Lewer, H. W. ed. (1908). *A Book of Simples*. (1700–1750). London: Sampson Low, Marston & Co. Ltd.

Lewis, W. (1753). *The English Dispensatory Improved*. London: J. Nourse.

Leyel, Hilda. *The Magic of Herbs*. London: Jonathan Cape, 1938.

Leyser, H. (1996). *Medieval Women*. London: Phoenix.

Lloyd, G. E. R. (1983). *Hippocratic Writings*. London: Penguin Classics.

Luft, D. (2020). *Medieval Welsh Medical Texts*. Vol. I. Cardiff: University of Wales Press.

Lyle, T. J. (1932). *Physio-Medical Therapeutics Materia Medica and Pharmacy*. London: National Association of Medical Herbalists.

Mabey, R. ed. (1988). *The Gardener's Labyrinth*. Thomas Hill. Oxford: Universities Press.

Mackie, J. D. (1962). *The Earlier Tudors. 1485–1558*. Oxford: Clarendon Press.

Magnusson, M. (1977). *BC The Archaeology of the Bible Lands*. London: The Bodley Head Ltd.

Mattingly, H. trans., *Tacitus on Britain and Germany*. Middlesex: Penguin Books, 1948.

Maulucci, F. P. *The National Archaeological Museum of Naples*. Naples: Carcavallo.

"Medical Act 1858." Legislation.gov.uk, July 31, 1979. https://www.legislation.gov.uk/ukpga/Vict/21-22/90/contents.

Mesue, J. (1581). *Opera de Medicamentorum*. Venice.

Meyrick, W. (1790). *The Family Herbal or Domestic Physician*. Birmingham: Thomas Pearson.

Miller, A. (1976). *Shaker Herbs. A History and a Compendium*. New York: Clarkson N. Potter Inc.

Miller, J. (1722). *Botanicum officinale*. London: Bell.

Miller, J. I. (1998). *The Spice Trade of the Roman Empire*. Oxford: Clarendon Press.

Mills, S. (1991). *Out of This Earth*. London: Viking Arcana.

Mills, S. and Bone, K. (2000). *Principles and Practice of Phytotherapy*. Churchill Livingstone.

Milton, G. (1999). *Nathaniel's Nutmeg*. London: Sceptre.

Mingren, W. "The Incredible Medical Interventions of the Monks of Soutra Aisle." Ancient Origins Reconstructing the story of humanity's past, June 22, 2018. https://www.ancient-origins.net/ancient-places-europe/incredible-medical-interventions-monks-soutra-aisle-003285.

Minnitt, S. and Coles, J. (1996). *The Lake Villages of Somerset*. Glastonbury Antiquarian Society, Somerset Levels Project and Somerset County Council Museums Service.

Moloney, M. *Irish Ethno-Botany and the Evolution of Medicine in Ireland*. Litter Press.

Moody, J. ed. (2001). *The Private Life of an Elizabethan Lady*. Stroud: Sutton Publishing.

North, W. ed. (1892). *Cooley's Cyclopaedia of Practical Receipts and Collateral Information*. London: J. & A. Churchill.

Nunn, J. F. (1996). *Ancient Egyptian Medicine*. London: British Museum Press.

Oberstockstall, T. von. trans. (2013). *The Virtuous Book of Distillation*. Laurens Andrews London. 1527. The Restorers of Alchemical Manuscripts Society Digital.

O'Brian, P. (1993). *H.M.S. Surprise*. London: Harper Collins.

"Oldest Woman Ever." Guinness World Records. Accessed July 31, 2023. https://www.guinnessworldrecords.com/world-records/oldest-person.

Orme, N. and Webster, M. (1995). *The English Hospital 1070–1570*. London: Yale University Press.

O'Malley, C. D. (1964). *Andreas Vesalius of Brussels 1514–1564*. University of California Press.

Parkinson, J. (1976). *A Garden of Pleasant Flowers*. New York: Dover Publications, Inc.

Pasca, M. et al. (1990). *Salerno School of Medicine*. Regione Campania—Assessorato al Turismo.

Pavord, A. (2009). *Searching for Order*. London: Bloomsbury.

Payne, R. trans. (1966). *Hortulus* Walahfrid Strabo. Pennsylvania: The Hunt Botanical Library.

Pechey, J. (1694). *The English Herbal of Physical Plants*. London.

Peplow, E. and R. (1988). *In a Monastery Garden*. Devon: David and Charles.

Pharmacopoeia Collegii Regii Medicorum Edinburgensis. Edinburgh: Hamilton, Balfour, et Neill, 1756.

Pharmacopoeia Londinensis of 1618. (Facsimile) Wisconsin: Madison State Historical Society, 1944.

Phelps Brown, O. (1878). *The Complete Herbalist*. London: Published by the author.

Pitman, V. (2006). *The Nature of the Whole. Holism in Ancient Greek and Indian Medicine*. Delhi: Motilal Banarsidass Publishers Private Ltd.

Plat, Sir, H. (1955). *Delightes for Ladies*. (1609). London: Crosby Lockwood.

Pollington, S. (2000). *Leechcraft*. Norfolk: Anglo Saxon Books.

Priest A. W. and L. R. (2000). *Herbal Medication*. Essex: The C.W. Daniel Co. Ltd.

Pryce, D. ed. (1957). John Baptista Porta, *Natural Magic*. New York: Basic Books Inc.

Pryor, F. (2003). *Britain BC*. London: Harper Collins.

Pryor, F. (2006). *Britain in the Middle Ages*. London: Harper Press.

Pughe, J. trans. (1989). *The Herbal Remedies of the Physicians of Myddfai*. Dyfed: Llanerch Enterprises.

Quincy, J. (1736). *A Complete English Dispensatory*. 10th edition. London: Thomas Longman.

Rawcliffe, C. (1997). *Medicine and Society in Later Medieval England*. Stroud: Sutton Publishing.

Reynolds, P. (1979). *Iron Age Farm. The Butser Experiment*. London: British Museum Publications.

Riddle, J. (1997). *Eve's Herbs*. Cambridge Mass: Harvard University Press.

Riddle, J. (2011). *Dioscorides on Pharmacy and Medicine*. Austin: University of Texas Press.

Robinson, M. (c1872). *The New Family Herbal and Botanic Physician*. Halifax: William Nicholson and Sons.

Roller, D. W. *The Geography of Strabo: An English Translation, with Introduction and Notes*. E-book.

Rosenman, L. D. (1999). *A Medieval Surgical Pharmacopoeia and Formulary*. 1170–1325. San Francisco: Rosenman.

Rovelli, C. (2023). *Anaximander and the Nature of Science*. London: Penguin Books.

Saad, B. and Said, O. (2011). *Greco-Arab & Islamic Herbal Medicine*. New Jersey: John Wiley & Sons.

Salmon, W. (1694). *Pharmacopœia Bateana*. London: Smith and Walford.

Scarborough, J. "The Life and Times of Alexander of Tralles" *Expedition Magazine* 39 2 (1997): *Expedition Magazine*. Penn Museum http://www.penn.museum/sites/expedition/

Scott, M. ed. (1986). *An Irish Herbal*. K'Eogh. (1735). Northants: The Aquarian Press.

Scudder, J. M. (2020). *The Eclectic Practice of Medicine*. Hardpress publishing.

Scullard, H. H. (1979). *Roman Britain.-Outpost of the Empire*. London: Thames and Hudson.

Scurrah, J. W. (1905). *The National Botanic Pharmacopoeia*. Bradford: National Association of Medical Herbalists.

Sherley-Price, L. trans., Bede. *A History of the English Church and People*. Middlesex: Penguin Books, 1975.

Singer, P. N. trans. (1997). *Galen. Selected Works*. Oxford: University Press.

Sitch, B. "DNA and the Roman Army in Britain." Ancient Worlds, August 19, 2015. https://ancientworldsmanchester.wordpress.com/2013/03/04/dna-and-the-roman-army-in-britain/.

Smith, E. (1739). *The Compleat Housewife*. (London: J. and J. Pemberton).

Spazzapan, G. B. (1992). *Il Cinquantesimo libro sulla storia di Salerno il meglio e di più*. Istituto Grafico Editoriale Italiano.

Spencer, W. G. trans. (1971). *Celsus De Medicina*, I Books 1–1V. London: William Heinnemann Ltd.

Spencer, W. G. trans. (1989). *Celsus De Medicina*, II Books V–V1. London: William Heinnemann Ltd.

Spindler, K. (1994).*The Man in the Ice*. London: Weidenfeld & Nicolson.

Stapley, C. ed. (2004). *The Receipt Book of Lady Anne Blencowe*. Basingstoke: Heartsease Books.

Stapley, C. (2021). *The Tree Dispensary. The Uses, History and Herbalism of Native European Trees*. Lewes: Aeon Books.

Sumner, J. (2019). *Plants Go to War*. North Carolina: McFarland & Co. Inc.

Talbot, C. H. (1967). *Medicine in Medieval England*. London: Oldbourne.

Teetgen, A. (1916). *Profitable Herb-Growing and Collecting*. London: George Newnes Ltd.

The Medical Herbalist. Vols, 1. 1925, 6. 1930, & 8. 1932.

The Proprietor. (1782). *The Westminster Magazine*. Vol. X. London: John Walker.

Thomson, A. T. (1826). *The London Dispensatory*. 4th edition. London: Longman, Rees, Orme, Brown, and Green.

Thompson, C. J. S. (1929). *The Mystery and Art of the Apothecary*. Philadelphia: Lippincott.

Thompson, S. (1848). *The Poor Man's Friend*. 12th edition. Halifax: Thompson.

Thornton, R. (1810). *A New Family Herbal*. London: Richard Phillips.

Tobyn, G. (1977). *Culpeper's Medicine*. Dorset: Element.

Tobyn, G. et al. (2011). *The Western Herbal Tradition*, London Churchill Livingstone.

Tournefort, Monsieur. (1730). *The Compleat Herbal*. Vol. II. London: Walthoe, Wilkin, Bonwicke, Birt, Ward & Wicksteed.

Turnbull, W. (1800). *The Naval Surgeon*. London: B. Mc Millan.

Tusser, T. (1984). *Five Hundred Points of Good Husbandry*. (Original 1573). Oxford: University Press.

Ulrich, L. T. (1991). *Good Wives*. New York: Vintage Books.

Ulrich, L. T. (1991). *A Midwife's Tale*. New York: Vintage Books.

Urban, S. (1738). *The Gentleman's Magazine and Historical Chronicle*. Vol. XV. London: Edward Cave.

Urban, S. (1788). *The Gentleman's Magazine and Historical Chronicle*. Vol. XV. London: Edward Cave.

Urban, S. (1753). *The Gentleman's Magazine and Historical Chronicle*. Vol. XV. London: Edward Cave.

Urban, S. (1745). *The Gentleman's Magazine and Historical Chronicle*. Vol. XV. London: Edward Cave.

Urban, S. (1746). *The Gentleman's Magazine and Historical Chronicle*. Vol. XV. London: Edward Cave.

Urban, S. (1761). *The Gentleman's Magazine and Historical Chronicle*. Vol. XV. London: Edward Cave.

Urdang, G., Introduction. (1944). *Pharmacopoeia Londinensis* of 1618, (Facsimile), (Wisconsin: Madison State Historical Society).

Ussery, H. E. (1971). *Chaucer's Physician*. Louisiana: Tulane University.

Vaisrub, Samuel. "Ancient Jewish History—Medicine." Medicine. Accessed April 22, 2023. https://www.jewishvirtuallibrary.org/medicine.

Van der Veen, M. et al. (2007). *The Archaeobotany of Roman Britain: current state and identification of research priorities.* Britannia. Vol. 38, The Society for the Promotion of Roman Studies.

Wacher, J. (1979). *The Towns of Roman Britain.* Batsford Ltd.

Wade, W. (1794). *Catalogus systematicus plantarum indigenarum in comitatu dubliniensi inventarum.* Dublin.

Waite A. E. trans. (1992). *The Hermetic and Alchemical Writings of Paracelsus the Great.* U.S.A: The Alchemical Press.

Walker, David. Rep. *Report on the Regulation of Herbal Medicines and Practitioners.* London: UK Government, 2015. https://www.gov.uk/government/uploads/system/uploads/attachment_data/file/417768/Report_on_Regulation_of_Herbal_Medicines_and_Practitioners.pdf

Wallis Budge, E. A. (2020). *Syrian Anatomy, Pathology, and Therapeutics* Vol. I. Alpha Editions.

Warde, W. and Anglosse, R. trans. (2000). *The Secretes of Maister Alexis* 1558–1569. Oxford: Atenar.

Warwick, T. ed. (2016). Wesley J. *Primitive Physic.* 1743. New edition.

Wear, A. (2000). *Knowledge & Practice in English Medicine,* 1550–1680. Cambridge: Cambridge University Press.

Webb, W. H. ed. (1916). *Standard Guide to Non-Poisonous Herbal Medicine.* Southport: Webb.

Whiteman, R. (1996). *Brother Cadfael's Herb Garden.* London: Little, Brown and Co.

Willich, A. F. M. (1800). *Lectures on Diet and Regimen.* 3rd edition. London: Longman and O. Rees.

Wilson, R. (2002). *A Guide to the Roman Remains in Britain.* London: Constable.

Wood, M. (1983). *In Search of the Dark Ages.* London: BBC.

Wood, R. (2005). *The Wooden Bowl.* Ammanford: Stobart Davies Ltd.

Woodville, W. (1790). *Medical Botany.* 3 vols + Supplement. London: James Phillips.

Woolley, B. (2004). *The Herbalist.* London: Harper Collins.

Wren, R. C. (1998). *Potter's New Cyclopaedia of Botanical Drugs & Preparations.* Saffron Walden: C. W. Daniel Co. Ltd.

Zhang, Y. ed. (2021). *Pharmacognosy.* Virginia: Cognella Academic Publishing.

GLOSSARY OF HERBS

Common to Latin Names and Plant Index

Acacia 37, 74, 355

Acacia Gum, see Gum Arabic

Aconite, *Aconitum* spp. 36, 94, 321, 323

Adders tongue, *Ophioglossum vulgatum* 245

Agrimony, *Agrimonia eupatoria* 22, 57, 113, 119, 120, 123, 245, 250, 299, 330, 355

Alder, *Alnus* spp. 249

Alecost, *Tanacetum balsamita* 119, 130

Alehoof, *Glechoma hederaceae* 119

Alexanders, *Smyrnium olusatrum* 90

Alkanet, *Alkanna tinctoria* 93

Allspice, *Myrtus pimento* 297

Aloes, *Aloe vera* and other spp. (socotrine often preferred) 94, 107, 112, 191, 207, 209, 229, 230, 273, 297, 357, 358

American mandrake, *Podophyllum peltatum* 250, 321

Ammi visnaga see Bishop's weed

Angelica, *Angelica archangelica* 237, 238, 248, 260, 268, 357

Aniseed, *Pimpinella anisum* 210, 215, 228, 229, 245, 268, 272, 328

Arnica, see Wolf's bane

Ash, *Fraxinus excelsior* 119, 169

Astragalus membranaceous see Milk vetch

Autumn crocus, *Colchicum autumnale* 121, 357

Wild rosemary, *Ledum palustre* 250
Wild strawberry, *Fragaria vesca* 124, 205, 206, 244, 259
Wild thyme, *Thymus serpyllum* 22, 120, 122, 215, 354, 358
Willow, *Salix alba,* and other spp. 17, 20, 238, 357
Wintergreen, *Gaultheria procumbens* 250
Witch hazel, *Hamamelis virginiana* 250
Woad, *Isatis tinctoria* 22, 358
Wolf's bane, *Arnica montana* 321
Wood chervil, *Anthriscus* spp. 120
Woodruff, see Sweet woodruff
Wormwood, *Artemisia absinthium* 93, 113, 119, 124, 125, 127, 129, 169, 171, 172, 176, 177, 178, 201, 244, 246, 272, 282, 330, 354, 357
Yarrow, *Achillea millefolium* 22, 39, 119, 120, 169, 176, 177, 238, 245, 248, 270, 297, 299, 312, 330;356, 357, 358
Yellow flag, *Iris pseudacorus* 174
Yellow gentian, *Gentiana lutea* 282
Yellow wild indigo, *Baptisia tinctoria* 325
Yew, *Taxus* spp. 123, 124
Zedoary, *Curcuma zedoaria* 112, 260

Latin to Common Names

Abies spp., Fir
Acacia Arabica, Gum Arabic
Achillea millefolium, Yarrow
Aconitum napellus, and other spp., Aconite
Aframomum melegueta, Grains of paradise
Agrimonia eupatoria, Agrimony
Agrostemma githago, Corncockle
Ajuga reptans, Bugle
Alcea rosea, Hollyhock
Alnus spp., Alder
Alkanna tinctoria, Alkanet
Allium porrum, Leek
Allium sativum, Garlic
Aloes, Aloe spp. (socotrine often preferred)
Alpinia galangal, Galingale (Galangal)
Althaea officinalis, Marshmallow
Ammi visnaga, Bishop's weed
Anacyclus pyrethrum, Pellitory of Spain
Anchusa officinalis, Bugloss
Andrographis paniculata, King of bitters
Anethum graveolens, Dill

Angelica archangelica, Angelica
Anthemis cotula, Mayweed
Anthemis nobilis, Roman chamomile
Anthriscus cerefolium, Chervil
Anthriscus sylvestris, Wood Chervil
Apium graveolens, Wild celery
Aquilaria agallocha, Lignum aloes
Aralia nudicaulis, sweet root
Aralia racemosa, Spikenard
Arctium lappa, Greater burdock
Arnica montana, Wolf's bane
Artemisia abrotanum, Southernwood
Artemisia absinthium, Wormwood
Artemisia dracunculus, Tarragon
Artemisia vulgaris, Mugwort
Asclepias syriaca, Milkweed
Asperula odorata, Sweet woodruff
Asplenium scolopendrium, Hart's tongue
Astragalus gummifer, Gum tragacanth
Astragalus membranaceous, Milk vetch
Atriplex hastata, Orache
Atropa belladonna, Belladonna
Avena sativa, Oats
Baptisia tinctoria, Yellow wild indigo
Berberis vulgaris, Barberry
Betula spp., Birch
Borago officinalis, Borage
Boswellia spp. *olibanum*, Frankincense
Brassica nigra, Black mustard
Caffea Arabica, Coffee
Calamintha sativa, Calamint
Calendula officinalis, Marigold
Calluna vulgaris, Heather
Capparis spinosa, Caper
Capsella bursa-pastoris, Shepherd's purse
Capsicum baccatum, C. annuum, Cayenne pepper
Carlina vulgaris, Carline thistle
Carum carvi, Caraway
Cassia senna, Senna alexandrina, Senna
Caulophyllum thalictroides, Blue cohosh
Centaurea cyanus, Cornflower
Centaurium erythraea, European or lesser Centaury
Chelidonium majus, Greater celandine

Chenopodium album, Fat hen
Chionanthus virginicus, Fringetree
Chicorium endivia, Endive
Cichorium intybus, Chicory
Cimicifuga racemosa, Black cohosh
Cinchona spp., Jesuit's bark
Cinnamomum aromaticum, Chinese cinnamon, or Cassia
Cinnamomum camphora, Camphor
Cinnamomum spp., Cinnamon
Cirsium vulgare, Spear thistle
Citrus aurantium, Bitter orange, orange flowers
Citrus aurantium, Bitter orange
Citrus limonum, Lemon
Citrus medica, Citron
Citrus sinensis, Orange
Cochlearia armoracia, Horseradish
Colchicum autumnale, Autumn crocus
Commiphora spp., myrrh, (also balsam)
Cnicus benedictus, Carduus benedictus, Blessed thistle
Conium maculatum, Hemlock
Convolvulus arvensis, Black bindweed
Convolvulus scammonia, Scammony
Coriandrum sativum, Coriander
Corylus avellana, Hazel
Crataegus spp., Hawthorn
Crocus sativum, Saffron crocus
Croton eluteria, Cascarilla
Cucumis melo, Melon
Cucumis sativus, Cucumber
Cucurbita pepo, Pompion
Cuminum cyminum, Cumin
Curcuma longa, Turmeric
Curcuma zedoaria, Zedoary
Cydonia vulgaris, Quince
Cynoglossum officinale, Hound's tongue
Datura stramonium, Thorn-apple
Daucus carota, Wild carrot
Delphinium consolida, (staphisagria), Delphinium
Dianthus caryophyllus, Clove pinks
Dictamnus creticus, Dittany
Digitalis purpurea, Foxglove
Dioscorea communis, Black bryony berry
Dipsacus fullorum, Teasel

Doronicum spp., Leopard's Bane
Echium vulgare, Viper's bugloss
Elettaria cardamomum, Cardamom
Eruca sativa, Rocket
Eryngium maritimum, Sea holly
Eugenia caryophyllus, Cloves
Eupatorium perfoliatum, Boneset
Euphrasia spp., Eyebright
Ferula galbaniflua, Galbanum
Ficus spp., Fig.
Filipendula ulmaria, Meadowsweet
Foeniculum vulgare, Fennel
Folium indicum, Cinnamon leaf
Fragaria vesca, Wild Strawberry
Fraxinus excelsior, Ash
Fumaria officinalis, Fumitory
Galium aparine, Cleavers
Galium verum, Lady's bedstraw
Gaultheria procumbens, Wintergreen
Gelsemium sempervirens, False jasmine
Genista scoparia, G. vulgaris, Broom
Gentiana lutea, Gentian
Geum urbanum
Glechoma hederaceae, Alehoof
Glycyrrhiza glabra, Liquorice
Gnaphalium uliginosum, Cudweed
Guaiacum officinale, Tree of life, pockwood
Hamamelis virginiana, Witch hazel
Hedera helix, Ivy
Helleborus cyclophyllus
Helleborus niger, Black hellebore
Hordeum vulgare, Barley
Humulus lupulus, Hop
Hydrastis Canadensis, Golden seal
Hyoscyamus niger, (*H. albus*, and *H. aureus*), Henbane
Hypericum perforatum, St. John's wort
Hyssopus officinale, Hyssop
Inula campana, Spearwort
Inula helenium, Elecampane
Ipomoea purga, Jalap
Iris spp. *I. germanica, I. pallida*, Orris root
Iris pseudacorus, Yellow flag
Isatis tinctoria, Woad

Juglans cinerea, Butternut
Juglans nigra, Black walnut
Juglans regia, Walnut
Juniperus communis, Juniper
Juniperus Sabina, Savin
Knautia arvensis, Scabious
Lactuca virosa, Lettuce (wild)
Lauro cerasus, Black cherry
Laurus nobilis, Bay
Lavandula officinalis, Lavender
Ledum palustre, Wild rosemary
Leonurus cardiaca, Motherwort
Lepidium campestre, Pepperwort, dittander
Leucanthemum vulgare, Ox-eye daisy
Levisticum officinale, Lovage
Lignum vitae—see *Guaiacum officinale*
Lilium candidum, Lily (white)
Linum catharticum, Mountain flax
Linum usitatissimum, Flax, Linseed
Liquidamber styraciflua, Sweet gum
Lobelia inflata, Indian tobacco
Lupinus spp., Lupin
Lycopodium spp., clubmoss
Lycopus virginicus, Virginia water horehound
Malus sylvestris, Crab apple
Malva spp., Mallow
Mandragora officinarum, European Mandrake
Marrubium vulgare, White horehound
Matricaria recutita, German chamomile
Melissa officinalis, Lemon balm
Mentha spp., Mints
Mentha piperita, Peppermint
Mentha pulegium, Pennyroyal
Mentha spicata, Spearmint
Menyanthes trifoliata, Bogbean
Mespilus germanica, Medlar
Morus nigra, Mulberry
Myrica cerifera, Bayberry
Myrica gale, Sweet gale
Myrrhis odorata, Sweet Cicely
Myristica fragrans—see *Nux moschata*
Myrobalan Emblica officinalis, Indian gooseberry
Myroxylon balsamum, Balsam of Tolu

Myroxylon pereirae, Peruvian bark
Myroxylon peruiferum, Balsam of Peru
Myrtus communis
Myrtus pimento, Allspice, Jamaica pepper
Nardostachys jatamansi, Indian nard, or Indian Spikenard
Nasturtium officinale, Watercress
Nepeta spp., Catmint
Nicotiana tabacum, Tobacco
Nigella sativa, Black cumin
Nux moschata, Nutmeg
Nux vomica, Strychnine tree
Nymphaea odorata, Water Lily
Ocimum basilicum, Basil
Ophioglossum vulgare, Adders tongue
Origanum majorana, Marjoram (sweet)
Origanum vulgare, Oregano (Greek)
Paeonia spp., Peony
Papaver rhoeas, Poppy, (field)
Papaver somniferum, Opium Poppy
Parietaria officinalis, P. diffusa, Pellitory of the Wall
Petasites officinalis, Butterbur
Petroselinum crispum, Parsley
Phytolacca decandra, Pokeroot
Picea spp., Spruce
Pimpinella anisum, Aniseed
Piper cubeba, Cubeb
Piper longum, Long pepper
Piper nigrum, Black pepper
Pistacia lentiscus, Mastic
Plantago lanceolata, Ribwort plantain
Plantago major, Greater plantain, waybroad
Podophyllum peltatum, American mandrake
Polygonatum multiflorum, Solomon's seal
Polypody vulgare
Portulaca oleracea, Purslane
Potentilla erecta, Tormentil
Potentilla reptans, Cinquefoil
Primula veris, Cowslip
Prunella vulgaris, Self-heal
Prunus laurocerasus, Cherry Laurel
Prunus serotina, Wild cherry
Prunus spinosa, Blackthorn, sloe
Pterocarpus draco, Dragon's Blood

Punica granatum, Pomegranate
Quassia spp. bitterwood
Quercus spp., Oak
Ranunculus spp., Crowfoot
Raphanus sativus, Radish
Rhamnus catharticus, Purging buckthorn
Rheum palmatum, Turkey rhubarb, Rhubarb
Rhus copallina, Sumach
Ribes cynosbati, Prickly gooseberry
Rosa canina, Dog rose
Rosa centifolia, Cabbage rose
Rosa Damascena, Damask rose
Rosa gallica officinalis, Apothecary's rose
Rosmarinus officinalis, *Salvia Rosmarinus*, Rosemary
Rubia tinctorium, Madder
Rubus idaeus, Wild raspberry
Rubus spp., Blackberry
Rumex spp., Docks
Ruscus aculeatus, Butcher's broom
Ruta graveolens, Rue
Sagapenum, concreted juice of an unidentified Ferula plant
Salix spp., Willow
Salvia officinalis, Sage
Sanguisorba minor, Salad burnet
Sanicula europaea, Sanicle
Sambucus ebulus, Dwarf elder
Sambucus nigra, Elder
Santalum album, and other spp. Sanders, Sandalwood
Saponaria officinalis, Soapwort
Sassafras albidum, Saloop, ague tree
Satureja spp., Savory
Scrophularia nodosa, Figwort
Sempervivum tectorum, Houseleek
Serpentaria Virginiana, Virginia serpentary, Virginia snake root
Sinapis alba, White mustard
Smilax aristolochiifolia, Sarsaparilla
Smyrnium olusatrum, Alexanders
Solanum dulcamara, Nightshade
Solidago odora, American Golden rod
Solidago vulgare, European golden rod
Sonchus spp., Sow thistle
Sphagnum spp., Sphagnum moss
Stachys betonica, Betony

Stellaria media, Chickweed
Strychnos nux vomica, strychnine tree
Styrax benzoin, S. tonkinensis, Benzoin
Symphytum spp., Comfrey
Tamarindus indica, Tamarind
Tanacetum balsamita, Alecost
Tanacetum parthenium, Feverfew
Tanacetum vulgare, Tansy
Taraxacum officinale, Dandelion
Taxus spp., Yew
Teucrium chamaedrys, Germander
Thuja occidentalis, Northern white cedar
Thymus serpyllum, Wild thyme
Thymus vulgaris, Thyme
Tilia cordata, T. europaea, T. platyphyllos, Limeflower
Trigonella foenum-graecum, Fenugreek
Trillium pendulum, Beth root
Tropaeolum minus, Nasturtium
Tussilago farfara, Coltsfoot
Ulmus fulva, Slippery elm
Ulmus minor, Elm
Urginea maritima, Squill
Urtica dioica, Stinging nettle
Urtica pilulifera, Roman nettle
Urtica urens, Annual nettle
Vaccinium macrocarpum, Cranberry
Vaccinium myrtillus, Bilberry, whortleberry
Valeriana officinalis, Greek valerian
Vanilla planifolia, Vanilla
Veratrum album, White hellebore
Verbascum thapsus, and other species, Mullein
Verbena officinalis, Vervain
Veronica officinalis, Speedwell
Vicia sativa, vetch
Vinca spp., Periwinkle
Viola odorata, Violet
Viola tricolor, Heartsease
Viscum album, Mistletoe
Xanthoxylum fraxineum, X. americanum, X. clava-herculis, Prickly ash
Zingiber officinale, Ginger

INDEX

Printed in the USA
CPSIA information can be obtained
at www.ICGtesting.com
JSHW050005281123
52787JS00002B/2